PRACTICAL HANDBOOK *of*
NEBULIZER THERAPY

PRACTICAL HANDBOOK *of*

NEBULIZER THERAPY

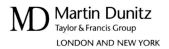

Martin Dunitz
Taylor & Francis Group

LONDON AND NEW YORK

© 2004 Martin Dunitz, a member of the Taylor & Francis Group plc

First published in the United Kingdom in 2004
by Martin Dunitz, a member of the Taylor & Francis Group plc,
11 New Fetter Lane, London EC4P 4EE

Tel.:   +44 (0) 20 7583 9855
Fax.:   +44 (0) 20 7842 2298
E-mail: info@dunitz.co.uk
Website: http://www.dunitz.co.uk

Although every effort has been made to ensure that all owners of copyright material have been
acknowledged in this publication, we would be glad to acknowledge in subsequent reprints or
editions any omissions brought to our attention.

Although every effort has been made to ensure that drug doses and other information are presented
accurately in this publication, the ultimate responsibility rests with the prescribing physician.
Neither the publishers nor the authors can be held responsible for errors or for any consequences
arising from the use of information contained herein. For detailed prescribing information or
instructions on the use of any product or procedure discussed herein, please consult the prescribing
information or instructional material issued by the manufacturer.

A CIP record for this book is available from the British Library.

ISBN 1 84184 293 1

Distributed in the USA by
Fulfilment Center
Taylor & Francis
10650 Toebben Drive
Independence, KY 41051, USA
Toll Free Tel.: +1 800 634 7064
E-mail: taylorandfrancis@thomsonlearning.com

Distributed in Canada by
Taylor & Francis
74 Rolark Drive
Scarborough, Ontario M1R 4G2, Canada
Toll Free Tel.: +1 877 226 2237
E-mail: tal_fran@istar.ca

Distributed in the rest of the world by
Thomson Publishing Services
Cheriton House
North Way
Andover, Hampshire SP10 5BE, UK
Tel.: +44 (0)1264 332424
E-mail: salesorder.tandf@thomsonpublishingservices.co.uk

Composition by EXPO Holdings, Malaysia
Printed and bound in Great Britain by The Cromwell Press Ltd

Contents

Section C. Practical Considerations

PREFACE

Why was this book written?

This book is the product of a close professional relationship between two pulmonary physicians (JB and ROD) and an aerosol scientist (JHD). The two pulmonary physicians have struggled for years to use inhalation devices, including nebulizers, to treat their patients, but they have realized that like most clinical colleagues they had limited understanding of the basic scientific principles underpinning such therapy. Furthermore, it became clear that many clinical trials of nebulizer use have been conducted in an unsatisfactory manner because of these problems. For example, many published studies of nebulized treatment have not stated which nebulizer system was used or how it was administered (which nebulizer device, driving source, face mask or mouthpiece, fill volume and the nebulization time, etc). As each of these factors can influence the dose delivered to the patient's lung (up to 10-fold variation between systems), the reader will understand that many published studies of inhaled medications may not be reproducible and, in some cases, the results may not be valid. The editors also realized that healthcare professionals have little access to practical guidance when they need to treat a specific patient with a specific nebulized drug.

The three editors of this book were the co-chairmen of a task force which was commissioned by the European Respiratory Society to produce guidelines for nebulizer use in Europe.[1] In preparing these guidelines, the editors organized a series of meetings of clinical and scientific experts in nebulizer use. These meetings allowed each group to understand better the needs of the other group and the detailed results of these discussions have been published in the *European Respiratory Review*.[2,3] However, it became clear to the editors that most 'front-line' healthcare staff, who use nebulizers to treat patients on a daily basis, would not be likely to have access to these documents and there was a clear need for a practical book for their use.

The main aims of the book are to help readers to understand the principles of nebulizer use and to provide practical support in treating and supporting patients who need to use nebulized therapy.

Who is the book aimed at?

We hope that the book will be of benefit to the following professional groups:

- Doctors (pulmonologists; general physicians/internists; intensivists; pediatricians; geriatricians; general practitioners; pharmacologists; research clinicians; commissioners of care; etc)
- Nurses (ward nurses; emergency department nurses; respiratory nurse specialists; primary care nurses (practice nurses in the United Kingdom); community nurses; pediatric nurses; intensive care unit nurses; research nurses; etc)
- Physiotherapists/respiratory therapists
- Pharmacists (hospital pharmacists; community pharmacists; research pharmacists; etc)
- Students (medical students; student nurses; pharmacy students; physiotherapy students)
- Pharmaceutical companies (for all staff involved in research or marketing of inhaled products)
- Aerosol scientists
- Health authorities; health maintenance organizations; insurers; other commissioners and providers of health care

How should this book be used?

Some readers may wish to read the book from the beginning through to the end but it is likely that most readers will dip into specific chapters that are of most relevance to their particular needs. For example, a new user of nebulizers may wish to read the sections on the science of nebulizer therapy, a few disease-specific chapters and one of the sections on the organization of services. For this reason, the book is divided into chapters to address the needs of specific readers. Some areas are covered in detail in one chapter but also mentioned in other chapters, often with reference to a specific situation. We hope that the table, which follows, will help to guide readers to the topics that are of most relevance or of most interest to them at any particular time; we also hope that readers will keep this volume in a convenient place and return to its pages from time to time to explore unfamiliar areas of nebulizer use or to refresh areas that they have studied previously.

How to find the information that you need quickly: use this table to find the chapters which cover the topics which are of interest to you. The main theme of each chapter is given in the chapter list but you will find that many chapters contain additional generic information which may be of value to you.

Topic	Chapter													
	1	2	3	4	5	6	7	8	9	10	11	12	13	14
What is a nebulizer?	*	*								*		*		
How does a nebulizer work?	*								*		*			
Types of nebulizer available	*		*						*			*	*	
How to make valid comparisons between different nebulizer devices		*							*					
How to use a nebulizer (general principles)	*											*		
Recent and future developments in nebulizer technology			*					*						
Indications for using a nebulizer				*	*	*	*	*	*	*	*	*		
Alternatives to using a nebulizer				*	*	*	*	*	*	*				
How to decide if a nebulizer is the best option for individual patients	*			*	*	*	*	*	*	*	*	*		
How to choose the right nebulizer for each patient	*			*	*	*	*	*	*	*	*	*		
How to assess and evaluate the response to nebulizer use				*	*	*	*	*	*	*				
How to use a nebulizer for specific medical conditions				*	*	*	*	*	*	*				
Aspects of nebulizer use in childhood							*	*	*	*		*		
How to select and use a nebulizer for diagnostic purposes									*					
How to educate patients and healthcare staff in nebulizer use					*					*			*	
How to clean, maintain, service and replace components of the nebulizer system											*			
How to deliver a local nebulizer service										*		*	*	*

Acknowledgements

Finally, the authors wish to thank all of the contributors for their hard work in producing such clear summaries of their areas of expertise and to our long-suffering families for putting up with yet another project!

References

1. Boe J, Dennis JH, O'Driscoll BR. European Respiratory Society guidelines on the use of nebulizers. *Eur Respir J* 2001; **18**:228–42.
2. Boe J, Dennis JH eds. European Respiratory Society nebulizer guidelines: technical aspects. *Eur Respir Rev* 2000; **10**:1–237.
3. Boe J, Dennis JH, O'Driscoll BR eds. European Respiratory Society nebulizer guidelines: clinical aspects. *Eur Respir Rev* 2000; **10**:495–583.

CONTRIBUTORS

Peter W Barry
Consultant in Paediatric Intensive
Care
and Honorary Senior Lecturer
Department of Child Health
Clinical Sciences Building
Leicester Royal Infirmary
Leicester, UK

Jacob Boe
Professor
Department of Respiratory
Medicine
Rikshospitalet, The National
Hospital
Oslo, Norway

Andrew Bush
Consultant Physician
Department of Paediatric
Respiratory Medicine
Royal Brompton Hospital
London, UK

Torsten Bauer
Abteilung fur Pneumologie,
Allergologie und Schlafmedizin
Schlafmedizin
Begmansheil-Universitatsklinik
Bochum, Germany

Jennifer Cleland
Clinical Lecturer/Coordinator,
Medical Interviewing and
Communication
Department of General Practice
and Primary Care
University of Aberdeen
Aberdeen, UK

John H Dennis
Reader in Aerosol Science
Department of Environmental
Science
University of Bradford
Bradford, UK

Patrice Diot
Centre Hospitalier Universitaire
Hopitaux de Tours
Service de Pneumologie
Hopital Brettonneau
Tours, France

Mary Dodd
Specialist Physiotherapy Clinician
North West Lung Centre
Wythenshawe Hospital
Manchester, UK

Jim Fink
Fellow, Respiratory Science
AeroGen, Inc.
Mountain View, CA, USA

Karen Heslop
Respiratory Nurse Specialist
Dept Respiratory Medicine
Royal Victoria Infirmary
Newcastle Upon Tyne, UK

Christer Janson
Associate Professor
Department of Medical Sciences
Respiratory Medicine &
Allergology
Uppsala University
Uppsala, Sweden

Jill Karpel
Professor of Medicine
Albert Einstein College of Medicine
Montefiore Medical Centre
New York, NY, USA

Louise Lannefors
Physiotherapist, Specialist in
Respiratory Diseases
Department of Respiratory
Medicine
Lund University Hospital
Lund, Sweden

Ronan O'Driscoll
Consultant Respiratory Physician
Hope Hospital
Salford, UK

Cora A Pieron
Honorary Research Fellow
Department of Environmental
Science
University of Bradford
Bradford, UK

David Price
GPIAG Professor of Primary Care
Respiratory Medicine
Department of General Practice
and Primary Care
University of Aberdeen
Foresterhill Health Centre
Aberdeen, UK

S Chris Stenton
Chest Unit
Royal Victoria Infirmary
Newcastle upon Tyne, UK

Ranjan Suri
Department of Paediatric
Respiratory Medicine
Royal Brompton Hospital
London, UK

Mike Thomas
GPIAG Research Fellow
Department of General Practice
University of Aberdeen
Aberdeen, UK

A Kevin Webb
Clinical Director and Professor
Bradbury Cystic Fibrosis Unit
Wythenshawe Hospital
Manchester, UK

SECTION A. TECHNICAL

1. THEORY AND SCIENCE OF NEBULIZER USE

John H Dennis

History of nebulized aerosol delivery

The history of drug inhalation is well documented.[1,2] The first described inhalation therapy, more than 4000 years ago, was with inhalation of smoke containing atropine from *Atropa belladonna* plant leaves, for treatment of the diseases of the throat and chest.[3] Ever since, sporadic reports of smokes and inhalation vapors appear in the medical literature throughout recorded history, perhaps the most notable being the use of Potters asthma cigarettes (containing shredded *Datura stramonium* leaves) which has been proven to cause a bronchdilatory effect analogous to the inhalation of ipratropium aerosol.[4] Today, by far the most common means of drug aerosol therapy delivery are pressurized metered dose inhalers (MDIs), with dry powder inhalers (DPIs) coming in second place.

Nebulizers did not appear as an inhalation therapy device until the steam driven devices of the early nineteenth century. Although various nebulizing devices have since been developed for generation of therapeutic and diagnostic aerosols, the current popularity of nebulized drug aerosols as a share of the modern drug aerosol market remains a distant third compared with pressurized MDIs and DPIs. However, nebulizers offer some drug inhalation therapy that may not be available as pressurized MDIs or DPIs (e.g. off-license use of intravenous drug solutions). Alternatively, some drug aerosols are simply more conveniently and efficiently delivered by nebulizer (e.g. for pediatric patients, ICU patients, emergency treatment, etc) due to the inherent simplicity of use and higher aerosol delivery rate of nebulizers compared with either pressurized MDIs or DPIs. Detailed information relating to the degree in which nebulizers are used today in modern medicine is not available; however, estimates summarized by Muers[1] suggest that although nebulizers are in third place in drug aerosol delivery, they still account for substantial amounts of healthcare spending. In the United Kingdom (UK) alone, some 40 000 nebulizer compressors were in use for adult domiciliary nebulized aerosol treatment delivering drugs costing in the order of £50 million (US $75 million – Figures from 1997) per annum nationally. In other words, roughly US $1.50 per head of population per year. One would expect the same order of costs to exist in most Western national healthcare systems.

Aerosol size and respiratory tract deposition

The word 'aerosol' originates from the Greek *aero* (air) and *sol* (solution), and describes figuratively a suspension of fine particles that are small enough to remain in air for a considerable length of time. These aerosols are usually defined at the upper end by a maximum of 100 μm (0.1 mm). Any larger than this, the particle is no longer aerodynamic and will fall so quickly it cannot be considered an aerosol. At the lower end of the size spectrum, particles cease to become aerosol at about 0.01 μm. Much below this size the particles are really single molecules – consider that the diameter of a benzene ring (C_6H_6) is about 0.001 μm (or 1 nm, nanometer) and the reader can appreciate that the nominally adopted 0.01 μm size for the lower end of aerosol definition is describing small airborne units – any smaller and the particle enters the realm of large airborne molecules.

However, it is not only the size that is important in considering how aerosol particles interact with the human respiratory tract. Other aspects such as particle shape and density are also important. The physics of particle–air interaction gets complicated, but a system has been devised which simplifies the discussion. The aerodynamic properties of aerosol particles are determined by particle size, shape and density, and govern their interaction with air. These properties are difficult to predict, but may be measured and expressed as an aerodynamic equivalent diameter (AED). This is defined as the diameter of a hypothetical sphere of unit density having the same aerodynamic properties as the aerosol irrespective of the geometric shape, size and density.

The respiratory tract has evolved as a natural barrier to intercept the majority of inhaled naturally occurring aerosols before they can penetrate, and, perhaps, damage the peripheral tissues of the lung. Aerosol particles may be removed from inhaled air by three principal mechanisms (Figure 1.1). Impaction occurs when the air stream in which an aerosol is suspended changes direction at high speed, such as at the bifurcation of

4

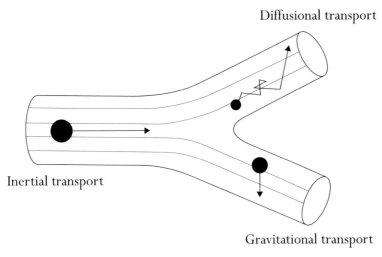

Figure 1.1 *Schematic illustration of the principal mechanisms of particle deposition onto airway surfaces. (Adapted from Heyder et al. Lung Biology in Health and Disease Series, Vol. 162. Marcel Dekker, 2000, 303–37.[5])*

larger airways. While the air stream flows around the obstruction, the greater inertia of a particle may force it to collide with the bronchial wall. Sedimentation of aerosol particles onto the respiratory surfaces is the result of settlement due to gravity, and occurs largely after entry to the smaller airways and alveolar spaces. Inertial and gravitational mechanisms of aerosol deposition are enhanced if particles increase in size within the respiratory tract after inhalation due to hygroscopic growth of individual particles. Diffusion, which is the third major mechanism (see Figure 1.1) is the natural entropic tendency of aerosol particles to drift randomly within the suspension medium – some particles making chance contact with the respiratory wall. Although these processes of respiratory deposition are largely dictated by the aerodynamic properties of the inhaled aerosol and the geometry of the airways, other factors, particularly the breathing pattern, are also important.[6] There is a fourth mechanism termed interception, which occurs when only a small part of an aerosol particle makes chance contact with a bronchial wall; because the contact is secure the particle is retained. This is particularly important in the deposition of fibers (e.g. asbestos) but less so with the spherical droplets produced by nebulizers. Regardless of method, once deposited within the respiratory tract, an aerosol particle has virtually no chance of re-entrainment due to the retentive nature of the moist respiratory passages.

The general pattern of deposition of inhaled particles in the respiratory tract has been long established (Figure 1.2). As inhaled air travels down the respiratory tract, the airways become progressively narrower, but more numerous. The velocity of air flow decreases markedly as it travels down the respiratory tract because the total cross-sectional area of the airways increases substantially. Thus, the speed of inhaled air is greatest in the central airways and it is here that large particles (>5 μm AED) are progressively more likely to be removed by impaction. Within the peripheral airways consisting of smaller bronchi, bronchioles and gas exchanging tissues, smaller particles are removed by interception, sedimentation and diffusion. Generally speaking, the smaller the particle, the greater its chance of peripheral penetration and retention. However, for very fine particles (<0.5 μm AED), there is increasing chance they may avoid deposition

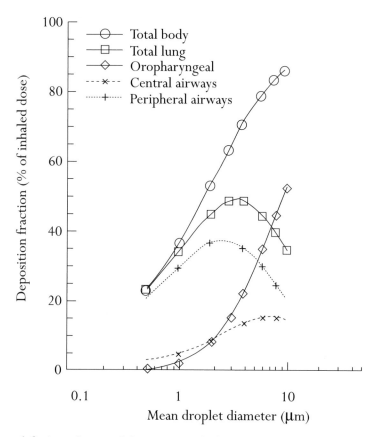

Figure 1.2 *Aerosol size and deposition in the human respiratory tract. (Adapted from Rudolph G. J Aerosol Sci 1990; 21:S306–406[7] with permission from Elsevier.)*

altogether and be subsequently exhaled. It is for these reasons that the optimal deposition in the lower respiratory tract and lung parenchyma occurs with aerosol particles in the size range of 1–5 μm.[7]

However, it must be stressed that these figures represent generalizations of a complex relationship. This relationship, between aerosol size and respiratory tract deposition and function of aerosol size depicted in Figure 1.2, must be used as a general guide only. It is common for clinicians to forget that these curves are generally representative of young healthy adults. Other factors besides size also influence the site of respiratory tract deposition of inhaled nebulized aerosol such as patient age, disease state and characteristics of inhalation.[6,8]

On reflection, the human respiratory tract has evolved an efficient system for protection against incursion of unwanted inhaled particles. Much above 5–10 μm aerosols impact in the upper respiratory tract and are removed quickly by the mucociliary escalator and much below 1 μm inhaled particles are likely to be exhaled without deposition. The challenge to the clinician is to deliver an aerosol with a narrow size range of only a few micrometers (1–5 μm) for effective treatment. The challenge presented by this narrow range is a particularly important consideration with nebulized aerosols as these particles are comprised of relatively volatile aqueous solutions or suspensions and, as will be discussed below, have a dynamic size dependent on the extent of particle shrinkage due to evaporation.

Science of nebulized aerosol

Broadly speaking, there are two basic designs of drug nebulizer – jet and ultrasonic. Jet nebulizers operate using compressed air while ultrasonic nebulizers operate using vibrating piezo-electric crystals. New nebulization technologies (particularly ultrasonic) are emerging and are discussed in detail in Chapter 3. In any case, with either of the basic conventional nebulizer designs, there is a great range of differences in aerosol output and aerosol size. This section will introduce the reader to the fundamental aspects of nebulizer design and attempt to generalize the features that influence nebulizer performance. It must be said at the outset, that it is inappropriate to choose a theoretical nebulizer design that is the best for all applications. Patient needs, desired doses and target areas require such a diverse range of desired performance, that it really is not possible for any one nebulizer to accommodate all applications. The search for the 'ideal' nebulizer is, in the author's opinion, a common misunderstanding by many in the clinical, pharmaceutical and scientific communities.

All drug nebulizers work by transforming aqueous drug solutions or suspensions from a liquid to an aerosol state and thereby allowing a dose of the solute (i.e. drug) to be inhaled and deposited in the respiratory tract. By controlling the rate (or amount) of drug aerosol and its particle size, a desired dose of drug can be delivered to the intended site of action in the respiratory tract, thereby minimizing dosage and systemic distribution, and any side effects. In describing the dose made available to the patient, two dimensions of nebulizer output need to be considered: (i) the quantitative amount of aerosol produced, and (ii) the size distribution of the inhaled

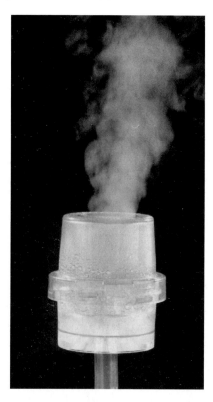

Figure 1.3 Photograph of a typical constant output nebulizer. Note the large amount of deposited sprayed droplets, which have impacted onto the interior surfaces within the nebulizer before being returned to the main reservoir. Aerosol droplets released from the nebulizer dissipate and evaporate the further they travel from the point of release. This phenomenon is due to evaporation of the droplets when exposed to ambient air.

aerosol cloud. While the first describes the total dose available for inhalation, the latter describes its potential respiratory tract penetration and deposition site(s).

Jet nebulizers

Jet nebulizers operate by forcing compressed air through a narrow orifice (Figure 1.3). Negative pressure created by the expanding jet leaving the orifice draws liquid (Bernoulli effect) up a feeder tube, the lower end of which is immersed in the main nebulizer reservoir. Migration of liquid from the reservoir to the air jet is enhanced in many nebulizer designs by a capillary effect within the feeder tube. In any case, liquid leaves the upper end of the feeder tube and enters the air jet as a 'stream' where it is rapidly broken up both by primary impaction against a strategically placed impaction plate (Figure 1.4) and by air turbulence within the nebulizer jet. The resulting

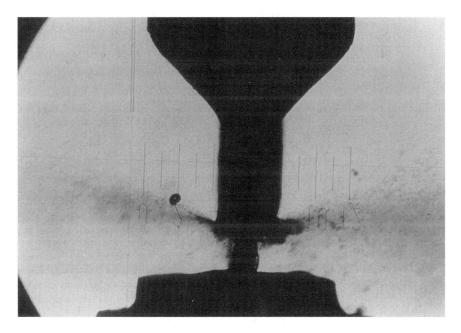

Figure 1.4 *Magnified image of the nebulized jet stream impacting on the primary impaction plate in a Pari nebulizer (courtesy of Pari GmbH).*

droplet spray within the nebulizer offers an extremely large surface area from which solvent water quickly evaporates to saturate the decompressed air within the nebulizer. The importance of evaporation in understanding nebulizer performance is only beginning to be realized.

The primary spray within the nebulizer contains a great range of droplet sizes, from the very small (<1 μm) to the very large (>100 μm). The larger the droplets in the spray, the more momentum they have, and the more likely they are to impact on interior surfaces of the nebulizer where they then fall back to the nebulizer reservoir. This can be seen in any operating nebulizer and is visually evident in Figure 1.3. The reflux action occurs at a rapid rate. The primary spray in most nebulizers is emitted within the nebulizer at a rate over 100 times greater than the rate of aerosol release (personal observation). The reader can check this by allowing a nebulizer with a few milliliters of water to operate without its 'top' (although the resulting spray can make a bit of a mess!).

This high rate of solution reflux implies that any given drug inside the nebulizer can be 'refluxed' hundreds of times, during the course of nebulizer treatment – hence the tendency when nebulizing large fragile molecules such as proteins to lose some or all of their tertiary structure and 'denature', which leads to search for alternative nebulizer designs for the effective delivery of proteins. In any case, decompressed nebulized air leaves the nebulizer a given flow rate, usually 5–7 l/min. This released air flow contains the smallest of the droplets generated inside the nebulizer, the bulk of the remaining spray having impacted on the interior surfaces which act as baffles filtering out all but the smallest of the nebulized droplets. It is this aerosol that is made available for patient inhalation. The factors which determine the overall performance of a given jet nebulizer design include the velocity of the air jet (which is defined by the jet diameter and flow rate); the volume flow of reservoir liquid drawn into the air jet (which relies on the design of the feeder tube system); the generation of droplet size range within the primary droplet spray (that depends on a combination of factors including the velocity of the entrained liquid stream in the air jet and the force with which it is impacted onto the primary impaction plate) (see Figure 1.4). The rate of output and particle size of aerosol droplets released from the nebulizer are defined by all of these factors as well as the particular design of the baffle structures within the nebulizer. Fundamentally, an important consideration in considering overall nebulizer performance is its 'residual volume' which can be defined as the minimum volume of liquid required by a nebulizer design to facilitate the nebulization process. Most readers will have observed nebulizers operating – at some point the liquid in the nebulizer drops to such a low level that it ceases to operate effectively, is heard to 'splutter' and stops releasing an aerosol cloud. This volume is sometimes referred to as the 'dead' volume or the 'residual' volume.

With any nebulizer, the rate of aerosol release (times the treatment time) defines the total available dose of aerosol while the size of the droplets in the released air stream defines the potential site of aerosol deposition within the respiratory tract.

Nebulization seems a relatively simple and convenient process, and most readers would like to think that it is also relatively easily understood. If it were only that simple! The author invites the reader to consider that there is considerable confusion in assessing nebulizer performance. The reader is asked to think carefully about what really occurs with nebulized aerosol output. Most nebulizer designs only allow about half of the aerosol to be delivered to the patient; the remainder either drifts into the ambient environment (often presenting unwanted drug aerosol contamination of home or hospital) or is collected in a scavenging filter (often at significant expense compared to costs of the nebulizer itself). This is perhaps the single greatest area where the efficiency of future nebulizer designs can improve. In addition, aerosol that can be inhaled, can also be sufficiently large as to deposit on valves or poorly designed tubing and t-pieces connecting the nebulizer to the patient.

With regard to understanding nebulized aerosol size, this too is not as simple as it appears, and it would benefit the reader to think carefully about what can happen to nebulized droplet size after release from the nebulizer, but before being inhaled by the patient. Most readers will have noticed that released nebulized aerosol cloud will waft around in the air space above a nebulizer for a short while before disappearing (see Figure 1.3). The aerosol cloud is dense at the point of release, and with distance (or time) from release, fades away until it 'disappears'. This disappearance is due to droplets evaporating their water solvent to ambient air. As they evaporate, they decrease in size. Ultimately, water solvent from each droplet will evaporate completely, until the droplet either disappears entirely (which is the case with pure water droplets) or whatever dry solute was in the solution is left as a residue (this might comprise some amounts of sodium chloride (NaCl), drug and whatever other excipient(s) were present in the formulation).

In other words, the particle size of the droplet is only stable if it is contained and shrouded in a saturated air stream, such as the initial air stream emitted from the jet nebulizer. When the droplets mix with ambient air, they evaporate. This evaporation will continue until either the droplets lose all their water solvent and dry completely or until the ambient air they are mixed with becomes saturated by absorption of the droplet's own water solvent. This is a key factor to consider when interpreting nebulized aerosol size. However, it is often overlooked and represents a fundamental mis-understanding of nebulizer operation. The important implication of this process is when a patient inhales from a nebulizer. One must consider care-fully to what degree the nebulized air stream (which saturated with mois-ture and containing stable droplets) will be forced to mix with ambient air (which may be anywhere between 20–80% saturated with water vapor, percent relative humidity, depending on the local climate). The effect of droplet evaporation, post production and release in ambient air, has a huge and largely unrecognized effect on the nebulized droplet size that is actually delivered to the patient and therefore defines the likely site of deposition in the patient's respiratory tract.

This effect can be readily estimated by simple theoretical calculations depicted in Table 1.1. For example, consider two patients, each using a commonly available constant output nebulizer design: that year's 'chosen' brand. One patient is an adult, the other a child. Each patient needs the same drug (e.g. an antibiotic) delivered to a general respiratory tract target site (e.g. peripheral and mid-bronchial). Each patient nebulizer is charged with a 2 ml 'fill', which is allowed to run until 'dryness' (usually 5–10 min), a typical application in most hospitals. We know from experi-ence and theory, that the child's lungs behave differently from the adult's, but nonetheless, were told by the nebulizer manufacturer that the aerosol droplets from their nebulizer have a size of 4 μm, and an output rate of 0.3 ml/min. As we shall see later, the method of measurement is critical, but for this example let us assume size was determined conveniently by laser diffraction, and output determined by weight loss. Both patients have beds in comfortable hospital wards – implying an ambient environment around 18 °C/68 °F and 50% relative humidity. Estimating by theoretical calcula-tion the quality of aerosol these two patients get is an interesting exercise and is summarized in Table 1.1.

Here, the different inhalation rates of the adult and child patients, as well as the condition of the ambient air, have a profound effect on particle size. The same nebulized aerosol therapy presented to an adult and a child (as in this example) would be expected to deliver fundamentally different aerosol. The adult's rate of inspiration entrains significant amounts of ambient air, which absorbs water to reach saturation from the nebulized aerosol released into the t-piece. This will inevitably result in a considerable reduction in

Table 1.1 The effect of evaporation on nebulized aerosol droplet size.
The calculations below assume a simple evaporative model for adult vs child
patients, using a typical and commonly available constant output nebulizer
design. Representative data is used, which assumes a nebulizer flow of 6l/min,
producing total nebulizer aerosol output of 0.1 ml/min (100 μl/min) containing
droplets with a initial Diameter of 4 μm. Adult and child patients inhale air at
average flow rates of 15 l/min and 7.5 l/min, respectively. In this example, from an
initial droplet size of 4 μm, the droplets inhaled by adults are seen to decrease to
2.6 μm (nearly half) due to the effect of evaporation on the nebulized droplet when
mixed with ambient air. The child, who entrains very little ambient air compared to
the adult, will theoretically inhale virtually unadulterated droplets of 3.8 μm
diameter. The magnitude of the evaporative effect would be influenced by ambient
temperature and humidity. The warmer and drier the environment, the greater the
evaporation, and the smaller the resulting nebulized droplet inhaled by the patient.[9]
Of course, the same amount of drug solute will be present, though it will necessarily
exist in a more concentrated state within the inhaled nebulized droplet. Further, the
lower the rate of nebulized aerosol output, the greater the evaporative effect.

			Adult	Child
A	Typical average flow rate of inhaled air during tidal breathing	ESTIMATE	15 μl/min	7.5 l/min
B	Typical air flow rate driven through nebulizer	ESTIMATE	6 l/min	6 l/min
C	Entrained ambient make-up air	A – B	15 – 6 = 9 l/min	7.5 – 6 = 1.5 l/min
D	Amount of water vapour contained per l of air at 100% RH and 18 °C	PHYSICAL CONSTANT	16 μl water vapour per l air	16 μl water vapour per l air
E	Calculated amount of water vapour at typical ambient conditions of 50% RH and 18 °C	D ÷ 2	8 μl water vapour per l air	8 μl water vapour per l air
F	Calculated amount of water vapour to be absorbed into ambient air entrained by patient during inhalation	C × E	9 l/min × 8 μl water vapour/l air = **72 μl** water vapour/min	1.5 l/min × 8 μl water vapour/l air = **12 μl** water vapour/min
G	Typical nebulizer aerosol output rate	ESTIMATE	100 μl/min	100 μl/min

Table 1.1 *(Continued)*

			Adult	Child
H	Calculated rate of aerosol output volume, after taking into account evaporation of water vapour to inhaled ambient air	G – F	100 μl/min – 72 μl/min = 28 μl/min	100 μl/l air – 12 μl/min = 88 μl/min
I	Initial droplet size produced by nebulizer	ESTIMATE	4 μm	4 μm
J	Volume of initial droplet size	radius is 2 μm, 4/3 pi r^3	33.5 um³	33.5 um³
K	Calculated volume of evaporated inhaled droplet	J × H/G	33.5 um³ × 0.28 = 9.3 um³	33.5 um³ × 0.88 = 29.5 um³
L	Calculated radius of evaporated droplet	$r = \sqrt[3]{(V \div pi \times \frac{3}{4})}$	1.3 μm	1.9 μm
M	Calculated diameter of droplet inhaled by patient taking into account evaporative effect.	D = 2 × r	2.6 μm	3.8 μm

particle size – in this example nearly half, from 4 μm down to 2.6 μm MMAD (Mass Median Aerodynamic Diameter). The child's lower rate of inspiration would result in entrainment of less ambient air, and therefore less evaporation of nebulized droplet solvent, and in the typical example above, the particle size is virtually unaffected (from 4 μm to 3.8 μm).

The reader is invited to consider their own experience with nebulized drug aerosol treatment, and perhaps do some basic maths themselves to explore the effect of evaporation in their own circumstances – nebulizer system, patient groups and ambient conditions. The importance of the likely confounding effect on the understanding and delivery on nebulized therapy cannot be overemphasized. The confusion in this area will remain until sensible standards are developed and adopted guiding nebulizer manufacturers to quote more informed and realistic information in describing the performance of their devices.

There are three jet nebulizer designs – constant output, breath-enhanced, and dosimetric.[10] The constant output design described above is the most commonly available nebulizer design. Here the nebulizer operates at the same speed throughout treatment, releasing aerosol into a t-piece during both patient inhalation and expiration. There are two other general nebulizer design concepts, breath-enhanced and dosimetric. All three are shown schematically in Figure 1.5. Breath-enhanced designs operate by allowing air inhaled by the patient to be drawn through the nebulizer, thus 'enhancing' the rate of air and aerosol output from the nebulizer during inhalation. On expiration, the output from this nebulizer falls back to a lower rate. Interestingly, because the entrained ambient air is drawn through the nebulizer itself, the evaporation of solvent to saturate this entrained air (discussed above) still occurs, but water vapor is drawn from the large reservoir within the nebulizer rather than the small volume contained in the released droplets as is the case with constant output nebulizers. This is extremely important, as it implies that the droplet size from breath-enhanced nebulizers is inherently stable. It does not change. It is not affected by either ambient air conditions, nor by characteristics of a particular patient's inhalation rate. However, there is a slightly increased rate of solute concentration within the reservoir of a breath-enhanced nebulizer. The extent of this will vary with ambient conditions, rates of air flow, etc. However, this is not nearly as important a confounding factor as post production evaporation of nebulized droplets.

Dosimetric nebulizers represent a third general category of nebulizer design. In theory, these release aerosol only to the patient during inhalation. During exhalation, patient breath-hold or pause in treatment, the dosimetric nebulizer does not release aerosol. Surprisingly given their apparent efficiencies, dosimetric nebulizer designs such as the AeroEclipse (Trudell Medical International, Canada), Circulaire (Westmed, USA) and Halolite (Profile Therapeutics, UK) seem to attract little attention. Whether this is due to weaknesses in the individual design of each and/or relatively high costs is unclear.

Ultrasonic nebulizers

Ultrasonic nebulizers are a separate design category from jet nebulizers. To date, they have not matched the popularity of jet nebulizers which is less than 1% of jet nebulizers. The reasons for this are not clear, but are believed

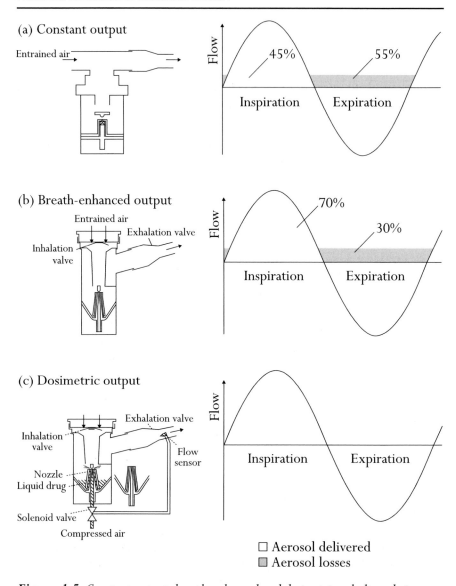

Figure 1.5 *Constant output, breath-enhanced and dosimetric nebulizer designs. (Adapted from Knoch and Sommer.* Eur Resp Rev *2000; 10: 183–6.[11])*

to be due primarily to historical problems of poor design, limitations in electronics, heating of drug liquids and higher costs. Various new examples of conventional designs are being developed such as AeroSpin (Lifecare Hospital Supplies Ltd, UK) which demonstrates promising results. None of the available conventional ultrasonic nebulizers have attracted much attention.

Having said this, it is largely the ultrasonic and ultrasonic-like technology that is providing the design platform for many of the new generation nebulization devices. Most of these new designs are taking advantage of technological advances in microelectronics and microtechnologies. Some of these new designs are introduced and discussed in Chapter 3. However, detailed information on the design and function of traditional ultrasonic nebulizers is beyond the scope of this chapter, and the reader is directed to comprehensive reviews elsewhere.[12]

References

1. Muers MF. Overview of nebulizer treatment. *Thorax* 1997; **52**(Suppl 2):S25–S30.
2. O'Callaghan C, Nerbrink O, Vidgren MT. The history of inhaled drug therapy. In: Bisgaard H, O'Callaghan C, Smaldone G eds. *Drug Delivery of the Lung*. New York: Marcel Dekker, 2002, 1–20.
3. Muthu DC. *Pulmonary tuberculosis: its etiology and treatment – record of twenty-two years observation and work in open-air sanatoria*. London:Bailliere, Tindal and Cox, 1922.
4. Elliott HL, Reid JL. The clinical pharmacology of a herbal asthma cigarette. *Br J Clin Pharmacol* 1980; **10**:487–90.
5. Heyder H, Svartengren MU. Basic principles of particle behavior in the human respiratory tract. In: Bisgaard H, O'Callaghan CO, Smaldone GC eds. *Drug delivery to the lung*. New York: Marcel Dekker, 2002, 303–37.
6. Smaldone GC, LeSouf PN. Nebulization: the device and clinical considerations. In: Bisgaard H, O'Callaghan C, Smaldone G eds. *Drug Delivery of the Lung*. New York: Marcel Dekker, 2002, 269–302.
7. Rudolph G, Kobrich R, Stahlhofen W. Modelling and algebraic formulation of regional aerosol deposition in man. *J Aerosol Sci* 1990; **21**:S306–S406.
8. Nikander K, Denyer J. Breathing patterns. *Eur Respir Rev* 2000; **10**:576–9.
9. Dennis JH, Stenton SC, Beach JR et al. Jet and ultrasonic nebuliser output: use of a new method for direct measurement of aerosol input. *Thorax* 1990; **45**:728–32.
10. Dennis JH. Drug nebuliser design and performance: breath enhanced jet vs constant output jet vs ultrasonic. *J Aerosols Med* 1995; **8**:277–80.
11. Knoch M and Sommer E. Jet nebuliser design and function. *Eur Resp Rev* 2000; **10**:183–6.
12. Rau JR. Design principles of liquid nebulization devices currently in use. *Respir Care* 2002; **47**:1257–78.

2. QUALITY CONTROL AND STANDARDS IN NEBULIZER PERFORMANCE AND USE

John H Dennis and Cora A Pieron

Introduction

Prescription drugs including oral and intravenous medications, as well as inhaled aerosol from pressurized metered dose inhalers (MDI) and dry powder inhalers (DPI) undergo clinical trials in an effort to prove safety and efficacy. This is not the case with the many drugs used for nebulization that are prescribed off-license and bypass regulatory requirement. The specific focus of this chapter, and the general focus of this book, is to address the issues surrounding off-license nebulizer use and provide effective guidance to clinicians.

Nebulizers are regarded as cheap and convenient plastic devices that readily generate an aerosol (see Figure 1.3) containing whatever drug solution or suspension that is placed in them for delivery to the respiratory tract. Nebulized drug delivery to the lungs has been used for centuries in medical research, and has been commercially available throughout the twentieth century.[1-4] However, the delivery of nebulized drug aerosols is to date still uncontrolled and poorly understood by the clinical community. Rarely is the nebulizer delivery device specified in the prescription. Rather, only the drug solution 'volume and concentration' are specified. This leaves open the choice of which nebulizer device to use for the delivery of the off-license drug aerosol. The decision is often left to the local doctor or nurse – or perhaps more disturbingly, which nebulizer device to use is decided by a hospital clerk who may choose a device which will become the hospital's standard nebulizer for that period of time (usually decided on price or effective marketing material). This nebulizer is often chosen with little or no objective justification other than manufacturer's claims about its performance or, more often, simply the low cost of a particular nebulizer brand. The reader should recognize that there is a large range of differences in the performance of nebulizers. If, for example, a similar 2 ml drug concentration was placed in all available nebulizer devices, the dose of nebulized aerosol delivered to the patient would vary more than ten-fold.[5] The lack of regulation and understanding in matching the prescribed drug with the nebulizer delivery device implies that the quality, consistency and control of the delivered dose of nebulized drug aerosol are poor.

There are two main types of nebulizer, including jet (or pneumatic) nebulizers and ultrasonic nebulizers. Each type can in turn have different operating characteristics,[6] and as described in Chapter 1, can be categorized in terms of their overall performance as one of three designs: constant output, breath-enhanced, or dosimetric nebulizers.[5] Each nebulizer brand has specific characteristics that define its aerosol output including total rate of aerosol output, rate of aerosol delivered to the patient, residual or dead volume, and particle size characteristics. Some nebulizers are most efficient at delivering small droplets to the peripheral lung; others are better suited to deliver larger particles in the upper airways. Some nebulizers, in the authors' opinion, are not suited for drug aerosol delivery at all. But how is the clinician to know which nebulizer to use? How is the clinician to know which out of a range of nebulizers is best for a particular patient or patient group? What criteria can the clinician use to make an informed decision?

There are many different methods published to measure the 'performance' of a particular nebulizer design.[7-9] For instance, measurement of aerosol output using weight loss has been undertaken for decades and is still commonly used. However, weight loss measures both aerosol output and evaporated solvent – and evaporated solvent typically accounts for half of the weight lost over a period of nebulization. In some particularly inefficient nebulizers, evaporation can account for more than 75% of the weight loss.[10] Alternatively, total aerosol output can be estimated by measuring the amount of drug 'solute' left in the nebulizer cup. While this can provide a measure of the total drug aerosol emitted and is not confounded by evaporative losses, it does not reflect the aerosol delivered to the patient, as most nebulizers only allow inhalation of 40–70% of the emitted dose by the patient. A similar problem is embodied in methods that collect all emitted aerosol on a filter followed by subsequent analysis of the filtered residue. Thus, although all these methods produce data, the results do not reflect the situation in vivo. This, in the authors' opinion, makes them weak methods on which to base a nebulizer standard, as results are divorced from the clinical setting.

Measuring aerosol particle size is equally confusing. Application of the high flow cascade impactor, commonly used to size aerosol from pressurized MDIs and DPIs, can drastically distort the aerosol size by causing full evaporation of the nebulized aerosol. In contrast laser diffraction sizing of droplets using scattered light cannot take into account the solute concentration induced by post-production evaporation of nebulized aerosol – a phenomena inherent in all constant output nebulizer designs. For both aerosol output and aerosol size, different results are possible from the same nebulizer depending on the method used for measurement.

The relative merits of different methods used to assess in vitro nebulizer performance have been debated in the literature for decades, often by individuals or small groups with a greater or lesser amount of training in aerosol and clinical sciences. From all the different views, one common message emerges: that the method used to assess performance of a given nebulizer should ideally reflect the amount and size of nebulized aerosol received by the patient.[11] In other words, the in vitro test should reflect the in vivo delivered dose. While this is a common and desired objective, over the past 50 years individual researchers have not naturally regressed to a commonly accepted nebulizer test method – such is the politics and reality of academic science. Because nebulized drugs have largely escaped regulatory control, it has been no particular national or international group's responsibility to examine the science and produce 'standard' in vitro assessment methods. At least, this was the situation up to the early 1990s. In 1994, the United Kingdom (UK) standards body the 'British Standards Institute' (BSI) made the first ever attempt at standardizing test methods through the publication of a British Standard.[12,13]

While British Standard BS 7711 part 3 specified methods that are now known to have significant limitations (Box 2.1), the very existence of the published standard became a focal point for debate and progress. In the late 1990s, the European Standards Organization addressed the issue of standardizing in vitro methods to assess nebulizer performance more comprehensively, by a 'critical mass' of aerosol scientists, clinicians, pharmaceutical scientists and nebulizer manufacturers. These efforts culminated in the development of new nebulizer in vitro test methods published as a European Standard, EN 13544-1.[15]

This chapter summarizes standardization issues inherent in the in vitro measurement of nebulizer performance, and presents the basic scientific and

---

Box 2.1 Strengths and weaknesses of British Standard BS 7711

Strengths of BS 7711 part 3

Issue	*Comment*
1. First formal national standard relating to jet nebulizers	Focused attention on assessment of nebulizer performance and provided a platform for debate and technical research and development
2. Adopted a chemical tracer rather than weight loss to evaluate nebulizer performance	Standard practice relied on weight loss which grossly overestimated true aerosol output due to concurrent evaporation to compressed and ambient air

Weaknesses of BS 7711 part 3

Issue	*Comment*
1. No use of breathing pattern in assessing nebulized aerosol inhaled	This is particularly important for assessing the performance of breath-enhanced and dosimetric nebulizer designs
2. Does not extend to ultrasonic nebulizers	Modern designs of ultrasonic nebulizers have solved many of past technical limitations and are expected to become more common as their advantages are recognized in the healthcare market (e.g. OMRON, Kyoto, Japan)
3. Relies on laser diffraction to estimate particle size parameters	Laser sizing takes no account of solute concentrating effects, particularly in the smaller particles, and provides a volume size distribution which will invariably be larger than the solute size (dry particles) distribution which is of far greater clinical relevance and interest
4. Applies laser diffraction to size a 'standing cloud'	Nebulized aerosols are largely aqueous and prone to rapid evaporation once in contact with drier ambient air, such as the air entrained over constant output or through breath-enhanced nebulizers

(Adapted from Dennis JH et al. *Eur Respir Rev* 2000; **19**:178–82.[14])

---

clinical principles underlying the European Standard. It also introduces the basic principles underlying the clinical nebulizer guidelines recently published by the European Respiratory Society, and describes how it usefully adopted the standard testing regimes formalized in the publication of the European Standard.

Standardization of methods to assess nebulizer aerosol output and size

There is a view that 'standardization' of an area may inhibit development and force regression to a mean – essentially making things more similar, making them a standard size, shape, color, or in the case of nebulizers, similar in terms of performance as measured by aerosol output and aerosol size. This is not the intended interpretation of standardization in this chapter.

There are many different types of nebulizer designs and brands, with a wide range of aerosol output and size performances. The authors regard this as a good thing because different drug solutions and suspensions are targeted to different parts of the airways. Further, different aerosol doses and droplet sizes are required for different patient–drug groups. Therefore, a variety of nebulizers are needed for pediatric and adult patients, and intensive care and home care. Clearly a wide range of nebulizer design and performance are required to fulfill this need, ideally every nebulized aerosol therapy being matched to a particular window of nebulizer performance. However, difficulty arises when clinicians (nurses, doctors, physiotherapists, etc) are faced with this great range of devices and manufacturers' claims of performance characteristics. How should a clinician make the choice of which nebulizer system is best suited to their patient (or patient group) for effective delivery of a particular drug?

In choosing the 'ideal' nebulizer for delivery of a particular drug the clinician should try to account for various factors including the intended site of aerosol deposition in the upper and/or lower respiratory tract. This, in turn, largely defines the required aerosol size depending on the patient's age and disease state, desired aerosol dose, total treatment time, compliance with the treatment, etc. In addition, there may be cost constraints on the clinician limiting the choice available in the market place. At the present time, a major difficulty is that the information on nebulizer performance is not presented to the clinician in any meaningful way.

The information on nebulized aerosol output and size may be entirely missing or only loosely described in marketing jargon using terms like: the 'best' performing nebulizer ... clinically proven ... preferred by over 90% of users, etc. These terms are often quoted without any real scientific justification behind the claim being made and they often do not stand up to scrutiny. Of course, not all nebulizer manufacturers are so vague in describing performance of their devices. Many manufacturers will actively promote, or at least have available, technical supporting literature. However, these performance data can also be obtained using a wide variety of laboratory methods.

However well informed the clinician, the manufacturer's performance data presented are very dependent on the method by which they were obtained. For this reason, a manufacturer's output data may become nearly meaningless. Aerosol output measured by weight loss, solute loss, etc may be done with or without breath simulation. Aerosol size measured by a laser sizer does not incorporate any simulated patient inhalation flow (which markedly affects the inhaled droplet size in many nebulizers, Table 1.1). Cascade impaction using methods developed and suited to high flow inhalation maneuvers seen with DPI and pressurized MDIs results in gross distortion of the droplet size delivered to the patient.

Yet, the manufacturer's information, if and when available, is often the only information available to the clinician to help make an educated guess for which device to adopt for nebulized delivery of an off-license drug. As recognized experts in the field, the authors often find it extremely difficult to determine relative performance from different sources of published data without undertaking further laboratory in vitro tests. It must be difficult in the extreme – if not impossible – for the average clinician, who is not an expert in the area of nebulizer design and function, to make an informed decision on which device might be best for their patient group.

The focus here is to present a case for establishing and accepting a common set of measurement methods to assess nebulized aerosol output and size. In so doing, the authors hope to convince the reader that the introduction and widespread adoption of 'standardization' of in vitro methods used to measure nebulized aerosol output and size would be beneficial to both the patient and the carer, and very likely the pharmaceutical and nebulizer device manufacturing industries as well.

Standardization of in vitro methodology should greatly help clinicians when they need to decide on the most appropriate nebulizer delivery device for their patient groups. If standardization of the in vitro assessment of nebulized aerosol output were to occur, then a commonly derived data set between all nebulizers could be more easily interpreted and the best choice made.

Standardization of in vitro performance measures can only serve to improve patient safety and drug efficacy. Moreover, in the long term, standardization of in vitro performance can help provide a more solid foundation for development of better nebulizer technologies as manufacturers can be assured that the market place is better prepared to recognize and appreciate the real benefits of any new technology. At the present time, if a manufacturer produced a better nebulizer, how would the clinician know? It would just get absorbed in the market place as yet another 'best performance' nebulizer claim with perhaps a few supporting papers written by individuals with personal bias and affiliation. It is for these reasons that standardization is required.

The European Standard for nebulizers

The European Standard developed over a period of six years, involving all European national standards bodies (e.g. the UK's BSI, the Netherlands TNO, etc) working within the European Committee for Standardization (Comité Européen de Normalisation CEN), the European umbrella organization. Most European scientists and clinicians with a serious interest in nebulizer testing and clinical application were involved either directly or indirectly in the development of this standard, which was published in 2001.[15] As stated before for the first time, a 'critical mass' of clinical and scientific experts were brought together to focus on how best to 'standardize' the measurement of nebulizer 'performance'. Although the European Standard on nebulizers addresses a number of regulatory issues, most are beyond the scope of this chapter. What is important here is that the European Standard facilitated the gradual evolution and development of in vitro testing methodologies that were thoroughly discussed and evaluated prior to acceptance by the European clinical and scientific aerosol community. Detailed aspects of the European Standard have been described elsewhere.[16,17] The more important general principles are introduced and summarized below.

Nebulizer versus nebulizer system

The European Standard recognizes that different nebulizers will deliver different doses of drug to the same patient – even if all conditions are controlled, such as breathing pattern, volume fill of drug solution or suspension, etc. This is because some nebulizers are inherently more efficient than others. For example, consider the most common nebulizer design, the constant output nebulizer which likely accounts for more than 70% of the nebulizers in home and hospital use today. A constant output nebulizer emits aerosol at a constant rate until the volume of drug solution remaining in the nebulizer cup is so small that the nebulizer ceases to function. The rate of aerosol output is constant – regardless of whether the patient is inhaling, breath holding, or exhaling. This implies that for at least half the duration of the operation the nebulizer is emitting aerosol into the general hospital or home environment. Not only is this extremely wasteful, it is a significant source of unwanted airborne pollution. Breath-enhanced nebulizers, on the other hand, release more aerosol during patient inhalation than during breath-hold or exhalation and are thus inherently more efficient. Dosimetric nebulizers are theoretically the most efficient. Dosimetric nebulizers waste no aerosol to the environment (in theory) as aerosol is only released during patient inhalation so the entire emitted dose is delivered to the patient.

However, it is not only the nebulizer design which is important in establishing the relative performance of the nebulizer, the characteristics of the nebulizer itself can be critically important. In general with a jet nebulizer, the greater the flow of compressed air through the nebulizer, the greater the aerosol output and, usually, the smaller the particle size. So the compressor becomes an integral part of the nebulizer 'system'. Another important part of the nebulizer system which can significantly influence the quantity and quality of nebulized aerosol delivered to the patient is the mouthpiece, its use and design – for example, whether the mouthpiece is valved for exhalation or non-valved. Alternatively, the mouthpiece might be replaced by a facemask, which will greatly reduce the amount of drug effectively delivered to the patient.

The European Standard recognizes the importance of the 'nebulizer system' rather than simply the nebulizer itself. For this reason, the European Standard specifies that nebulizer manufacturers should test performance of the system as they intend it to be used. So, for example, if a nebulizer manufacturer sold their nebulizer sometimes with a mouthpiece and sometimes with a facemask, then each of these two nebulizer systems would need to be tested for aerosol output and size using the European Standard methods. Similarly if the nebulizer was recommended for use with different compressed air flows, the manufacturer is required to test each nebulizer system with the range of recommended air flows – the minimum and maximum, as well as typical average air flow rates. Although these permutations can result in a significant range of testing parameters, each permutation relates to a specific clinical condition of use for which the manufacturer is targeting their nebulizer product. Adoption of a nebulizer system concept will dissuade manufacturers or researchers to publish performance information on a given nebulizer without also making reference to the system in which it was tested.

Effect of drug preparation on nebulizer performance

One area the European Standard avoids is testing all nebulizer designs for their ability to nebulize all drugs. Most drugs commonly prescribed are solutions of an active drug compound in a water-based system that also contains excipients and usually some concentration of sodium chloride (NaCl). Some drugs are suspensions and are present in small, nearly colloidal, suspensions of individual solid particles within an aqueous solution, again, usually with excipients including some concentration of NaCl. Most drug formulations intended for nebulization (by design or prescribed off license) behave much like a simple salt solution. Admittedly, a few drug solutions/suspensions do not because they are extremely viscous, or froth or foam during reflux in the nebulizer, or have some other physical characteristics that result in atypical behavior. However, they are the exceptions. The European Standard recognizes that testing all forms of drug solutions and suspensions on all of the nebulizer system combinations would place an unreasonable burden on resources. The practice adopted within the European Standard was to adopt a single test solution for each nebulizer system permutation – a low concentration of sodium fluoride (NaF). Sodium fluoride was chosen for a number of reasons: it has similar properties to NaCl which is commonly used in nebulized drug formulations; it is relatively unique in most laboratory environments so contamination from other sources is minimized; and finally, analysis of NaF concentrations using electrochemistry (a method similar to pH measurement) is relatively simple, low cost, and sufficiently sensitive for analysis.

Measuring aerosol output and aerosol size using the methods embodied within the European Standard

Aerosol output

The standard methodology adopted in the European Standard for measuring aerosol output is described schematically in Figure 2.1. The nebulizer system under test is fitted to a breath simulation device and a low resistance electrostatic filter simulating the patient is placed between this and the

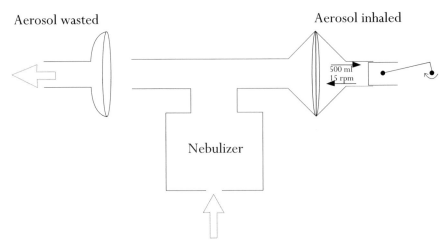

Figure 2.1 *Schematic of CEN (European Committee for Standardization) methodology to measure nebulized aerosol output. 'Inhaled' aerosol output is subject to sinus flow breath simulation and aerosol is collected onto low resistance electrostatic filters. Aerosol contains trace concentrations of sodium fluoride which can subsequently be desorbed and quantified electrochemically. (Adapted from Boe J et al.* Eur Respir J *2001;* **18**:228–42.[17])

nebulizer system being tested. The intention here is that aerosol collected on this filter will represent aerosol delivered to the patient under clinical conditions. The breathing cycle adopted within the European Standard is a simple sinus flow pattern of 15 cycles/min and 500 ml/cycle. This pattern was adopted because it is a relatively simple pattern to simulate and reproduce within a standard. Other breathing patterns were considered (square waves, various inspiratory–expiratory ratios, etc) but none was thought more appropriate as a single measure than the simple sinus flow pattern. While this pattern is specifically defined in the European Standard, the method used can be adapted to virtually any other breathing pattern. Whatever the breathing pattern, the nebulizer is filled with a volume of test liquid that contains a trace amount (1%) of NaF. With the breath simulation device running and an electrostatic filter in place, any aerosol generated by the nebulizer system that is drawn into the breathing system (the analogy of being 'inhaled' by a patient) is collected on the filter. The fluoride residue on the filter can be subsequently quantified.

Aerosol size
The standard methodology adopted in the European Standard for measuring aerosol particle size is described schematically in Figure 2.2. Here a low

28

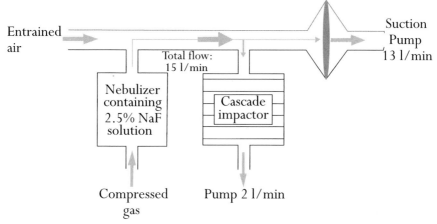

Figure 2.2 *Schematic of CEN (European Committee for Standardization) methodology to measure nebulized aerosol particle size. A constant inhalation of 15 l/min is drawn over (or through) the nebulizer. Nebulized aerosol containing a NaF solute tracer mixes with this entrained air. A low flow cascade impactor (Marple 290X Series Low Flow Multiple Stage Cascade Impactor, Westech Instruments Services, Upper Stondon, UK) samples aerosol at 2 l/min from this flow, and impacted aerosol can subsequently be desorbed and analyzed from each size fraction from which the normative and cumulative particle size distributions can be derived. (Adapted from Boe J et al.* Eur Respir J *2001;* **18**:228–42[17] *with permission from European Respiratory Society Journals Limited.)*

flow cascade impactor is placed in line with the nebulizer system, again containing a trace (2.5%) concentration of NaF. Instead of using the dynamic air flow pattern of a breathing machine, a constant simulated 'inhalation' flow of 15 l/min is applied, which was thought to represent a typical midflow inhalation speed. The cascade impactor samples a 2 l/min (2/15) fraction of this total inhaled flow. Again, the fluoride residue drawn into the low flow cascade impactor is deposited on the interior stages of the cascade according to the size of the droplets generated. The fluoride residue can be subsequently quantified and the relative amounts found on each stage can be compiled. Table 2.1 presents a sample set of cascade impactor data, which can then be used to derive cumulative and normative size distributions such as those depicted in Figure 2.3.

Clinical relevance of the European Standard in vitro methods

It is not known how well the currently drafted European Standard EN 13544-1 test conditions will predict clinical use. This can only be established once appropriate studies have compared in vitro output and size

Table 2.1 Worked example of data obtained from a low flow cascade impactor.

A Stage	B µg Drug (SampleA1)	C log₁₀(Gstage 1) − log₁₀(Gstage2) (Δlog (Dp))	D B ÷ C (Conc/Δlog (Dp))	E √(Gstage 1 × Gstage 2) geometric mean Dp (GMD (µm))	F Dstage ÷ (Dtotal/100) (conc/Δlog (Dp)) normalized	G Cut-point from manual (Dp (µm))	H Cumulative sums from column I (% <Dp)	I Bstage ÷ Btotal × 100% (V/Vtot (%))
MMAD 3.9 Top	1.36					50	98.491 74	1.508 262
Stage 1	1.43	0.853 316	1.675 815	32.634 34	1.057 587	21.3	96.905 84	1.585 893
Stage 2	1.94	0.364 08	5.328 501	17.755	3.362 753	14.8	94.754 35	2.151 492
Stage 3	7.80	0.412 245	18.9 208	12.043 26	11.940 69	9.8	86.104 03	8.650 327
Stage 4	13.4	0.490 623	27.312 22	7.668 116	17.236 41	6	71.243 21	14.860 82
Stage 5	24.3	0.538 997	45.083 78	4.582 576	28.451 83	3.5	44.294 11	26.9491
Stage 6	21.6	0.814 508	26.519 08	2.329 163	16.735 87	1.55	20.339 36	23.954 75
Stage 7	11.7	0.510 826	22.9041	1.200 625	14.45 45	0.93	7.363 868	12.975 49
Stage 8	4.64	0.581 356	7.981 343	0.695 414	5.036 93	0.52	2.218 033	5.145 836
Final	2.00	0.732 368	2.730 868	0.360 555	1.723 418	0.25	0	2.218 033
	90.17		158.4565		100			100

Column A identifies the different stages; column B the amounts of drug or salt assayed by the HPLC on each stage; columns C–F contain calculations on how to process the size distribution data; column G the cut-point of each stage from the Graseby 298 operating manual; column H the cumulative summation of material (derived from column I) which allows plotting of the cumulative distribution curve against size fraction; column I the proportion of the aerosol on each stage (derived from column B). MMAD, mass median aerodynamic diameter; HPLC, high performance liquid chromatography; Dp, droplet diameter. (Table and formula is adapted from the manufacturer's operating manual for the Graseby 298 impactor running at 2 l/min.[18])

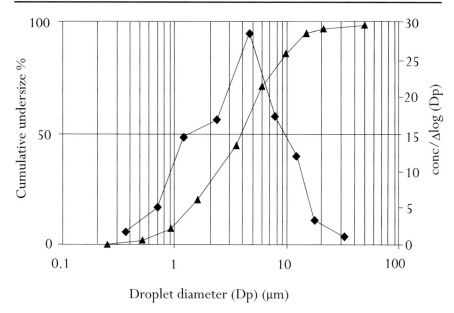

Figure 2.3 *Cumulative (▲) and normative (♦) distribution curves obtained from data in Table 2.1. Aerosol was collected and size assessed using the low flow cascade impaction method specified in EN 13544-1. The MMAD (median mass aerodynamic diameter) of 3.9 µm (Table 2.1) is derived from the cumulative plot as the size in µm intersecting the 50% cumulative undersize. (Data: courtesy CA Pieron.)*

measurements against in vivo lung deposition from a variety of nebulizer devices. However, the European Standard in vitro methods were developed with the agreement of a number of leading nebulized aerosol scientists and clinicians in Europe and were deliberately tailored so they could meet the needs of type testing within a European Standard as well as being as clinically relevant as practicable. Preliminary work relating draft in vitro methods embodied in the European Standard with in vivo measures of aerosol deposition seem promising (Figure 2.4)[19] though more research is needed in this area. If the European Standard in vitro methodology were to provide good estimates of in vivo deposition, then the in vitro methods could be used to guide clinical users when deciding which nebulizer systems may be best suited for different patient groups. If the correlation is shown to be poor the in vitro methods can be examined and modified in subsequent standards to provide a better and more clinically representative measure of nebulized aerosol output.

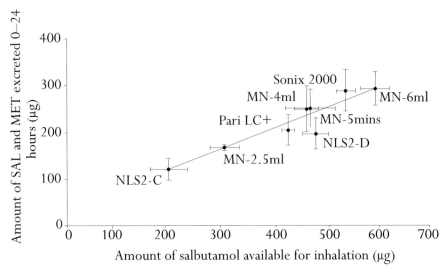

Figure 2.4 *Correlation between an early draft of the in vitro methods used in the European Standard (x-axis) with in vivo deposition (y-axis) measured by urinary salbutamol from eight nebulizer systems with different design and performance characteristics. SAL, salbulamol; MET, sulphate ester conjugate. (Adapted from Silkstone VL et al. J Aerosol Med 2002; **15**:251–60.[19])*

European Respiratory Society guidelines on the use of nebulizers

The in vitro methods embodied in the European Standard to estimate nebulizer performance are already being used to improve clinical practice. To appreciate inherent advantages in the standardization of in vitro nebulizer performance, the following section introduces and describes basic principles underlying the clinical nebulizer guidelines recently introduced by the European Respiratory Society (ERS).

The ERS commissioned a Task Force in the mid-1990s to review the scientific and clinical principles of nebulized therapy and to produce a set of guidelines (evidence-based whenever possible) for users of nebulized treatment in Europe. The aims were to produce a set of clinical guidelines to improve clinical practice in the use of nebulized therapy throughout Europe. The Task Force through a series of three interactive workshops developed the ERS guidelines; each workshop was conducted with about 25 invited experts from the field of nebulizers. The ERS nebulizer guidelines were published in 2001.[17]

The most important aim of the guidelines was to increase efficacy and patient safety by recommending systems by which nebulizers could be chosen and used. The guidelines were aimed at a wide group of healthcare professions practicing in very different healthcare systems throughout Europe. Although the immediate target audience included pulmonary physicians the message was also aimed at all healthcare workers involved in treating patients with nebulized medication. The guidelines provided recommendations based on scientific and clinical evidence and also identified areas of ignorance where present practice is based on tradition or opinion rather than scientific evidence. It was also hoped that by identifying the gaps in the present knowledge, the guidelines would spur on clinical scientists to undertake new trials to guide future practice. The full details of the background to the content of the guidelines can be found in published supplements from the technical[20] and clinical[21] workshops as well as in the ERS guidelines themselves.[17]

The specific part of the ERS nebulizer guidelines most relevant to this chapter is the technical reliance on the methods embodied in the European Standard. The European in vitro methods offer, for the first time, opportunity to obtain a set of aerosol output data for each nebulizer sold in the European market. In other words, a comprehensive set of nebulizer performance data that has been commonly derived from the same in vitro methods. Hopefully, each set of nebulizer performance data will closely reflect the in vivo performance. Further, the ERS clinical guidelines have adopted the distinction embodied in the European Standard on the difference between a nebulizer and a nebulizer system, and the clinical guidelines rely on data obtained from complete nebulizer systems.

The availability of clinically representative in vitro systems has led to the establishment and implementation of standard operating practices as a means of improving the efficacy of nebulized drug therapy. These are embodied in the ERS clinical guidelines and are worth summarizing in this chapter.

Type testing using the European Standard within the ERS clinical guidelines

Nebulizer manufacturers are now required to test each of their nebulizer systems with a reference solution according to the European Standard. This will result in standardized information being supplied with every nebulizer and will include:

1. Description of the nebulizer system that includes the flow rates and volume fills at which tests were made.
2. Rate of aerosol output and total aerosol output.
3. The droplet size distribution curve from which the median size (mass median aerodynamic diameter, MMAD) and spread (geometric standard deviation, GSD), and % aerosol mass within any given range can be obtained, i.e. >5 μm, 2–5 μm, <2 μm.

As mentioned above, the in vitro methods on which the European Standard is based are designed to reflect clinical conditions as closely as possible. The consistency of methods to obtain this in vitro information through the European Standard will essentially provide a type test for each nebulizer system. This will allow meaningful comparison of relative performances of different nebulizer systems which, in turn, can be used to guide the optimal use of different nebulizer models in clinical practice.

There are some important limitations in interpreting test data supplied by manufacturers complying with the European Standard. The first is that data supplied by the manufacturers relate only to drug solutions that have properties similar to saline. Test data cannot be readily extended to suspensions (e.g. budesonide) or to solutions that have a significantly greater viscosity than saline (e.g. some antibiotics). The second is that the rates and amounts of aerosol delivery have been obtained using a simulated adult healthy breathing pattern and these cannot be readily transferred to pediatric applications or to diseased adults. However, the test methods adopted within the European Standard are sufficiently flexible to accommodate additional test configurations.

Characteristics of good and bad nebulizer systems

Nebulizer systems have a wide range of performance and how good or bad an individual system is depends on what it is intended for. For example, if a system were required to deliver the maximum amount of 'useful' aerosol (droplets between 0.5 μm and 5 μm) in the minimum amount of time, with the least inconvenience, then the characteristics of a 'good' system would include:

- Fast rate of nebulization – implying that the maximum amount of nebulized aerosol is potentially available to the patient over any given time.
- Minimum waste of drug aerosol – implying that maximum amount of aerosol released is delivered to the patient and not emitted to the environment.
- Low residual volume – implying that more of the volume fill will be delivered to the patient as aerosol.
- Well defined droplet size distribution.

If, however, the same system were required to deliver only a modest volume of drug aerosol then the system above becomes 'bad', because such an efficent system of delivery will deliver an unnecessarily large aerosol dose with possible increased local and systemic side effects.

The ERS guidelines recognize that consideration must be given to matching nebulized drug delivery to the performance of nebulizer systems. This requirement will vary according to the needs of different patient groups or stage of the disease under treatment. The two main factors to take into account are:

1. How much nebulized drug is ideally required for delivery to the patient; and
2. The aerosol size required to deliver nebulized droplets to the site of action. Small aerosols (<5 μm) will deposit peripherally whereas droplets around 5 μm will mainly deposit in airways that are more central.

The ERS guidelines recognize that little clinical evidence exists to answer these questions and it is therefore difficult to choose the ideal nebulizer system for a given application. This being the case, the ERS guidelines recommend that a scheme is developed to define the best available nebulizer system for various therapies, in order to reduce variability in nebulized dose delivery and thereby improve clinical practice.

How to select the optimal system for a given patient group or for specific usage

Healthcare systems throughout Europe currently have some system by which nebulized drugs are prescribed for each clinical application. In addition, all prescribers and users of nebulized therapy usually have experience of using one (or more) nebulizer systems for each clinical application. Local practices differ greatly, possibly even within an institution.

It was therefore recommended in the ERS nebulizer guidelines that a Standard Operating Practice (SOP) be adopted for each nebulizer system in use. This would provide a baseline for determining the clinical effectiveness of that nebulizer system for each given application. In turn, this could then be used to assess potential improvements to the nebulizer system.

Implementation and use of the Standard Operating Practice to improve the efficacy of nebulized drug therapy

To standardize the way current nebulizer systems are used

If health practitioners can agree an SOP for the way in which nebulizer systems are used locally, then they can be sure that future clinical outcomes are patient specific, rather than due to a significant change in drug output from the nebulizer. Nebulizer manufacturers can provide advice on the optimum operating parameters for a particular nebulizer.

To assess drug output from the current nebulizer system

The scarcity of useful in vitro data describing nebulizer system performance has perhaps contributed to arbitrary choice of nebulizer systems. However, the standardization of nebulizer aerosol output and size measurements made possible through the European Standard allows any given SOP to be reassessed. For a specific clinical application, the SOP can be used in conjunction with data from the manufacturer to allow the dose delivered using this SOP to be derived. This dose can be the total output, or can be modified by the fraction of the aerosol in the optimal size range, to give a 'useful' dose. If appropriate, one should also consider the potential systemic exposure arising from drug not in the 'useful' range, either by (a) being too large, being swallowed and subsequently orally available, or (b) depositing in an inappropriate region of the lung, and being directly absorbed into the systemic circulation with minimal local efficacy. Based on this approach, potential modification to the existing SOP can be assessed to see whether drug delivery can be further optimized by a change in one of the operating parameters, e.g. gas flow rate.

To evaluate alternative nebulizer systems

This information can be re-evaluated over time, as more efficient or cheaper nebulizers emerge. Consideration can then be given to altering prescription convention and/or adopting alternative nebulizer systems whose nominal delivered dose and droplet size (available from the manufacturer using the same standard in vitro data) may be better suited to that given clinical application. However, any changes to SOP should be supported by appropriate follow-up of outcomes such as clinical benefits or side effects. It is recommended that the effect of significant changes to nebulizer usage be monitored by the appropriate follow-up of clinical outcomes.

Future developments in nebulized drug delivery

The ERS guidelines anticipated that technical advances in microtechnology and other areas would drive improvements in nebulizer design. These advancements in performance are being embodied in the next generation of nebulizers,[22] which are beginning to enter the market and will compete alongside more traditional jet and ultrasonic nebulizers. Some of this new nebulizer technology is introduced and discussed in Chapter 3.

At the very least, improved nebulizer technology offers significant improvements in efficiency in nebulized drug delivery. While these systems offer the potential to improve the quality of nebulized drug therapy, there are risks if they were adopted with insufficient consideration of the consequences of improvements in efficiency. However, if local practices adopted the above recommendations of instituting and reviewing SOPs, new and improved nebulized therapies could be safely integrated with net benefits to patients requiring nebulized drug therapy. It is likely that newer, more efficient systems will deliver inhaled drugs more effectively and thus reduce the wastage and cost associated with inefficient systems. Clearly, standardization of the measurment of in vitro performance is required to make safe and best use of these new nebulizer technologies.

Summary

Standardization of the in vitro methods to measure nebulizer performance would greatly reduce confusion and improve safety and efficacy of nebulized aerosol therapy. A new European Standard has been recently published which specifies in vitro methods for measuring and reporting nebulizer performance that is expected to correlate closely with in vivo nebulizer dose and size. The independent development of the ERS nebulizer guidelines takes advantage of the European Standard and relies on the latter's in vitro methods to develop and recommend a common-sense strategy to improve clinical practice in the use of nebulized therapy throughout Europe.

Both the European Standard and ERS guidelines on the use of nebulizers are, by definition, intended to influence and improve the standard of nebulized aerosol therapy care in Europe. In practice, the in vitro methods described are universal. So, too, are the recommendations to improve clinical practice. This is the authors' message to readers: that although the standardization issues have been tackled in Europe they apply equally in North America and elsewhere. If there is no good reason to adopt alternative in vitro methods for assessing nebulizer performance, then the methods embodied in the European Standard can be adopted in North America, or perhaps even adopted (with or without refinements) at a higher level by the International Standards Organization (ISO). This evolution would allow for any required changes and improvements to the European in vitro assessment methods that might become evident with time.

Some standardization in assessing in vitro nebulizer performance in North America is inevitable, and very much required. However, the nebulizer manufacturing industry is very small in comparison to the pharmaceutical industry and can ill-afford a plethora of testing regimes. In the authors' opinion, there should be only one recognized standard for in vitro assessment of nebulized aerosol. Developing a separate standard set of in vitro methods for North America defeats the purpose and would only serve to confuse the issue. It is the authors' hope that North American standards bodies look closely at the methods adopted in Europe, and consider two options. First, and perhaps most simply, the in vitro methods accepted in Europe could be simply adopted in entirety in North America. Second, if fundamental problems with the European methods were discovered, or alternative methods were found to be more closely correlated with in vivo response, then dialog and cooperation between interested organizations in North America, Europe and elsewhere could agree a new set of methods embodied in an International Standard. Either way, a single set of in vitro methods would result which could be used in the absence of clinical trials to guide nurses, physiotherapists, doctors and other clinicians in the most appropriate choice of nebulizer for their patients.

The worst case scenario would be that more than one set of in vitro methods are adopted in different countries which yield a variety of results for different nebulizer systems. This would act to retard progress and increase confusion and must be avoided.

At the present time, it is difficult if not impossible to compare meaningfully in vitro data due to confusion in methodology and understanding of nebulizer operation. If a single in vitro method like the European Standard EN 13544-1 standard was widely adopted then output figures between different nebulizer systems could be compared and evaluated by users.

References

1. Muers MF. Overview of nebulizer treatment. *Thorax* 1997; **52**:S25–S30.
2. O'Callaghan C, Nerbrink O, Vidgren MT. The history of inhaled drug therapy. In: Bisgaard H, O'Callaghan C, Smaldone GC eds. *Drug Delivery to the Lung*. New York: Marcel Dekker, 2002:1–18.
3. Mercer TT. Production of therapeutic aerosols: principles and techniques. *Chest* 1981; **80**:S813–S817.
4. Wright BM. A new nebulizer. *Lancet* 1958; **ii**:24.
5. Dennis JH. Drug nebuliser design and performance: breath enhanced jet vs constant output jet vs ultrasonic. *J Aerosol Med* 1995; **8**:277–80.
6. Hess DR. Nebulizers: principles and performance. *Respir Care* 2000; **35**:609–22.
7. Dolovich M. Assessing nebulizer performance. *Respir Care* 2002; **47**:1290–1304.
8. Beach JR, Young CL, Avery AJ et al. Measurement of airway responsiveness to methacholine: relative importance of the precision of drug delivery and the method of assessing response. *Thorax* 1993; **48**:239–43.
9. Smaldone GC, LeSouef P. Nebulization: the device and clinical considerations. In: Bisgaard H, O'Callaghan C, Smaldone GC eds. *Drug Delivery to the Lung*. New York: Marcel Dekker, 2002:269–302.
10. Dennis JH, Stenton SC, Beach JR et al. Jet and ultrasonic nebulizer output: use of a new method to measure aerosol output directly. *Thorax* 1990; **45**:728–32.
11. Smaldone GC. Drug delivery via aerosol systems: concept of 'aerosol inhaled'. *J Aerosol Med* 1991; **4**:229–35.
12. British Standard 7711 Part 3: Respiratory Therapy Equipment: Part 3, Specification for gas-powered nebulizers for the delivery of drugs. London: The Stationery Office, 1994.
13. Dennis JH. Standardisation in drug nebulisers: BS7711 Part 3. *J Aerosol Med* 1995; **8**:313–15.
14. Dennis JH, Pieron CA, Nerbrink O. Standardis in assessing in vitro nebulizer performance. *Eur Respir Rev* 2000; **19**:178–82.
15. European Standard EN 13544-1. Respiratory Therapy Equipment Part 1. Nebulizing Systems and their Components. 2001.

16. Dennis JH. A review of issues relating to nebulizer standards. *J Aerosol Med* 1998; **11**(Suppl 1):S73–S79.

17. Boe J, Dennis JH, O'Driscoll BR. European Respiratory Society Guidelines on the use of nebulizers. *Eur Respir J* 2001; **18**:228–42.

18. Graseby Operating Manual Series 290 Maple Personal Cascade Impactors. *Bulletin No. 2091.M.-3-82.*

19. Silkstone VL, Dennis JH, Pieron CA, Chrystyn H. An investigation of in-vitro/in-vivo correlations for salbutamol nebulized by eight systems. *J Aerosol Med* 2002; **15**:251–60.

20. Boe J, Dennis JH eds. European Respiratory Society nebulizer guidelines: technical aspects. *Eur Respir Rev* 2000; **10**.

21. Boe J, Dennis JH, O'Driscoll BR eds. European Respiratory Society nebulizer guidelines: clinical aspects. *Eur Respir Rev* 2000; **10**.

22. Dennis JH, Nerbrink O. New nebulizer technology. In: Bisgaard H, O'Callaghan C, Smaldone GC eds. *Drug Delivery to the Lung*. New York: Marcel Dekker, 2002:303–34.

3. NEW DEVELOPMENTS IN NEBULIZER TECHNOLOGY

John H Dennis

Introduction

So many new nubulizer technologies are being concurrently developed around the world at present that it is inconceivable they will not significantly impact on the drug aerosol delivery market in the very near future. This chapter presents specific examples of developments from the Netherlands, United States of America (USA), Germany, and Japan although there are still other technologies that have not yet been made public. Some of these new nebulizer technologies are in the latter stages of basic research and development in industrial and/or academic laboratories while others have evolved into working prototypes. The more advanced examples of new nebulizer technology are fully developed and now being released in the market place. It is an exciting time in the history of nebulizer technology. Just how fast the introduction of these various technologies is with regard to their economics, uptake by the clinical community and the extent of anticipated integration with pharmaceutical partners remains to be seen. This chapter describes these new generation of nebulizer technologies and evaluates implications from their introduction in regards to patient safety and drugs efficacy.

In the author's view, nebulizers are as efficient as other common means of drug aerosol delivery. Conversely, the author believes that the traditional nebulizer can be described as being 'equally inefficient' as modern pressurized metered dose inhalers (MDIs) and dry powder inhalers (PDIs). All of these deliver only around one-fifth of the available drug dose effectively to the patient – the remaining 80% being of no therapeutic value.

Traditional nebulizers typically waste the majority of the drug fill as residue in the nebulizer cup after treatment, and generally waste about half the aerosol released to the ambient environment. Pressurized MDIs used without spacer lose the majority of the drug dose by impaction at extreme velocity in the patient's mouth and throat, as well as residue left in the device itself. Pressurized MDIs used with a spacer are better as they replace the aerosol lost to throat deposition with aerosol lost to deposition within the spacer device – at least here it has no unwanted swallowed systemic effect. DPIs in theory offer higher efficiencies, though in practice patients have difficulty achieving the 'correct' inhalation air flow maneuver for optimum dispersion and release of the drug aerosol – this reduces the overall efficiency of DPIs to that typical of traditional nebulizers and pressurized MDIs without spacer. Of course these views are controversial and represent liberal generalizations of relatively complex fields. However, these generalizations are presented to ask the reader to consider the relative merits of traditional aerosol delivery devices: pressurized MDI (with and without spacer), DPI and nebulizer.

Of these three basic technologies, the traditional drug aerosol market seems to have regressed over the past decades to traditional bulk volume production of the pressurized MDI. This device is conveniently portable, traditional and well established, and seems to be the cheapest device to manufacture. In contrast, nebulizer systems are substantially more expensive due to the compressor systems required for operation while DPIs face costly formulation challenges. Hence, both DPIs and nebulizers are more expensive than pressurized MDIs. This is the current state of play and none of the presently available technologies represent the 'ideal' drug delivery system.

The ideal drug aerosol delivery system

The ideal drug aerosol delivery system, from the universal perspective, would include the following features:

1. Delivers a safe and therapeutically useful drug aerosol dose.
2. Delivers a safe and therapeutically useful aerosol dose across a wide range of drug preparations.
3. Delivers the desired drug aerosol dose across a wide range of patient and disease groups.
4. Easy to use (for all including young and old).
5. Portable (small and light).
6. Silent and inconspicuous.
7. Smart (signals indicating when: not functioning properly; dose delivery is complete; patient compliance monitor, etc).

8. Cost effective.
9. No wasted aerosol (occupational and environmental hazard from release of wasted drug aerosol).
10. No significant wasted residual drug left in device after use.
11. Environmentally friendly [no damaging propellants such as chloro-fluro-carbons (CFCs) and hydrofluroalkanes (HFAs)] and ideally recyclable.

This is a long list of 'ideal' features. Because different patient groups will require varying drug aerosol doses with different drug aerosol size ranges it is unlikely that one 'ideal' device is possible – although conceivably could be possible if the device could be set or programmed for different needs. It is clear that neither pressurized MDIs nor DPIs meet all of these criteria, despite the enormous amounts of pharmaceutical funding which have been devoted to these devices over the past 3 decades. The funding devoted to traditional pressurized MDIs and DPIs by the pharmaceutical industry is grossly disproportionate to the funding given to developing nebulizer technology. However, given the apparent 'dead end' encountered in further efficiency gains from pressurized MDIs and DPIs, over the past 10 years or so, funding and efforts in research and development of nebulizer technology has been gaining ground with notable successes. It is in the future development of new nebulizer technologies that the author believes the greatest gains are and will be made approaching the 'ideal' drug aerosol delivery technology.

New developments in generic nebulizer technology

Nebulizer technology of the future promises a leap forward in delivery efficiency. Over the past decade there has been a progressive trend led by nebulizer device manufacturers to develop nebulizer technology which could offer advantages in drug delivery performance – not only compared to traditional inefficient nebulizer designs, but also which would perform better than pressurized MDIs and DPIs. These nebulizer designs are being called the 'next generation' drug aerosol delivery devices and are only now being introduced to the market place as commercial devices. They are expected to be more expensive than most other drug delivery platforms, they must compete with each other as well as the traditional systems.

New generation devices incorporating specific drug formulations (non-generic): Respimat (Boehringer Ingelheim, Ingelheim, Germany) and AERx (Nektar Therapeutics, Bradford, UK)

Some next generation nebulizer technologies are already advanced, and been clinically proven and licensed by device manufacturers with pharmaceutical partnerships. AERx and Respimat are examples of the efficiency and elegance of new nebulizer technology that seem far superior to conventional nebulizer, pressurized MDI or DPI drug aerosol delivery systems.[1] Respimat is a compact propellant-free multidose nebulized aerosol (soft mist) inhaler that employs a spring to force drug solutions (including bronchodilators and corticosteroids) through a nozzle, which generates a slow-moving nebulized aerosol. Deposition studies indicate Respimat can consistently deliver 39–44% of the dose to the lung.[2] The AERx device uses sophisticated electronics to deliver aerosol drugs – including insulin, rhDNase (recombinant human deoxyribonuclease), and opioids – from a single dose blister using an integral, disposable nozzle array. The AERx electronics control dose expression and titration, timing of aerosol generation with patient inhalation, and provide feedback to the patient to control optimum inhalation technique. Lung deposition with AERx is reported to be 50–80% of the available dose.[3]

Both the AERx and Respimat devices have been developed and licensed only for delivery of specific drugs, and are not being introduced or marketed as devices for delivery of off-license drugs as are the traditional 'generic' nebulizers.

New general purpose nebulizer technologies

This section introduces and reviews four new nebulizer technology platforms that have and are being developed, it is anticipated, for aerosolization and delivery of generically available drug solutions and suspensions. As they are introduced in the market place they will offer a far more efficient 'substitute' for the conventional inefficient nebulizer. The expected increased efficiency of drug aerosol delivery gives rise to implications for patient safety – particularly in regard to effective delivery of higher doses, which require careful consideration in their adoption and use within the clinical community. Given the potential widespread introduction and off-license use of more efficient nebulizer technology platforms delivering drug aerosol, the chapter concludes with a discussion of how use of standardized in vitro methods could help control risks in regard to patient safety and drug efficacy.

MedSpray: medical spray chip inhalers

MedSpray develops and manufactures non-electrical medical spray chips for the generation of mono-dispersed aerosols. These chips form the basis for a technology platform on which new types of nebulizers/inhalers are being designed. These devices will result in important improvements and innovations for inhalation therapy, all based on the characteristics of the chips that form the aerosols. Any target drugs can be used, provided that the formulation is liquid and to a certain extent particle free (which may preclude the use of some suspensions).

In the last few decades, it has become accepted that control over particle size, size distribution and dose influences total drug deposition in the lung, and, hence, drug intake. Clinical experiments using mono-dispersed aerosols show a 5–10 times dose reduction for the same therapeutic effect and hence a reduction in side effects.[4,5] Pulmonary drug delivery technologies today are required to exhibit many features: mono-dispersed droplets with MMAD (mean median aerodynamic diameter) in the 1–5 μm window, flexible dosing, ease of use, portability, low cost, low energy input and a performance independent of the drug solution and inhalation flow.[6,7]

As described in Chapter 1, in traditional nebulizer devices the droplet size distributions of aerosol for inhalation are determined by three major mechanisms. A primary mechanism breaks up a liquid drug formulation into droplets and determines the primary droplet size distribution. A secondary mechanism, evaporation (and to a lesser extent coalescence) has a major effect. Thirdly, baffles or other size discriminating structures inside the nebulizer are used to filter and return larger aerosols to the main reservoir in order to achieve release of narrow size distributions of nebulized aerosol for delivery to the patient. The manufacturers of the MedSpray device argue that their technology simplifies the primary aerosol generation process by generating mono-dispersed aerosols directly from the spray chip and preserving these characteristics.

MedSpray chips utilize micro-machined nozzle structures that transform liquid drugs directly into flows of mono-dispersed droplets. Here the effect of Rayleigh break-up of small diameter liquid jets is exploited (Figures 3.1 and 3.2). Miniaturization of plain orifice nozzles down to micron scale reveals excellent break-up, fully controlled by chip geometry and Rayleigh

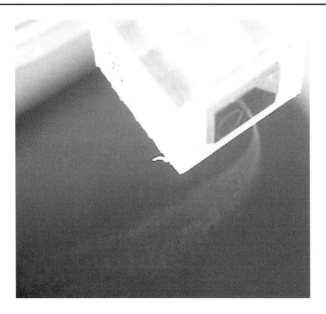

Figure 3.1 *MedSpray: medical spray chip generating a mono-dispersed spray with median aerodynamic diameter (MMAD) of 5 μm.*

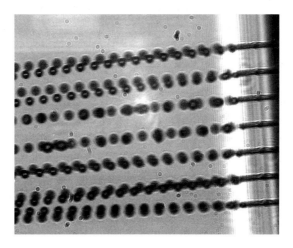

Figure 3.2 *MedSpray: high speed photograph of aerosol generated at 0.5 bar near the point of break-up. The nozzle orifice diameter here is 10 μm.*

effect alone, while inertia and gravity forces play a minor role, at transnozzle pressures below 5 bar.[8–11]

The inhaler devices based on the technology exploit the advantages of the spray chip technology. Nebulizers become non-electrical and look like MDIs. The chips are small, so devices are portable and fit into a

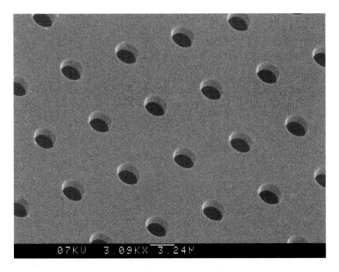

Figure 3.3 *MedSpray: SEM (scanning electron microscope) photograph of a micro-engineered nozzle array with a pore size of 2 μm.*

pocket easily. The Rayleigh break-up process itself is not influenced by drug properties, inhalation flows or environmental properties, yielding stable droplet size distributions. The generated droplet size depends exclusively on nozzle dimensions enabling individual therapy, comparable to selecting needle sizes. Finally the atomization process is very efficient with respect to energy consumption; a pressure of 5 bar is needed to form micro-jets; the break-up itself requires no energy. Degeneration of drug molecular structure by high shear, high temperature or high-energy input is avoided.

The most important aspect in the success of the development and widespread adoption of the MedSpray device may be cost. The manufacturing technology enables processing of millions of orifices in parallel, lowering the cost per orifice dramatically (Figure 3.3). This results in a low cost per product and enables disposable products to eliminate cleaning procedures. Advancements in the new technologies of microlithography, surface and bulk micromachining and wafer scale assembly have enabled the necessary miniaturization of dimensions. So far the manufacturer reports no indications that would limit further miniaturization of the device.

However, the MedSpray device is currently still in the research and development phase. Only time will tell whether a commercial product emerges. Although this is likely, it is not yet clear whether this technology will be developed for use as a general purpose nebulizer device for delivery of off-license drugs and/or development for delivery of specific drug formulations, as has become the case with AERx and Respimat.

Pari:eFlow™ electronic inhaler

Pari's new electronic inhaler, eFlow™ (Pari GmbH, Stanberg, Germany), combines a new technology for aerosol generation with the advantages of established nebulizer therapy, namely inhalation during spontaneous tidal breathing and the possibility to use a variety of standard nebulizer medications with a single device. Silent, small and lightweight the eFlow™ provides a high degree of mobility to patients. Easy handling and efficient cleaning should help to improve compliance. The device has been designed to avoid the need for hand–lung coordination and includes useful feedback mechanisms to enhance patient acceptance and adherence to therapy. Additional attributes are high dose accuracy and reproducibility[12] and a gentle aerosolization process that makes it suitable for fragile drug compounds.[5] Distinct design parameters of the atomizing head and driving circuit allow tailoring of the droplet size distribution and other delivery characteristics to meet the requirements of various applications in pulmonary and nasal drug delivery.

The core element of the new device is a circular perforated membrane, which is caused to vibrate by means of a ring shaped piezo-electric actuator. The actuator is driven by a battery or mains operated electronic circuit. The vibrating motion of the membrane generates an alternating pressure field which forces the liquid through an array of microholes in the membrane thus creating a fine and dense aerosol cloud of low velocity.[13]

Low power consumption of the whole set-up enables miniaturization of the components and the device. Almost the entire drug volume can be nebulized into respirable droplets, thus providing a highly efficient therapy.[13] Sensors are integrated to prevent operational failure and safe operation.[14] The output rate and particle size distribution can be optimized for distinct drug formulations and various applications by adjusting the hole diameters in the membrane and to allow for a faster treatment compared with conventional nebulizer therapy.[15–17]

The eFlow™ device consists of two major components (Figure 3.4): a control unit containing the electronics and batteries and a nebulizer which can either be operated while attached to the control unit or via a connection cable. The liquid reservoir is designed for efficient supply of variable drug volumes (0.5–5 ml) to the membrane with virtually no residue left after each treatment. All parts of the nebulizer can be cleaned in warm water and detergent,

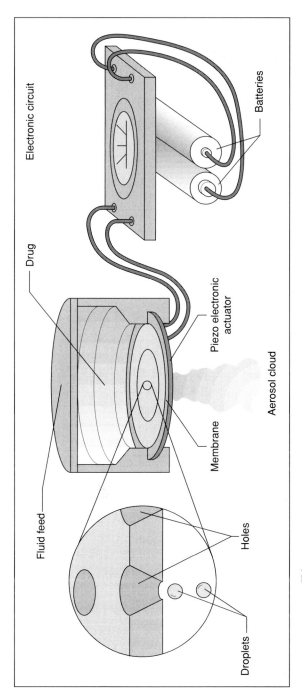

Figure 3.4 Pari:eFlow™ *design components. (Courtesy of Pari GmbH.)*

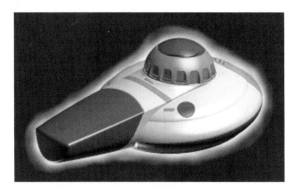

Figure 3.5 *Pari:eFlow™. Impression of the final product. (Courtesy of Pari GmbH.)*

disinfected in a vaporizer or by boiling in a waterbath containing a fraction of white vinegar, and sterilized in an autoclave (121 °C). Figure 3.5 presents an impression of the finished form of prototype of the Pari:eFlow™ device.

An inhalation treatment lasting for a few minutes has some advantages over administering the drug in one or two single breaths as provided by MDIs or DPIs. During spontaneous breathing the aerosol can deeply penetrate the lungs and develop a sustaining effect whereas with a single breath maneuver the risk is much higher that only an insufficient amount of drug reaches its target. Like traditional nebulizers, eFlow™ actively generates a slowly moving aerosol cloud, i.e. throat deposition is minimized and inhalation can be performed with minimal inspiratory force. The narrow droplet size distribution of the eFlow™ and the resulting high respirable fraction (up to 95%) further reduces oropharyngeal deposition and associated side effects by gastrointestinal absorption. In vitro delivery efficiency has been demonstrated up to 75% of the loaded dose.[13]

The eFlow™ can be used for both standard nebulizer medications and new or reformulated drug compounds, including suspensions[17] and proteins.[18] The increased delivery efficiency enables use of low fill volumes resulting in a significant reduction of treatment time compared with standard nebulizer therapy, thus increasing quality of life.

Omron MicroAIR U22

Although ultrasonic nebulizer technology is not new in itself, an ultrasonic nebulizer that works reliably with both solutions and suspensions would be new, as many past devices have suffered from electronic faults, heating of the medicant, inablity to nebulize suspensions, as well as producing droplets too large for penetration to the lower respiratory tract.

Omron Japan has developed ultrasonic nebulizer technology that has overcome previous limitations. The first commercial product, the NE-U03, was launched in 1994[19] and the design has since been rapidly developed and refined to emerge as a more compact model now branded as the Omron U22 (Figures 3.6 and 3.7). Power is supplied by two AA batteries.

The Omron U22 has been independently tested and found to have a relatively high rate of aerosol output with an extremely low residual volume (around 0.1 ml) compared to the traditional jet nebulizer. The maximum fill volume is 7 ml. The average particle size from the U22 is reported by the manufacturer to be within the respirable range (3.9 μm MMAD). Further, the Omron U22 device has been shown to operate effectively with most medications including solutions, suspensions, and heat sensitive medications such as antibiotics demonstrate no deterioration of chemical structure.[20] The medication bottle assembly (Figure 3.7) including the mesh and transducer can be removed and opened for cleaning and the metal mesh can be boiled.

The Omron device in its final form (U22) has one-button operation and is normally intended to be used in a continuous mode although it can also be used in an intermittent mode with patient interaction (stopping and starting the aerosol generator during inhalation). The design of the liquid feed in the U22 allows it to be used in a supine position, which has traditionally been a problem with ultrasonic nebulizers.

Like the Pari device (above) or the Aerogen (Mountain View, CA, USA) device (below), what is most impressive when using these next generation nebulizers such as the Omron U22 is that they are inherently silent during operation. This allows much more discreet use in the home, school or workplace compared to the traditional compressed air powered jet nebulizer.

Aerogen aerosol devices

Aerogen's OnQ™ Aerosol Generator is an electronic micropump, which efficiently aerosolizes a broad range of drugs in solution or suspension, including small molecules, proteins, peptides and macromolecules. The OnQ™ Aerosol Generator is approximately 3/8 in in diameter and wafer thin (Figure 3.8), and is comprised of a domed aperture plate containing approximately 1000 tapered apertures, surrounded by a vibrational element. When electrical energy is applied, contraction and expansion of the vibrational element causes the domed aperture plate to move up and down (about 1 μm) several thousand times per second, drawing liquid medication through the narrow end of the apertures to produce a low velocity aerosol. Because of the low power requirement, temperature

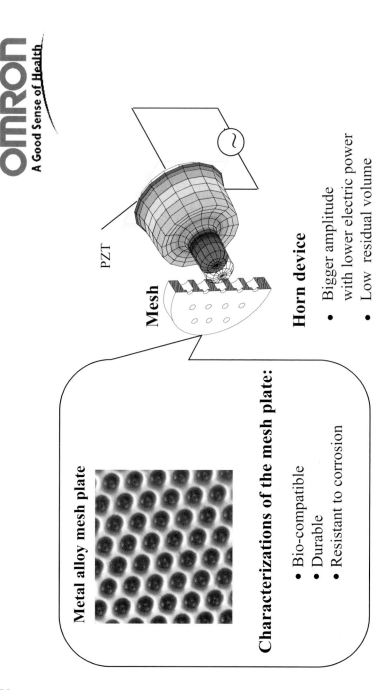

Figure 3.6 *MicroAIR U22: principle of operation. Piezo-electric transducer (PZT) vibrates with ultrasonic frequency. These axial vibrations 'squeeze' liquid medication through small holes in metal-alloy mesh. Medication leaves the mesh as a fine aerosol. (Courtesy of Omron, Japan.)*

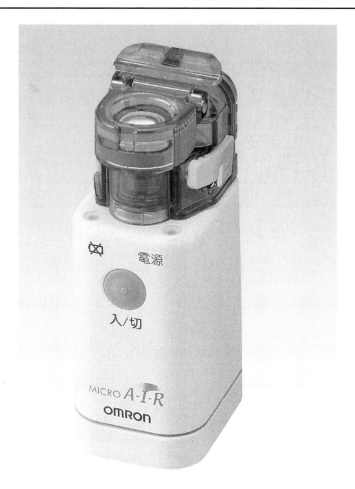

Figure 3.7 *Omron U22. Photograph of the commercial device. (Courtesy of Omron, Japan.)*

increase of the medication is minimal, reducing the risk of denaturing proteins and peptides. The aerosol droplet size and fine particle fraction are directly related to the exit diameter of the apertures, which may be modified for specific clinical applications. The Aerosol Generator is also very efficient; a single drop of 16 μl placed on the aerosol generator can produce up to 15 μl of aerosol, with as little as 1 μl of residual volume. The current devices that incorporate the OnQ™ Aerosol Generator are shown in Figure 3.9.

Aerogen Aeroneb nebulizers
The Aeroneb portable nebulizer system, which has been commercially available since June 2000, is a silent, portable nebulizer system (see Figure 3.9)

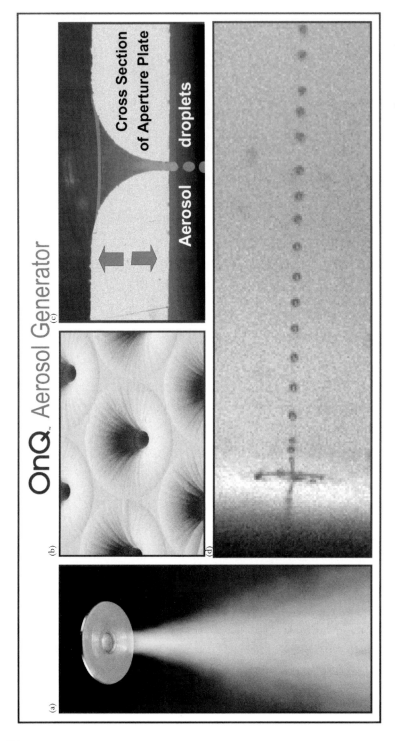

Figure 3.8 *(a) The Aerogen Aerosol Generator with (b) a microscopic view of tapered apertures and (c) cross-section of aperture plate. (d) High speed microscopic photograph of aerosol generated from a single aperture.*

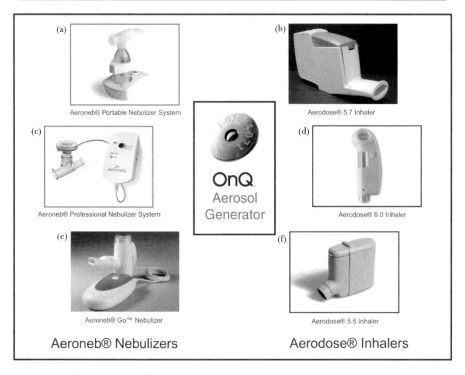

Figure 3.9 *Examples of commercial nebulizers (a,c,e) and breath actuated inhalers (b,d,f) utilizing Aerogen's aerosol generator (center). The Aeroneb portable nebulizer (a) was the first generation home nebulizer. The Aeroneb Professional (c) was designed for aerosol delivery during mechanical ventilation and general use in the acute and critical care settings. The Aeroneb Go (e) is the second generation home nebulizer. The Aerodose 5.7 inhaler (b) is a clinical device supporting both tidal breathing and deep breath with breath-hold patterns. The Aerodose 6.0 inhaler (d) is a second generation titratable device for delivery of insulin. The Aerodose 5.5 (f) was the first generation clinical inhaler.*

that aerosolizes general purpose nebulizer solutions as a fine-particle, low velocity aerosol. The Aeroneb consumes low power (1 watt), and this allows it to operate from a portable battery pack using AA batteries, or alternatively from an AC power supply or a car cigarette lighter. Droplet size distribution is reported to range between 1 μm and 5 μm MMAD, with over 80% mass of the drug in the respirable range. Current nebulizers typically require a minimum reservoir volume of 0.5–1.0 ml to be operational, so some drug remains in the system after nebulization is complete. The Aeroneb nebulizes virtually the entire drug solution, minimizing waste and increasing drug aerosol delivery.

The Aeroneb Go is the next generation successor of the original Aeroneb nebulizer, promising to offer improved performance: faster treatment time, greater inhaled mass, longer battery life, and reduced costs (taken from manufacturer's marketing material).

The Aeroneb professional nebulizer was designed specifically for use in the hospital setting, and mechanical ventilation in particular, and released in 2002. The Aeroneb Pro is a multiple patient, autoclavable nebulizer that generates aerosol continuously during mechanical ventilation, without modifying ventilator volumes and pressures. The device can be refilled and operated without interrupting ventilation, and has been demonstrated to be greater than four-fold more efficient than standard jet nebulizers in adults and 20-fold more efficient in neonates during mechanical ventilation (taken from manufacturer's marketing material). The nebulizer comes with a number of accessories that allow its use in a range of ventilator circuits, and off the ventilator, with mask or mouthpiece, for ambulatory applications such as the emergency room.

The Aeroneb Pro clinical nebulizer is a CE marked device which provides optimized phasic aerosol generation for use in clinical studies in which delivered efficiencies past the endotracheal tube of 50–90% are desired.

Aerogen inhalers

The Aerodose inhalers are small handheld, battery operated delivery systems that use the same OnQ™ Aerosol generator, but include additional features such as synchronized aerosol generation with inspiration (see Figure 3.9), automatic end of dose, dose tracking, and proprietary dosage forms such as BFS (blow-fill-seal) single dose and titratable multidose containers. Each Aerodose inhaler is designed for delivery of a specific drug, and can be pre-programmed to operate in tidal breathing, which is ideal for small children and for doses of greater than 150 μl, or SDB-BH (slow deep breath, breath-hold) maneuver, for small doses in a manner similar to that of an MDI or DPI. Performance of the Aerodose inhaler shows excellent efficiency across a broad range of patient inspiratory volumes, and dose-to-dose reproducibility. Three Aerodose inhalers are shown in Figure 3.9.

Ideal drug nebulizer design

To the author's knowledge, full evaluations of the new nebulizer technologies have not been completed – either because the final production version is not yet available or, if so, the devices simply have not been fully independently tested – or if they have, the data have not yet been made public. It is clear that some of the emerging technologies will satisfy most, if not all, of the criteria of an ideal drug delivery system. The technologies described above have the potential to be very small and portable operating on low power supplied by disposable (or rechargeable batteries). All these new devices are silent in operation due to the energy efficient mechanism of aerosol generation, after all unwanted noise is a characteristic of an inefficient system's energy loss. Further, because all these systems will produce a 'low velocity' aerosol that can be entrained in the patient's inhalation cycle, this implies that the aerosol will penetrate the upper respiratory tract (unlike pressurized MDI ballistic velocity and mouth/throat impaction).

Some of these technologies have a fundamental design limitation of producing aerosol constantly, both during inhalation and exhalation. This is unfortunate, as it implies that efficiency of aerosol delivery drops by a factor of 2 simply due to drug aerosol wasted to the environment. Besides the cost and inefficiency implication, aerosol wasted to the hospital ward or home presents unwanted contamination of that ambient environment. However, not all the designs described above have this limitation. Certainly, most need not be limited and improvements on the existing 'design' of each will constantly develop with time. In the author's opinion, the near future (i.e. between now and 2005) should witness widely available new nebulizer technology, which incorporates all the features of the ideal nebulizer. Whether or not the resulting devices are 'cost effective' will depend on market forces. The initial research and development costs coupled with the market demand and production numbers will inevitably be a large factor influencing the end-user cost of these devices. Having said this, the significant number of concurrently developing new nebulizer technologies promise a competitive market to reduce costs.

Summary and conclusions

Manufacturers of pressurized MDIs continue the uphill struggle to overcome technological problems in propellant reformulation and seem destined to require a spacer and/or breath actuated system to achieve reasonable efficiency in aerosol delivery – especially in patients with poor coordination. Both pressurized MDIs and DPIs have a potentially greater dependence on active patient cooperation and coordination than many of the new nebulizer technologies introduced above. While DPIs seem to offer more efficient drug aerosol delivery compared to MDIs for most applications, difficulties and expense of DPI drug formulation and technical difficulties in designing effective aerosol release mechanisms have proven to be a disadvantage compared to the apparent ease of formulation and delivery of nebulizer solutions.

Over the past decade, rapid technological development in nanotechnology, micro-electronics and advanced battery technology have driven development of new nebulizer technologies which will provide far greater efficiency of aerosol drug dose delivery than traditional nebulizers. The full impact of the new nebulizer technologies introduced and described in this chapter is not yet known but should offer realistic and more efficient alternatives to pressurized MDI and DPI aerosol delivery systems.

It was the intention of this chapter to introduce some of the new technologies which are emerging and/or have emerged in recent years, and to discuss their obvious advantages over conventional nebulizer systems. Specific output information from these devices and their relative performance compared to each other and conventional nebulizers, pressurized MDI/DPI systems is deliberately excluded. This omission is partly because no definitive and objective testing has been undertaken on them, so the data are hard to quote objectively. Further, some technologies are still in (albeit advanced) stages of research and development while others are fully developed and are now being sold – this makes meaningful comparison impossible. The author recommends interested readers get in touch directly with the manufacturers to obtain detailed information on design, costs and output efficiencies of their respective devices.

Despite these limitations, it is clear that some of the new technology should enable therapy to proceed more efficiently. Higher outputs imply a faster rate of drug aerosol delivery. Lower residual volumes imply higher delivered doses. Increased portability and quiet operation imply better patient compliance that, again, will inevitably increase delivered nebulized aerosol doses. New devices like Respimat and AERx will undergo the same regulatory procedure as DPIs and pressurized MDIs, as they are drug/device specific. The outcome will benefit the end user, as the dosing properties, accuracy and clinical efficacy will be proven. However, the new technologies introduced above are expected to be supplied as device only (i.e. without an integrated drug formulation) and as such are exempt from regulatory involvement. This new nebulizer technology presents greatly improved convenience, output rates, doses, and even dose accuracy of drug aerosol delivery compared to traditional nebulizer technology. To ensure continuation of appropriate drug aerosol delivery, care must be taken in clinical practice when transferring patients from less efficient traditional nebulizers to the increasingly more efficient new nebulizer technologies.

Safety and efficacy are particularly problematic given commonly used methods of prescribing drugs for delivery by nebulizer, as the relative efficiency of the nebulizer delivery system is not taken into consideration.

Given the lack of formal regulatory control over separate supply of drug and device in relation to nebulized drug delivery, it seems appropriate for respiratory societies, at both national and international level, to take further interest in the development and pending integration of new nebulizer technologies. New generation of nebulizer technology requires a more comprehensive study and dissemination of in vitro test results to characterize performance. Clinicians could then use standardized and clinically representative in vitro-based assessments of nebulizer performance in deciding which system is most appropriate for their application.

Nebulized drug delivery is possibly the most confused area of clinical practice, largely as a result of little or no regulatory control and poor understanding of the fundamentals of nebulized aerosol science amongst the clinical community. New nebulizer technology offers greater convenience and portability, and a significant increase in aerosol dose delivery. On one hand, this new, more efficient, technology offers obvious benefit to patients. On the other hand, adoption of this new and improved nebulizer technology without due consideration of the consequences of increased dosing presents potential risk to patients. Only if drug regulatory bodies and/or academic societies help manage the transition from the inefficient traditional nebulizers (20% efficiency) to new generation nebulizer devices (80%+ efficiency) will the benefits of new generation nebulizer technology be fully realized.

Acknowledgements

The author is grateful for product information from nebulizer manufacturers including Jeroen Wissink (MedSpray Xmems BV), Martin Knoch (Pari GmbH), Kei Asai and Ruud Boxstart (Omron Japan and Omron Europe), and Angela Strand and Jim Fink (Aerogen Inc).

References

1. Geller DE. New liquid aerosol generation devices: systems that force pressurized liquids through holes. *Respir Care* 2002; **47**:1392–404.
2. Newman SP, Brown J, Steed KP, Reader SJ, Kladders H. Lung deposition of fenoterol and flunisolide delivered using a novel device for inhaled medicines: comparison of

Respimat with conventional metered-dose inhalers with and without spacer devices. *Chest* 1998; **113**:957–63.

3. Gonda I, Fiore M, Johansson E et al. Bolus delivery of morphine solutions with the AERx pain management system. *J Aerosol Med* 1999; **12**:114.

4. Zanen, P. Aerosol formulation and clinical efficacy of bronchodilators, Thesis University Utrecht, 1998.

5. Colbeck, I. *Physical and chemical properties of aerosols*. London: Thomson Science, 1998.

6. Corkery, K. Inhalable drugs for systemic therapy. *Respir Care* 2000; **45**:831–5.

7. Frijlink HW, De Boer AH. Afleversystemen en formuleringen voor pulmonaal gebruik, Farmaca met een luchtje? *Anselmus Colloqium* 2001; 38–61.

8. Rayleigh, Lord. On the instability of jets. *Proc London Math Soc* 1878; **10**:4–13.

9. Lefebvre AH. *Atomization and sprays*. New York: Hemisphere Publishing Corporation, 1989.

10. Wissink JM. Smart micromachined nozzles for mono disperse aerosol generation using low pressure Rayleigh break-up. Respiratory Drug Delivery Conference VIII, Tuscon (Arizona), 2002.

11. Rijn van CJM. *Nano and micro engineered membrane technology*. 2002.

12. Schuschnig U, Keller M, Lintz F-C et al. Customisation of the eFlow™ electronic inhaler to target pulmonary delivery of aztreonam formulations for the treatment of lung infections. Drug Delivery to Lungs Conference XIII, London, December 2002; 12–13.

13. Stangl R, Luangkhot N, Liening-Ewert R, Jahn D. Characterising the first prototype of a vibrating membrane nebulizer. Respiratory Drug Delivery Conference VII, Palm Harbor (Florida), May 2000; 14–18.

14. Borgschulte M, Stangl R. The use of sensors in inhalation systems. Drug Delivery to Lungs Conference XIII, London, December 2002; 12–13.

15. Luangkhot N, Jauernig J, Balcke A et al. Characterisation of salbutamol solution compared to budesonide suspensions consisting of submicron- and micrometer particles in the PARI LC STAR® and a PARI Electronic Nebulizer (e-Flow) Prototype. American Association of Pharmacentical Scientists Annual Meeting, Indianapolis (Indiana), October 29–November 2, 2000.

16. Keller M, Lintz F-C, Walther E. Novel liquid formulation technologies as a tool to design the aerosol performance of nebulisers using an air jet (LC PLUS®) or a vibrating membrane principle (Flow™). Drug Delivery to Lungs Conference XII, London, December 2001; 13–14.

17. Keller M, Jauernig J, Lintz F-C, Knoch M. Nebulizer nanosuspensions: important device and formulation interactions. Respiratory Drug Delivery Conference VIII, Tucson (Arizona), May 2002; 12–16.

18. Smart J, Stangl R, Halsall I, Chrystyn H. TouchSpray™ technology: preliminary results from the in-vitro evaluation of insulin and albumin. Drug Delivery to Lungs Conference XII, London, December 2001; 13–14.

19. Noone PG, Regnis JA, Liu X et al. Airway deposition and clearance and systemic pharmacokinetics of amiloride following aerosolization with an ultrasonic nebulizer to normal airways. *Chest* 1997; **112**:1283–90.

20. Ito K, Kikuchi S, Yamada M, Torii S, Yoshida M. [Time course of drug concentrations in nebulizers and nebulized solutions]. [Article in Japanese] *Arerugi* 1992; **41**:772–7.

Section B. Clinical

4. ACUTE ASTHMA AND COPD EXACERBATIONS

Christer Janson and Jacob Boe

Introduction

Acute asthma and exacerbations of chronic obstructive pulmonary disease (COPD) are two of the most common reasons for emergency treatment at hospital casualty departments, and the management of patients with these conditions has been covered in a number of guidelines and reviews.[1–4] Nevertheless, several investigations have revealed that in clinical practice the management of acute asthma and COPD exacerbations is far from optimal.[5,6]

The underlying cause of asthma and COPD exacerbations varies. Airway infection is the most common trigger for both. Allergen exposure is a common cause for acute asthma whereas exposure to air pollutants may trigger both acute asthma and COPD exacerbations. In a recent case–control study of 60 adult patients hospitalized for acute asthma, Green et al reported a synergistic effect of allergen exposure and virus infections for being hospitalized with asthma.[7] Especially in asthma, an acute exacerbation is often an indication that the patient's current maintenance treatment is inadequate. Airway size is important with regard to the occurrence of obstructive airway diseases especially in childhood.[8–10] Children born with low lung function have recurrent attacks of acute bronchopulmonary obstruction in the early years.[8,9]

There are many similarities in the management of acute asthma and COPD exacerbations, but the expected outcome and the long-term prognosis is much better in asthma. This is also reflected in the statistics of hospitalizations, where better maintenance treatment resulted in decreased number of hospitalizations for asthma while the number for COPD increased (Figure 4.1).[11] Patients discharged after COPD exacerbations have a high relapse rate. In a Nordic study of hospitalized COPD patients 53% were readmitted within 12 months (Figure 4.2).[12] The rehospitalization rate after acute asthma is lower than after COPD exacerbations but Emerman et al found that 17% of patients sent home after emergency treatment of acute asthma had a relapse within 14 days.[13]

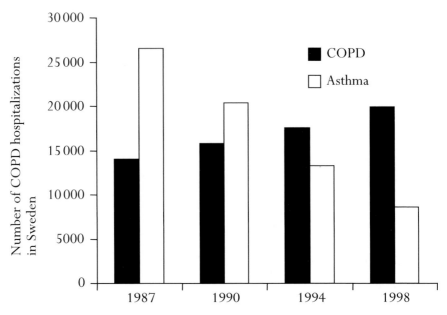

Figure 4.1 *Number of patients hospitalized because of COPD and asthma in Sweden in 1987–1997. (Adapted from the National Board of Health and Welfare, Stockholm, Sweden.[11])*

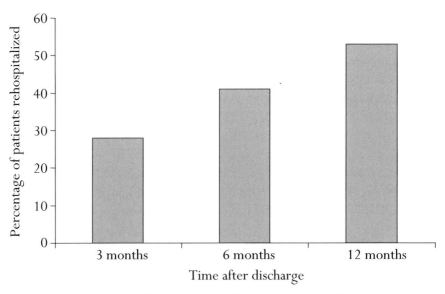

Figure 4.2 *Percentage of hospital-treated COPD patients from five Nordic university hospitals who were rehospitalized within 3, 6 and 12 months of discharge. (Adapted from Janson C et al.* Eur Respir Rev 2000; **10**:428–31[12] *with permission from the publisher.)*

Table 4.1 Characteristic features of asthma and COPD.

Asthma	COPD
Former allergen-induced attacks	Previous or present tobacco smoking
Case history with considerable variation	Older patients
Younger patients	Respiratory distress less than expected from occurrence of very low PEF values (less than 200 ml/min)
Other atopic disease	Combination of increased PCO_2 and normal pH when the patient is in a stable situation

COPD, chronic obstructive pulmonary disease; PEF, peak expiratory flow.

Assessment of patients with acute asthma and COPD exacerbations

Patients with acute airway obstruction should be assessed by a short history aiming at confirming the diagnosis (asthma or COPD). Features that might help to confirm the diagnosis are shown in Table 4.1. None of the features listed are specific to asthma or COPD, but their occurrence increases the probability of the respiratory distress being due to one of these conditions. The duration of the present exacerbation, possible triggers and the patient's current medication should also be checked (Table 4.2). A more detailed history can be obtained after the initial treatment has been given. A physical examination should be performed including measuring of respiratory frequency, heart frequency and lung function (see Table 4.2). Lung function is usually measured as peak flow since performing spirometry to obtain forced expiratory volume in one second (FEV_1) may be difficult in an emergency situation. In severe attacks arterial blood gases should be measured. If this is not possible pulse oximetry with SaO_2 recordings is an alternative even though this procedure gives no information on possible retention of carbon dioxide and acidosis.

Nebulizer versus other inhalation devices

Mild exacerbations of asthma and COPD can often be treated at home. In this setting, handheld inhalers (metered dose inhalers (MDIs) or powder

Table 4.2 Assessment of patients with acute asthma or COPD exacerbations before treatment.	
Patient history	Diagnosis: asthma or COPD? Duration of exacerbation? Trigger? Current treatment?
Physical examination	General condition? Cyanosis? Peripheral edema? Respiratory rate? Heart rate?
Peak flow	Compare with patient's best values or if unavailable compare with predicted values
Arterial blood gases	PaO_2, $PaCO_2$, pH
Pulse oximetry	SaO_2

COPD, chronic obstructive pulmonary disease.

dose inhalers) are recommended for administering inhalation therapy. However, in health centers or hospital-based care, nebulized therapy is the most common way of administrating inhalation therapy in acute asthma. An alternative route of administration is to give the inhalation treatment by an MDI attached to a spacer device. Studies comparing these two methods for inhalation therapy have almost exclusively looked at beta-2-agonist treatment. In a study of patients with acute asthma treated by an ambulance crew, Campbell et al found that 5 mg salbutamol via nebulizer was more effective than 5 mg terbutaline via a spacer inhaler or 200 mg salbutamol given by MDI.[14] Several other investigations have, however, found that treatment by MDI via a spacer and nebulized treatment are equally efficient.[15–17] The same conclusion was drawn in an extensive review in the *Cochrane Library*.[18] There are fewer data on the comparison of inhalation devices in COPD exacerbations. In a meta-analysis by Turner et al no significant difference was found between MDI and nebulized beta-agonist treatment in patients with acute airflow obstruction (asthma or COPD) (Figure 4.3).[19,20] The same result was found when analyzing only the subgroup of patients that had COPD exacerbations.

Inhaled therapy can also be administered by powder inhalers. Tønnesen and collaborators compared the efficacy of 2.5 mg terbutaline given twice with a dry powder device or with MDI with a spacer device.[21] The study

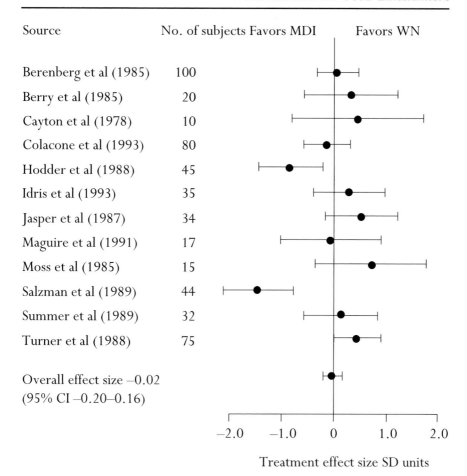

Source	No. of subjects	Favors MDI	Favors WN
Berenberg et al (1985)	100		
Berry et al (1985)	20		
Cayton et al (1978)	10		
Colacone et al (1993)	80		
Hodder et al (1988)	45		
Idris et al (1993)	35		
Jasper et al (1987)	34		
Maguire et al (1991)	17		
Moss et al (1985)	15		
Salzman et al (1989)	44		
Summer et al (1989)	32		
Turner et al (1988)	75		

Overall effect size −0.02
(95% CI −0.20–0.16)

−2.0   −1.0   0   1.0   2.0

Treatment effect size SD units

Figure 4.3 *Meta-analysis of studies comparing beta-2-agonist treatment with metered-dose inhaler (MDI) and wet nebulizer (WN) in subjects with acute asthma or COPD exacerbations. (Adapted from Muers MF et al.* Eur Respir Rev *2002; 10:511–15[20] with permission from European Respiratory Society Journals Limited.)*

comprised 62 patients with acute asthma. No difference in efficacy was found between these two different inhalation devices.

The reason why nebulization is the most often used method of inhalation in European hospitals is probably that it is regarded as more convenient for healthcare staff to administer because less patient education or cooperation is required.[22] Nebulizer treatment is, however, more expensive than treatment with handheld inhalers and early substitution of nebulizer therapy with MDI plus spacer therapy has the potential for considerable cost savings for hospitals.[23,24]

Drugs used in nebulizers

Beta-2-agonists

For at least two decades beta-2-agonists have been used as first-line therapy in acute asthma. The optimal route of administration of beta-2-agonists has been a matter of controversy,[25] but in the early 1990s several investigations showed that inhalation therapy is superior to intravenous therapy even in severe acute asthma.[26–28] No corresponding comparisons are available for COPD exacerbations but inhalation of beta-2-agonists is the recommended first-line treatment in acute exacerbations in all guidelines.[2,4]

Nebulized beta-2-agonists are generally well tolerated. When high doses of beta-2-agonists are nebulized a significant amount of the drug is, however, absorbed systemically,[29,30] and can cause systemic side effects (Box 4.1). Hypokalemia, which is one of the side effects of nebulized beta-2-agonist treatment has raised most concern. Usually, however, it is only a moderate decrease.[29,31] The mechanism behind the decrease is an increase in transport of potassium ions to the skeletal muscles and not a decrease of the total body potassium level. It is therefore uncertain whether the hypokalemia induced by beta-2-agonists can cause cardiac arrhythmias or any other clinically important metabolic event.

Many patients with acute asthma and COPD exacerbations have hypoxemia as a result of ventilation–perfusion inequalities in the lung. Beta-2-agonists have a vasodilatory effect which can lead to increased perfusion of poorly ventilated parts of the lung and thereby a temporary worsening of hypoxemia.[32] It is uncertain whether this has any clinical consequences, but it is recommended that oxygen should be given to all patients with severe acute asthma.[3] When treating COPD exacerbations monitored oxygen therapy is recommended (see below).[22]

Box 4.1 Systemic effects of nebulized treatment with high-dose inhaled beta-2-agonists.

Tremor
Tachycardia
Metabolic changes
   hyperglycemia
   hypokalemia
Decrease in the partial pressure of oxygen

Anticholinergics

Nebulized therapy with anticholinergics, especially ipratropium bromide, is widely used as an additional treatment to beta-2-agonist therapy. The scientific basis for this has been questioned as several studies have failed to show that adding anticholinergics leads to an improvement above that which can be achieved with beta-2-agonist treatment alone.[33,34] Other investigations have, however, found that anticholinergics improve the efficacy of acute asthma treatment. These investigations include a meta-analysis of five studies conducted during the 1980s[35] and a pooled analysis of data from over 1000 patients with acute asthma.[36] In the latter patients who were given nebulized 0.5 mg ipratropium in combination with 2.5 mg salbutamol had a slightly larger improvement in FEV_1 (40 ml) than patients treated with salbutamol alone. More important was that patients given the combination treatment had a reduced risk of admission to hospital (relative risk 0.80).[36] In a Cochrane review of treatment of acute asthma in children the combination of anticholinergics and beta-2-agonists was also found to be favorable compared to treatment with beta-2-agonists alone.[37]

In many of the studies one dose of a beta-2-agonist has been compared with the same dose of beta-2-agonist in combination with an anticholinergic. It may therefore be argued that doubling the dose of the beta-2-agonist may be as effective as the combination treatment. Results from two studies in the 1980s indicate, however, that combining adrenergic and anticholinergic agents is superior to doubling the dose of the adrenergic drug.[38,39] Combination therapy also probably has a more favorable effect to side effect ratio.

In contrast to the data from asthma studies, no additional effect has been found when adding anticholinergics to beta-agonists in COPD exacerbations (Figure 4.4).[40–42] The bronchodilatory effect of anticholinergics and beta-agonist appear to be similar in COPD exacerbations (Figure 4.4).[40] Anticholinergics have one advantage over beta-agonists in the sense that no hypoxia is seen with inhaled anticholinergic treatment.[43] It is therefore possible that beta-agonists could be substituted with anticholinergics at least in some patients with COPD exacerbations; for example, patients with COPD in combination with ischemic heart disease.[44] There is, however, less clinical and scientific experience with inhaled anticholinergics given as a single drug than with treatment with only beta-agonists in COPD exacerbations.[20]

Corticosteroids

Patients with acute asthma usually have increased airway inflammation[45] and treatment with corticosteroids as well as beta-2-agonist therapy is the

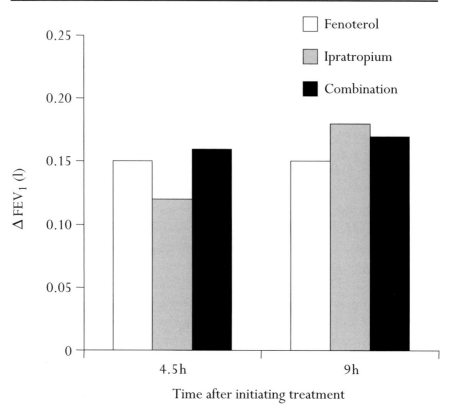

Figure 4.4 *Mean increase in FEV$_1$ after inhalation of fenoterol, ipratropium and the combination of both drugs in 51 patients with COPD exacerbations. (Adapted from Rebuck AS et al. Am J Med 1987; 82:59–64[40] with permission from the publisher.)*

most important pharmacological component of the treatment of acute asthma. Systemically administered corticosteroids have been found to decrease the risk of hospitalization[46] and oral treatment with steroids reduces the risk of readmission after discharge.[47] There is also evidence that systemic steroid treatment in COPD exacerbations increases lung function and reduces the relapse rate after discharge.[48–50] This should, however, be judged against the risk of side effects such as the development of osteoporosis in patients taking repeated oral steroid courses. Replacing systemically administered steroid treatment by inhaled treatment may reduce the risk of side effects especially in patients with frequent exacerbations. High-dose steroid treatment of acute asthma in the emergency room with a nebulizer or spacer has been tried but the results have been inconclusive.[51,52] There have, however, been some reports that after discharge high-dose treatment with inhaled steroids may be as effective as oral treatment.[53,54] No data are available on inhaled steroids in the treatment of acute exacerbations of COPD. Some studies have, however, found that maintenance treatment with inhaled steroids in patients with severe COPD decreases the risk of exacerbations.[55]

Other drugs for nebulization

Epinephrine is a drug that historically has been used extensively in the treatment of acute asthma. The use of intravenous or subcutaneous epinephrine is still indicated if the acute asthma attack is associated with an anaphylactic reaction.[3] The results of one study indicate that epinephrine injection may be of value to some patients who do not respond to inhaled beta-2-agonists.[56] Epinephrine can also be administered by nebulizer but the duration of the effect is much shorter than for beta-2-agonists.[57]

Infusions of magnesium have, in some studies, been found to result in greater bronchodilation than was achieved with only beta-2-agonist inhalation.[58,59] All studies, however, have not confirmed the value of this therapy.[60] In a study of 135 patients with acute asthma the patients who were treated with an infusion of 2 g $MgSO_2$ (magnesium sulfate) did not improve more than patients who were only treated with inhaled salbutamol and intravenous steroids.[61] In a subgroup analysis the authors did, however, find that in patients with an FEV_1 <25% of predicted ($n = 35$) $MgSO_2$ induced a larger improvement in lung function and these patients were less likely to be hospitalized. Magnesium can also be delivered by nebulizer. In a study of 33 adults with acute asthma Mangat et al found that serial nebulizations of four doses of 3 ml of 3.2% solution of $MgSO_2$ gave the same bronchodilatory response as four doses of 2.5 mg salbutamol.[62]

Inhalation of furosemide has been found to have a protective effect against bronchoconstriction.[63,64] The effect of nebulized furosemide has also been assessed in acute asthma.[65–67] In the most relevant of these studies the patients received 2.5 mg nebulized salbutamol and either 40 mg nebulized furosemide or placebo.[65] No difference was found between the treatment groups, but in a subclass analysis there were indications that the combination therapy was more effective in patients with an exacerbation of short duration (<8 hours).

At present, no nebulized drugs other than beta-agonists and anticholinergics are of proven value in COPD exacerbations.

Table 4.3 What to consider when choosing the delivery system for nebulizer treatment.

Nebulizer	Output
	Droplet size
	Residual volume
	CEN-evaluated nebulizer is recommended
Accessories	Mouthpiece or face mask
Driving gas	Oxygen or air
	Choose correct flow rate
Filling volume	Large volumes give less drug loss but longer nebulization time

CEN, European Committee for Standardization.

Delivery system

Apart from the choice of drug careful attention should be given to the different issues of how the drug is delivered. Some of these aspects are presented in Table 4.3.

Choice of nebulizer

It is important to have an effective nebulizer system and a system evaluated by the European Committee for Standardization (CEN) with good CEN performance (output and droplet size) is recommended. The target airway site is the central, and, to a lesser extent, the peripheral airways.[22] A droplet size of about 5 μm is therefore optimal.

The nebulizer could be equipped with a mouthpiece or a face mask. Theoretically a mouthpiece may be better as it avoids nasal deposition of drugs. A mouthpiece also decreases the risk of ocular complications with anticholinergic agents.[22] Some patients may, however, prefer a face mask, especially when acutely breathless. In such a situation the patients are likely to mouth-breathe and thus diminish the theoretical disadvantages of the face mask.

Driving gas

In most guidelines oxygen is recommended when treating acute asthma while air is the preferred driving gas in COPD exacerbations. Patients with COPD exacerbations should also be given oxygen, but this should be monitored. Monitored oxygen therapy is most easily accomplished by using air as the driving gas and giving oxygen through nasal prongs. The oxygen treatment is started with a low flow, 1–2 l/min, and the oxygen saturation is monitored with the aim to reach a SaO_2 of 90–91%. The patient should be closely followed to detect clinical signs of carbon dioxide retention such as drowsiness. As most emergency departments see patients with both acute asthma and COPD exacerbations it may be impractical to have two different nebulizer systems. In that case an air driven nebulizer with a mouthpiece in combination with oxygen given through nasal prongs may be the best solution. Patients with acute asthma can then be given oxygen with a high flow rate (6–8 l/min) while COPD patients are given monitored oxygen treatment as above.

In the future, driving gases other than oxygen and air may be used. Heliox, a mixture of helium and oxygen, is a low density gas and improves the deposition of inhaled particles when compared to air or oxygen. In a recent study Kress et al found that a group of patients who were given nebulized salbutamol with heliox had a larger increase in FEV_1 than patients nebulizing salbutamol with oxygen.[68]

Filling volume

The filling volume is a difficult issue when treating acute asthma and COPD exacerbations. With a lower filling volume the proportional loss of drug is larger.[69] The volume where a nebulizer ceases to function continuously and begins to 'sputter' varies between different models from 0.5 ml to as high as 1.5 ml.[22] This means that with a low filling volume the amount left in the nebulizer after the nebulization is complete is very high compared to when a higher volume is used. On the other hand, a high filling volume means a longer nebulization time which may be difficult for patients with acute airway obstruction. In order to reach a compromise between these two concerns a filling volume of 2–4 ml is often used.

Dose and dose intervals

There have been a number of investigations that have studied the efficiency of different doses and dose intervals in nebulized treatment. Most of these studies have looked at beta-2-agonist therapy. Schuh and collaborators found that in children with acute asthma frequent administration of a high dose of salbutamol (0.15 mg/kg every 20 min) was more effective than treatment with low doses of salbutamol (0.05 mg/kg).[70] Emerman et al on the other hand, found no difference in efficacy between 2.5 mg and 7.5 mg salbutamol every 20 minutes in adults with acute asthma.[71]

Investigations that have studied different dose intervals have also yielded conflicting results. Robertson and collaborators found that frequent nebulizations with low doses of salbutamol (0.05 mg/kg every 20 min) after an initial dose of 0.15 mg/kg was more effective than repeating the high-dose treatment every hour in children with acute asthma.[72] Papo et al, in another pediatric study, found that continuous nebulization of salbutamol 0.3 mg/kg per hour resulted in a more rapid improvement than intermittent therapy (0.3 mg/kg per hour).[73] In contrast, McFadden et al found that 5.0 mg salbutamol every 40 minutes was at least as effective as 2.5 mg salbutamol every 20 minutes.[74] Likewise, Reisner et al did not find any significant difference between patients treated with continuous nebulizations of salbutamol (7.5 mg/hour) compared with patients given intermittent treatment (2.5 mg every 20 min).[75]

Ward et al performed a cumulative dose–response study in six patients with acute asthma and found that 0.5 mg ipratropium bromide given by nebulizer produced a maximal increase in peak expiratory flow rate.[76]

In the European Respiratory Society (ERS) guidelines on the use of nebulizers it is recommended that adult patients with acute asthma and patients with exacerbations of COPD should be given a beta-2-agonist dose equivalent to 2.5–5 mg of salbutamol or 5–10 mg of terbutaline. A dose equivalent to 0.5 mg ipratropium bromide is recommended when administrating nebulized anticholinergic treatment.[22] The treatment should be repeated in line with what is shown in Figure 4.5.

In ambulances, the ERS guidelines recommend that nebulized bronchodilator therapy in a dose equivalent to 2.5–5 mg of salbutamol or 5–10 mg of terbutaline should be commenced as soon as possible for patients with acute asthma or acute exacerbations of COPD.[22]

Monitoring the effect of nebulization therapy

Peak flow measurements should be performed after administrating the nebulized treatment. The result of the peak flow measurements and the level of the patient's symptomatic improvement are used to decide whether the patient needs additional treatment or can be discharged. In the Global Initiative for Asthma (GINA) guidelines a peak flow returning to at least 80% of the

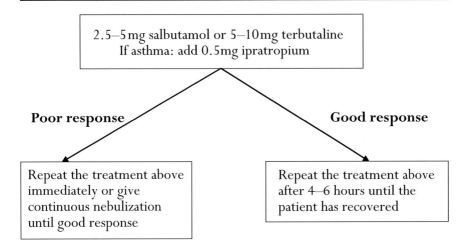

Figure 4.5 *Recommended doses and dose intervals of nebulized treatment of acute asthma and COPD exacerbations. (Adapted from Boe J et al. Eur Respir J 2001; 18:228–42[22] with permission from European Respiratory Society Journals Limited.)*

patient's normal best peak flow value is defined as a good response which may allow the patient to be discharged.[3] Increased heart rate (>100–110 beats/min) can be used as a measure of the component of stress occurring in acute asthma. Although the correlation between the degree of bronchial obstruction and heart rate may vary[77] (as heart rate is more dependent on psychological factors than bronchial obstruction) a decrease of heart rate following acute treatment, e.g. nebulizer treatment, indicates an improvement of the respiratory disorder. In severe exacerbations of COPD it is important to follow arterial blood gases. Patients in whom $PaCO_2$ increases or in those who are developing acidosis (pH <7.3) non-invasive or invasive ventilation should be considered. Pulse oximetry is useful when giving monitored oxygen therapy (see above) and can also be of some value when assessing the effect of treatment in patients who are unable to perform peak flow measurements.[78]

Clinical signs indicating potentially and immediately life-threatening respiratory distress are important to recognize as they influence choice of therapy (e.g. nebulizer treatment or immediate intubation/ventilation) at the time of hospital admission or during follow-up (Table 4.4).

Patients discharged from hospital after an acute asthma attack or an exacerbation of COPD should have an individualized written plan stating their subsequent therapy. This plan should include which measures to undertake in case of emergency. For those equipped with nebulizers at home see Chapters 5 and 11.

Table 4.4 Clinical signs indicating potentially or immediately life-threatening attacks.

Potentially life-threatening	Immediately life-threatening
Increasing dyspnea and rhonchi	'Silent chest'
Patient unable to talk fluently or to get up from chair/bed	Cyanosis
Heart rate more than 110 beats/min	Bradycardia
PEF less than 40% of predicted or best individual value	Exhaustion
PEF less than 200 l/min	Confusion Unconsciousness

Each of the signs indicate a potentially or immediately life threatening event.
PEF, peak expiratory flow.

Treatment other than inhalation

Apart from inhaled treatment, systemic corticosteroids are of proven value in the treatment of both acute asthma and COPD exacerbations (see above). Antibiotics are usually not needed in acute asthma except when there are clear signs of a bacterial infection. Broad spectrum antibiotics such as doxycycline or trimethoprim-sulfamethoxazole can be beneficial in patients with COPD exacerbations who, apart from worsening dyspnea and cough, also have increased sputum volume and purulence.[79]

Intravenous theophylline has traditionally been extensively used in the treatment of acute asthma and COPD exacerbations. Today this drug is used less frequently both because it has a narrow therapeutic range and can cause serious side effects and because a large number of studies have failed to show that theophylline has an additional effect above what can be obtained with inhaled therapy alone.[80,81]

Other potential systemic treatment alternatives for acute asthma and possibly COPD exacerbations are intravenous magnesium (see above) and, in the future, intravenous anti-leukotrienes.[82]

Summary

- Inhalation therapy given with a nebulizer and treatment by MDI with a spacer device appears to be equally efficient, but in some situations such as emergency treatment in ambulances nebulized treatment may be preferable.

- Inhaled beta-2-agonists together with systemically administered corticosteroids is the first-line treatment of both acute asthma and COPD exacerbations.
- There is evidence that the addition of an inhaled anticholinergic to beta-2-agonist therapy is more effective in treatment of acute asthma whereas no additional effect has been found when treating COPD exacerbations.
- Further studies are needed to evaluate the efficacy of inhaled steroids, epinephrine, magnesium and furosemide in the treatment of acute asthma and COPD exacerbations.
- Apart from the choice of drug, careful attention should be given to the different issues of how the drug is delivered, such as choice of nebulizer, driving gas and the filling volume of the drug solution.
- An initial dose of beta-2-agonist equivalent to 2.5–5 mg salbutamol is recommended in nebulization treatment of adults with acute asthma and in COPD exacerbations.
- Frequent nebulizations with low doses or continuous nebulization may be more effective than giving the same total dose as high-dose nebulization.

References

1. British Thoracic Society and Scottish Intercollegiate Guidelines Network. British Guideline on the Management of Asthma 1995: Review and position statement. *Thorax* 1997; **52**(Suppl 1):S1–S2.
2. British Thoracic Society. BTS guidelines for the management of chronic obstructive pulmonary disease. *Thorax* 1997; **52**(Suppl 5):S1–S28.
3. National Institutes of Health NHLaBI. Global Initiative for Asthma (GINA). Global strategy for asthma management and prevention 2002. www.ginasthma.com
4. National Heart LaBIWHO. Global strategy for the diagnosis, management, and prevention of chronic obstructive pulmonary disease (GOLD). NHLBI/WHO Workshop 2002. www.goldcopd.com
5. Kolbe J, Vamos M, Fergusson W, Elkind G. Determinants of management errors in acute severe asthma. *Thorax* 1998; **53**:14–20.
6. Hart SR, Davidson AC. Acute adult asthma – assessment of severity and management and comparison with British Thoracic Society guidelines. *Respir Med* 1999; **93**:8–10.
7. Green RM, Custovic A, Sanderson G et al. Synergism between allergens and viruses and risk of hospital admission with asthma: case–control study. *BMJ* 2002; **324**:763–6.
8. Martinez FD, Morgan WJ, Wright AL, Holberg CJ, Taussig LM. Diminished lung function as a predisposing factor for wheezing respiratory illness in infants. *N Engl J Med* 1988; **319**:1112–17.

9. Martinez FD, Morgan WJ, Wright AL, Holberg C, Taussig LM. Initial airway function is a risk factor for recurrent wheezing respiratory illnesses during the first three years of life. Group Health Medical Associates. *Am Rev Respir Dis* 1991; **143**:312–16.

10. Young S, Arnott J, Le Souef PN, Landau LI. Flow limitation during tidal expiration in symptom-free infants and the subsequent development of asthma. *J Pediatr* 1994; **124**:681–8.

11. National Board of Health and Welfare, Stockholm, 2000. Hälso-och sjukvårdsstatistisk årsbok 2000. Http://www.sos.se

12. Janson C, Haahtela T, Gislason T et al. Obstructive lung disease in patients within the hospital in the Nordic countries. *Eur Respir Rev* 2000; **10**:428–31.

13. Emerman CL, Woodruff PG, Cydulka RK et al. Prospective multicenter study of relapse following treatment for acute asthma among adults presenting to the emergency department. MARC investigators. Multicenter Asthma Research Collaboration. *Chest* 1999; **115**:919–27.

14. Campbell IA, Colman SB, Mao JH, Prescott RJ, Weston CF. An open, prospective comparison of beta 2 agonists given via nebuliser, Nebuhaler, or pressurised inhaler by ambulance crew as emergency treatment. *Thorax* 1995; **50**:79–80.

15. Colacone A, Afilalo M, Wolkove N, Kreisman H. A comparison of albuterol administered by metered dose inhaler (and holding chamber) or wet nebulizer in acute asthma. *Chest* 1993; **104**:835–41.

16. Idris AH, McDermott MF, Raucci JC et al. Emergency department treatment of severe asthma. Metered-dose inhaler plus holding chamber is equivalent in effectiveness to nebulizer. *Chest* 1993; **103**:665–72.

17. Parkin PC, Saunders NR, Diamond SA, Winders PM, MacArthur C. Randomised trial spacer v nebuliser for acute asthma. *Arch Dis Child* 1995; **72**:239–40.

18. Cates CJ, Rowe BH, Bara A. Holding chambers versus nebulisers for beta-agonist treatment of acute asthma (Cochrane Review). *Cochrane Database Syst Rev* 2002; CD000052.

19. Turner MO, Patel A, Ginsburg S, FitzGerald JM. Bronchodilator delivery in acute airflow obstruction. A meta-analysis. *Arch Intern Med* 1997; **157**:1736–44.

20. Muers MF, Wedzicha JA. Nebulizers in acute exacerbations of chronic obstructive pulmonary disease. *Eur Respir Rev* 2000; **10**:511–15.

21. Tønnesen F, Laursen LC, Evald T, Ståhl E, Ibsen TB. Bronchodilating effect of terbutaline powder in acute severe bronchial obstruction. *Chest* 1994; **105**:697–700.

22. Boe J, Dennis JH, O'Driscoll BR et al. European Respiratory Society guidelines on the use of nebulizers. *Eur Respir J* 2001; **18**:228–42.

23. Jasper AC, Mohsenifar Z, Kahan S, Goldberg HS, Koerner SK. Cost-benefit comparison of aerosol bronchodilator delivery methods in hospitalized patients. *Chest* 1987; **91**:614–18.

24. Summer W, Elston R, Tharpe L, Nelson S, Haponik EF. Aerosol bronchodilator delivery methods. Relative impact on pulmonary function and cost of respiratory care. *Arch Intern Med* 1989; **149**:618–23.

25. Janson C. The role of adrenergics in the management of severe acute asthma. *Res Clin Forum* 1993; **15**:9–14.

26. Swedish Society of Chest Medicine. High-dose inhaled versus intravenous salbutamol combined with theophylline in severe acute asthma. *Eur Respir J* 1990; **3**:163–70.

27. Janson C, Boe J, Boman G, Mossberg B, Svedmyr N. Bronchodilator intake and plasma levels on admission for severe acute asthma. *Eur Respir J* 1992; **5**:80–5.

28. Salmeron S, Brochard L, Mal H et al. Nebulized versus intravenous albuterol in hypercapnic acute asthma. A multicenter, double-blind, randomized study. *Am J Respir Crit Care Med* 1994; **149**:1466–70.

29. Janson C. Plasma levels and effects of salbutamol after inhaled or i.v. administration in stable asthma. *Eur Respir J* 1991; **4**:544–50.

30. Janson C, Herala M. Plasma terbutaline levels in nebulisation treatment of acute asthma. *Pulm Pharmacol* 1991; **4**:135–9.

31. Singhi SC, Jayashree K, Sarkar B. Hypokalaemia following nebulized salbutamol in children with acute attack of bronchial asthma. *J Paediatr Child Health* 1996; **32**:495–7.

32. Tal A, Pasterkamp H, Leahy F. Arterial oxygen desaturation following salbutamol inhalation in acute asthma. *Chest* 1984; **86**:868–9.

33. Karpel JP, Schacter EN, Fanta C et al. A comparison of ipratropium and albuterol vs albuterol alone for the treatment of acute asthma. *Chest* 1996; **110**:611–16.

34. FitzGerald JM, Grunfeld A, Pare PD et al. The clinical efficacy of combination nebulized anticholinergic and adrenergic bronchodilators vs nebulized adrenergic bronchodilator alone in acute asthma. Canadian Combivent Study Group. *Chest* 1997; **111**:311–15.

35. Ward MJ. Anticholinergics in acute severe asthma. *Res Clin Forum* 1990; **13**:75–80.

36. Lanes SF, Garrett JE, Wentworth CE, III, FitzGerald JM, Karpel JP. The effect of adding ipratropium bromide to salbutamol in the treatment of acute asthma: a pooled analysis of three trials. *Chest* 1998; **114**:365–72.

37. Plotnick LH, Ducharme FM. Combined inhaled anticholinergics and beta2-agonists for initial treatment of acute asthma in children. *Cochrane Database Syst Rev* 2000; CD000060.

38. Ward MJ, MacFarlane JT, Davies D. A place for ipratropium bromide in the treatment of severe acute asthma. *Br J Dis Chest* 1985; **79**:374–8.

39. Bryant DH. Nebulized ipratropium bromide in the treatment of acute asthma. *Chest* 1985; **88**:24–9.

40. Rebuck AS, Chapman KR, Abboud R et al. Nebulized anticholinergic and sympathomimetic treatment of asthma and chronic obstructive airways disease in the emergency room. *Am J Med* 1987; **82**:59–64.

41. Kuhl DA, Agiri OA, Mauro LS. Beta-agonists in the treatment of acute exacerbation of chronic obstructive pulmonary disease. *Ann Pharmacother* 1994; **28**:1379–88.

42. Weber EJ, Levitt MA, Covington JK, Gambrioli E. Effect of continuously nebulized ipratropium bromide plus albuterol on emergency department length of stay and hospital admission rates in patients with acute bronchospasm. A randomized controlled trial. *Chest* 1999; **115**:937–44.

43. Gross NJ, Bankwala Z. Effects of an anticholinergic bronchodilator on arterial blood gases of hypoxemic patients with chronic obstructive pulmonary disease. Comparison with a beta-adrenergic agent. *Am Rev Respir Dis* 1987; **136**:1091–4.

44. Au DH, Curtis JR, Every NR, McDonell MB, Fihn SD. Association between inhaled beta-agonists and the risk of unstable angina and myocardial infarction. *Chest* 2002; **121**:846–51.

45. Pizzichini MM, Pizzichini E, Clelland L et al. Sputum in severe exacerbations of asthma: kinetics of inflammatory indices after prednisone treatment. *Am J Respir Crit Care Med* 1997; **155**:1501–8.

46. Littenberg B, Gluck EH. A controlled trial of methylprednisolone in the emergency treatment of acute asthma. *N Engl J Med* 1986; **314**:150–2.

47. Chapman KR, Verbeek PR, White JG, Rebuck AS. Effect of a short course of prednisone in the prevention of early relapse after the emergency room treatment of acute asthma. *N Engl J Med* 1991; **324**:788–94.

48. Davies L, Angus RM, Calverley PM. Oral corticosteroids in patients admitted to hospital with exacerbations of chronic obstructive pulmonary disease: a prospective randomised controlled trial. *Lancet* 1999; **354**:456–60.

49. Wood-Baker R, Walters EH, Gibson P. Oral corticosteroids for acute exacerbations of chronic obstructive pulmonary disease. *Cochrane Database Syst Rev* 2001; CD001288.

50. Niewoehner DE, Erbland ML, Deupree RH et al. Effect of systemic glucocorticoids on exacerbations of chronic obstructive pulmonary disease. Department of Veterans Affairs Cooperative Study Group. *N Engl J Med* 1999; **340**:1941–7.

51. Afilalo M, Guttman A, Colacone A et al. Efficacy of inhaled steroids (beclomethasone dipropionate) for treatment of mild to moderately severe asthma in the emergency department: a randomized clinical trial. *Ann Emerg Med* 1999; **33**:304–9.

52. Dahlen I, Janson C, Bjornsson E et al. Inflammatory markers in acute exacerbations of obstructive pulmonary disease: predictive value in relation to smoking history. *Respir Med* 1999; **93**:744–51.

53. Levy ML, Stevenson C, Maslen T. Comparison of short courses of oral prednisolone and fluticasone propionate in the treatment of adults with acute exacerbations of asthma in primary care. *Thorax* 1996; **51**:1087–92.

54. Nana A, Youngchaiyud P, Charoenratanakul S et al. High-dose inhaled budesonide may substitute for oral therapy after an acute asthma attack. *J Asthma* 1998; **35**:647–55.

55. Burge PS, Calverley PM, Jones PW et al. Randomised, double blind, placebo controlled study of fluticasone propionate in patients with moderate to severe chronic obstructive pulmonary disease: the ISOLDE trial. *BMJ* 2000; **320**:1297–303.

56. Appel D, Karpel JP, Sherman M. Epinephrine improves expiratory flow rates in patients with asthma who do not respond to inhaled metaproterenol sulfate. *J Allergy Clin Immunol* 1989; **84**:90–8.

57. Coupe MO, Guly U, Brown E, Barnes PJ. Nebulised adrenaline in acute severe asthma: comparison with salbutamol. *Eur J Respir Dis* 1987; **71**:227–32.

58. Skobeloff EM, Spivey WH, McNamara RM, Greenspon L. Intravenous magnesium sulfate for the treatment of acute asthma in the emergency department. *JAMA* 1989; **262**:1210–3.

59. Noppen M, Vanmaele L, Impens N, Schandevyl W. Bronchodilating effect of intravenous magnesium sulfate in acute severe bronchial asthma. *Chest* 1990; **97**:373–6.

60. Tiffany BR, Berk WA, Todd IK, White SR. Magnesium bolus or infusion fails to improve expiratory flow in acute asthma exacerbations. *Chest* 1993; **104**:831–4.

61. Bloch H, Silverman R, Mancherje N et al. Intravenous magnesium sulfate as an adjunct in the treatment of acute asthma. *Chest* 1995; **107**:1576–81.

62. Mangat HS, D'Souza GA, Jacob MS. Nebulized magnesium sulphate versus nebulized salbutamol in acute bronchial asthma: a clinical trial. *Eur Respir J* 1998; **12**:341–4.

63. Yates DH, O'Connor BJ, Yilmaz G et al. Effect of acute and chronic inhaled furosemide on bronchial hyperresponsiveness in mild asthma. *Am J Respir Crit Care Med* 1995; **152**:2173–5.

64. Melo RE, Sole D, Naspitz CK. Comparative efficacy of inhaled furosemide and disodium cromoglycate in the treatment of exercise-induced asthma in children. *J Allergy Clin Immunol* 1997; **99**:204–9.

65. Tanigaki T, Kondo T, Hayashi Y et al. Rapid response to inhaled furosemide in severe acute asthma with hypercapnia. *Respiration* 1997; **64**:108–10.

66. Ono Y, Kondo T, Tanigaki T, Ohta Y. Furosemide given by inhalation ameliorates acute exacerbation of asthma. *J Asthma* 1997; **34**:283–9.

67. Pendino JC, Nannini LJ, Chapman KR, Slutsky A, Molfino NA. Effect of inhaled furosemide in acute asthma. *J Asthma* 1998; **35**:89–93.

68. Kress JP, Noth I, Gehlbach BK et al. The utility of albuterol nebulized with heliox during acute asthma exacerbations. *Am J Respir Crit Care Med* 2002; **165**:1317–21.

69. Clay MM, Pavia D, Newman SP, Lennard-Jones T, Clarke SW. Assessment of jet nebulisers for lung aerosol therapy. *Lancet* 1983; **2**:592–4.

70. Schuh S, Parkin P, Rajan A et al. High-versus low-dose, frequently administered, nebulized albuterol in children with severe, acute asthma. *Pediatrics* 1989; **83**:513–18.

71. Emerman CL, Cydulka RK, McFadden ER. Comparison of 2.5 vs 7.5 mg of inhaled albuterol in the treatment of acute asthma. *Chest* 1999; **115**:92–6.

72. Robertson CF, Smith F, Beck R, Levison H. Response to frequent low doses of nebulized salbutamol in acute asthma. *J Pediatr* 1985; **106**:672–4.

73. Papo MC, Frank J, Thompson AE. A prospective, randomized study of continuous versus intermittent nebulized albuterol for severe status asthmaticus in children. *Crit Care Med* 1993; **21**:1479–86.

74. McFadden ER, Jr, Strauss L, Hejal R, Galan G, Dixon L. Comparison of two dosage regimens of albuterol in acute asthma. *Am J Med* 1998; **105**:12–17.

75. Reisner C, Kotch A, Dworkin G. Continuous versus frequent intermittent nebulization of albuterol in acute asthma: a randomized, prospective study. *Ann Allergy Asthma Immunol* 1995; **75**:41–7.

76. Ward MJ, Fentem PH, Smith WH, Davies D. Ipratropium bromide in acute asthma. *BMJ (Clin Res Ed)* 1981; **282**:598–600.

77. McFadden ER, Jr, Kiser R, DeGroot WJ. Acute bronchial asthma. Relations between clinical and physiologic manifestations. *N Engl J Med* 1973; **288**:221–5.

78. Sole D, Komatsu MK, Carvalho KV, Naspitz CK. Pulse oximetry in the evaluation of the severity of acute asthma and/or wheezing in children. *J Asthma* 1999; **36**:327–33.

79. Saint S, Bent S, Vittinghoff E, Grady D. Antibiotics in chronic obstructive pulmonary disease exacerbations. A meta-analysis. *JAMA* 1995; **273**:957–60.

80. Parameswaran K, Belda J, Rowe BH. Addition of intravenous aminophylline to beta2-agonists in adults with acute asthma. *Cochrane Database Syst Rev* 2000; CD 002742.

81. Barr RG, Rowe BH, Camargo CA, Jr. Methyl-xanthines for exacerbations of chronic obstructive pulmonary disease. *Cochrane Database Syst Rev* 2001; CD002168.

82. Dockhorn RJ, Baumgartner RA, Leff JA et al. Comparison of the effects of intravenous and oral montelukast on airway function: a double blind, placebo controlled, three period, crossover study in asthmatic patients. *Thorax* 2000; **55**:260–5.

5. NEBULIZER USE IN CHRONIC ASTHMA AND OBSTRUCTIVE AIRWAY DISEASE

Jill P Karpel and Ronan O'Driscoll

Introduction

In the United States of America (USA) total healthcare costs for asthma were estimated to be $12.7 billion for 2001. Of this, $2.4 billion were attributed to treatment costs (Figure 5.1).[1] Despite current national and international guidelines recommending controller therapy with inhaled corticosteroids as first-line therapy, beta-agonists accounted for 53% of the total respiratory market (Figure 5.2)[2] with neublizers accounting for 16% (Figure 5.3). Similar figures have been published for patients with chronic obstructive pulmonary disease (COPD). As such, many patients with asthma and COPD are prescribed nebulizers at home as well as during exacerbations in the emergency department in the hospital.

Recent literature has focused on studies demonstrating that for both adults and children metered dose inhalers (MDI) with holding chambers, dry powder inhalers (DPI), and nebulizers provide equal efficacy in the acute and stable clinical settings.[4–6] Furthermore, we demonstrated that, for patients presenting with acute asthma, optimal dosing can be achieved with albuterol administered with a holding chamber at 60 minute intervals.[7] The majority of these studies have also suggested that there were significant cost savings associated with using handheld devices compared to nebulizers. Despite these reports, healthcare providers have been reluctant to abandon nebulizers and convert to other delivery systems with handheld devices.

Much of the confusion stems from different interpretations of the literature. The efficacy of drug delivery and, therefore, the ultimate outcome of therapy, for handheld devices is dependent on the patient's MDI technique, breathing pattern, airway anatomy, size, and physiology was well as the underlying chronic disease pathology. Alternatively, nebulizer devices can vary as much as >10-fold in the amount of aerosol delivered to the patient's airways. Different nebulizers can and do perform quite differently and are not held to the same government specifications as handheld devices.

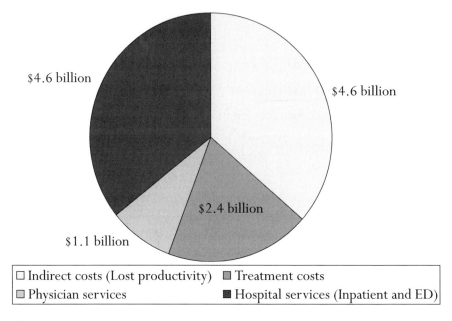

Figure 5.1

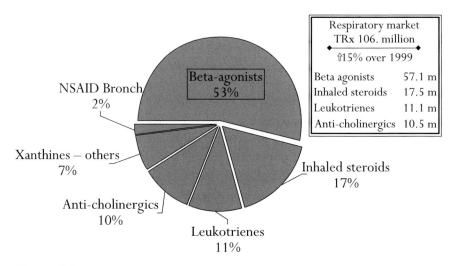

Figure 5.2

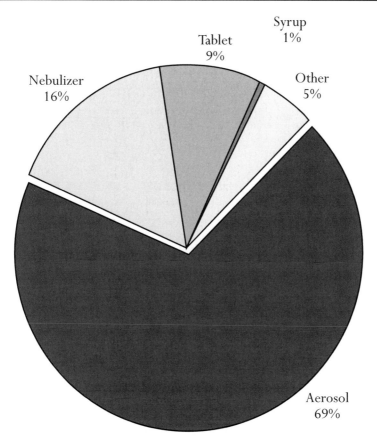

Figure 5.3

Additionally, there are few large, well controlled studies evaluating the use of nebulizers for patients with stable COPD and asthma.[8–12] Thus, individual clinical experience is often relied upon to make decisions concerning the use of nebulizers in the home setting.

To help identify which patients with asthma and COPD would benefit from nebulizer therapy, the European Respiratory Society (ERS) recently published guidelines on the use of nebulizers.[13] The aims were to:

1. improve clinical practice
2. enhance the safety and efficacy of nebulizer use
3. serve as an educational and scientific resource for healthcare professionals
4. stimulate future research by identifying areas of ignorance and uncertainty.

It is the purpose of this chapter to review the ERS guidelines and other pertinent literature to further our understanding of when to prescribe nebulizers for stable patients with asthma and COPD.

Why should nebulizers be used for chronic asthma and COPD?

There are several reasons why patients with asthma and COPD might benefit from nebulizers compared with handheld devices. These include:

- delivering a larger dose of medication
- delivering a medication not available in a handheld device
- patient preference
- physician preference
- home management of exacerbations
- effects on mucus secretion
- non-medical factors.

Delivering a larger dose of medication

For most patients who require inhalation therapy the most convenient and easiest method is to use an MDI and spacer device or DPI. However, if larger than usual doses of medications are required, a nebulizer can deliver a larger dose more conveniently than can be delivered by an MDI or DPI. This is the case for beta-agonists, anticholinergics, and inhaled corticosteroids. For example, 500 μg of ipratropium would require an average of 25 puffs of ipratropium delivered by MDI. A similar number of puffs would be required to deliver 2.5 mg of albuterol. For budesonide, 10 puffs would be required to deliver 2 mg. Therefore, in these clinical settings, a nebulizer would be more convenient as it would deliver the drug in 5–10 min. Additionally, prescribing 25 puffs using a handheld device would be a challenge for the patient to self-administer and one would question patient compliance with such treatment.

For beta-agonist treatment, the majority of patients demonstrate a relatively flat dose–response curve and therefore there is little reason to deliver large doses. Furthermore, the benefit of increased dosage is often exceeded by the adverse effects associated with high-dose beta-agonist treatment. However, Nisar et al, comparing 300 μg by MDI to 5000 μg delivered by nebulization, reported a 20% improvement with the larger nebulized dose for patients with COPD in support of higher dosage.[14] Similar findings have been reported by other investigators. For individual patients, a trial of high-dose therapy may be indicated with appropriate pulmonary function and symptom monitoring.

For anticholinergics, Gross and colleagues demonstrated that a maximal dose of ipratropium for patients with COPD was 500 μg.[15] Current MDIs deliver only 18–36 μg/puff. Again, for patients who respond to high-dose ipra-tropium, a nebulizer may be more convenient.

In some studies, combination therapy with an anticholinergic and beta-agonist may confer significant advantages in terms of improved pulmonary function and duration of action for patients with COPD.[16] Simultaneous administration of these drugs at higher doses delivered by an MDI combination inhaler may again benefit certain patients.

For chronic asthma, there are few available data to suggest that higher dosages of short-acting beta-agonists or combination therapy with an anticholinergic is of any clinical benefit. Data from a meta-analysis in the acute setting in emergency departments have suggested that combination therapy may benefit the most severely affected patients.[17] This currently cannot be extrapolated to the chronic stable asthma patient. For delivering inhaled bronchodilators, a meta-analysis of 16 clinical trials involving 686 children and 375 adults found no difference in pulmonary function or other outcomes when short-acting beta-agonists were administered via MDIs or nebulizers.[5]

There are some data comparing holding chambers with nebulizers for inhaled steroids in chronic asthma. Cates and co-workers performed a meta-analysis, finding two studies (63 adult subjects) suitable for analyses.[18] They reported that due to design differences they could not pool the studies, but one high quality study compared high-dose budesonide 2000–8000 μg delivered via Pari Inhaler Boy jet nebulizer (Pari Medical Ltd, West Byfleet, UK) with budesonide 1600 μg via a large volume spacer. The nebulizer group had higher morning peak flows (25 l/min; $p < 0.01$), higher evening peak flows (30 l/min; $p < 0.01$), fewer beta-agonist requirements and lower symptom scores compared to the holding chamber group. As this was the only double-blind study published, the authors concluded that this was an area worthy of future research. Another meta-analysis comparing 24 nebulizer with holding chamber trials using lower doses of inhaled corticosteroids found no difference between the delivery systems.[4] Other investigators have reported that oral corticosteroid dependent asthma patients were able to discontinue or substantially lower their dose of oral corticosteroids with the initiation of high-dose, nebulized budesonide.[19,20] These studies consisted of small numbers of subjects and were not blinded or placebo controlled. Thus, one may conclude that there may be an advantage to nebulizing high doses of inhaled steroids for certain asthma patients, but further study is clearly warranted. One should also be aware that nebulizing high doses of inhaled steroids has the potential risk of systemic absorption and may in fact not be substantially different than prescribing oral corticosteroids.

Children represent another population of asthma patients with different issues surrounding delivery of required medications. Despite this, in the results of three studies comparing the effectiveness of nebulizers with MDIs for beta-agonist use, no significant differences were demonstrated for bronchodilator delivery.[4] High-dose medication was not evaluated and children may be particularly sensitive to the adverse effects of high-dose beta-agonist therapy. No literature concerning high-dose inhaled corticosteroids in the pediatric population was available for review.

In summary, nebulizers may afford certain advantages over handheld devices when large dosages of medications are prescribed for patients with stable COPD and asthma. The ERS guidelines recommend that handheld inhalers be used for increasing doses of up to 1 mg of salbutamol and/or 160 μg of ipratropium or combinations of such therapy that could be given more conveniently with a nebulizer system.[13] Periodic re-evaluation of their continued efficacy should be undertaken to ensure improved pulmonary function and quality of life with minimal adverse effects.

Delivering medications not available in handheld devices

An obvious reason for using a nebulizer would be to deliver medications not available in handheld devices. For patients with asthma and COPD, there is one beta-agonist medication available only as a solution. This is levalbuterol, an isomer of racemic albuterol. It has been hypothesized that (S)-albuterol compromises the effectiveness of racemic albuterol since it can oppose the bronchodilatory effects of (R)-albuterol, be proinflammatory, and exhibit the potential to exacerbate airway reactivity to a wide variety of stimuli by enhancing bronchoconstriction.[21] Theoretically, the removal of (S)-albuterol should increase the potency of (R)-albuterol (levalbuterol).

In a study of 424 stable asthma patients (>12 years of age), Nelson randomized patients to receive either nebulized levalbuterol (1.25 mg), levalbuterol (0.63 mg), racemic albuterol (1.25 mg), racemic albuterol (2.5 mg) or placebo three times daily for 4 weeks.[22] All medications resulted in significant bronchodilation (forced expiratory volume in one second (FEV_1) >15%) compared to placebo. However, levalbuterol had the greatest and most prolonged effect on bronchodilation, particularly for those subjects who were the most obstructed (FEV_1 <60%). For all analysis, the rank order for efficacy was levalbuterol 1.25 mg, levalbuterol 0.63 mg, racemic albuterol 2.5 mg more than racemic 1.25 mg. Similar findings were reported for children aged 6–11 years with doses of levalbuterol ranging from 0.16–1.25 mg. Thus, levalbuterol which currently can only be administered with a nebulizer may be advantageous for some patients with chronic asthma. Additionally, levalbuterol is a sterile, additive-free unit-dose vial. The use of levalbuterol in acute exacerbations of asthma is still under investigation. Trials for patients with COPD are ongoing.[23] The role of the combination of nebulized levalbuterol and anticholinergics is potentially interesting.

Once daily nebulized long-acting beta-agonist solutions are also undergoing clinical trials. These would offer the convenience of once daily dosing, which would have potential value for patients with both asthma and COPD.

N-acetyl cysteine has occasionally been recommended as a mucolytic agent. There are no published clinical trials demonstrating its efficacy. Furthermore, it can induce bronchoconstriction. Therefore, in a recent meta-analysis, only oral mucolytic agents have been shown to result in a small reduction in acute exacerbations and total days of disability for patients with COPD.[24]

Other possible medications would include inhaled antibiotics. It would be anticipated that the need for such medication would imply a diagnosis such as bronchiectasis in addition to asthma or COPD. In conclusion, nebulizers may be of great value in administering selected medications which are not available in handheld delivery systems for specific indications.

Patient preference

Many patients request home nebulizers, particularly after having received treatment with nebulizers either in an emergency department or in hospital. This is usually because they perceived the nebulizer as being more effective or they have poor inhalation technique with handheld devices.[25] However, the majority of patients can be taught correct inhaler technique. For those patients who simply cannot use handheld devices due to physical impairments, the nebulizer is the device of choice to deliver necessary medications. There also appears to be a small group of adult patients who will not accept handheld devices and insist upon nebulizers. Education about devices should be offered to these patients, but for those who are insistent, nebulizers can be prescribed.

In study of 22 elderly patients with COPD or asthma (age 67 ± 2 years; mean FEV_1 46.5% predicted), treated with either MDI or a nebulizer and a multidrug inhalation regimen, patient preference was in favor of the nebulizer with regard to effectiveness and in favor of the MDI with regard to acceptability.[26]

Nebulizers may also be preferred by some parents with infants for whom the parents find nebulizers easier to use than face masks with attached MDIs.

There is some literature on home nebulizers and patient preference. Simpson and colleagues had 26 patients with severe COPD or asthma complete a standard questionnaire before and 2 months after starting home nebulized bronchodilator therapy.[27] Patients' perceived illness severity and their expectations for treatment were assessed in the first questionnaire and outcomes at 2 months. Prior to treatment, patients expected symptomatic improvement. Results demonstrated only marginal improvement and the authors concluded that patients had unrealistic expectations from the treatment.

In a study evaluating symptoms among patients with asthma, White and Sander reported that of 1230 pediatric and 604 adult asthma patients, 58–79% reported significant side effects from bronchodilaotors, and these were most common among nebulizer users of all ages and pediatric patients using oral medications. Bronchodilator use was reduced on their own by 25–30% and 14–24% skipped doses to avoid side effects.[28] Thus, it appears that patients using nebulizers appear to experience significant adverse effects from beta-agonist bronchodilators.

In conclusion, nebulizer therapy should be considered for those patients (adult or pediatric) who cannot or will not use handheld devices. Despite the fact that patients believe nebulizers are more effective, they experience more adverse effects from nebulized medication and do not necessarily achieve improved pulmonary function compared to handheld devices. Patient education is critical when prescribing nebulizers.

Physician preference

Physicians often prescribe nebulizers for those patients whom they perceive as having severe obstructive airways disease or frequent exacerbations that could be treated more effectively at home. Also, physicians will prescribe nebulizers if their patients strongly request one. There is no pertinent literature concerning physician preference or how they make decisions concerning delivery systems. However, of interest, White and Sander reported that only 4% of respondents to their survey about asthma and adverse effects of medication found their physicians 'caring/sympathetic, willing to listen or discuss their bronchodilator use, effects' etc.[28] Patients claimed physician responses were to change brands within the same class of drug, change dosages of the same drug, or tell patients to tolerate the adverse effects because the medication was necessary.

In a population of Scottish patients with COPD, Godden et al reported that the majority of patients with COPD and asthma who had home nebulizers did not understand the principle of nebulizer use and that over half the compressors were malfunctioning.[12] They suggested the need for more patient education and technical support. In a group of inner city children with asthma, Butz et al found nebulizer use to be higher than anticipated (33% of 686 children).[29] However, this was not associated with reduced morbidity. It was felt that the children were not being adequately monitored by their physicians and that anti-inflammatory therapy was not being appropriately prescribed.

Although many physicians prescribe nebulizers, it is clear from the literature that both physicians and patients need considerable education concerning delivery systems. It is the responsibility of the healthcare providers to understand the limitations and advantages of all the delivery systems and to communicate them effectively to their patients.

Treat exacerbations at home (reduce morbidty)

Many patients with COPD and asthma believe that home nebulizers will prevent them from having to go to the emergency department or hospital for exacerbations. There are some objective data to support this conclusion. Godden et al, in a study of the use of home nebulizers in Scotland in 405 patients with either COPD or asthma (185 with asthma and 208 with COPD), mean age 64.5 years, reported that the percentage of patients requiring hospital admissions for exacerbations of lung disease fell from 56% to 46% (p <0.01) with nebulizer use.[12] The number and duration of admissions were unchanged. Those whose duration of admission increased had more severely impaired lung function when the nebulizer was supplied, had lower activity scores and higher breathlessness scores at the time of interview. Of interest, 87% used their nebulizer at least once daily. Fifty-four percent reported adverse events related to the frequency of use and these were more common in the younger patients. Over the 2-year period these patients were followed, 29 patients (7%) died.

In a study of 32 patients with COPD and asthma using home nebulizers, it was reported that mortality was similar to a group of patients who chose MDI therapy (5-year survival 56% vs 53%). However, there was some evidence that hospital admissions were reduced.[8] The authors concluded that nebulizer therapy was safe and effective for a small number of carefully selected patients with severe asthma or COPD. It was recommended that these patients undergo rigorous home nebulizer assessment prior to initiating home nebulizer therapy. The protocol for this is described later in this chapter.

In a study whose objective was to investigate the benefit of home nebulizers dispensed to a group of patients under the age of 21 years, who were discharged from the hospital following an exacerbation of asthma, it was reported that 43 weeks after the home nebulizer was dispensed, an estimated average of 3.6 emergency department visits and 5.4 office/clinic visits for each patient were prevented by the home nebulizer.[30] The savings from the reduced visits were estimated to range from $855/$1710 or more. The majority of the patients felt that the home nebulizer was a 'good idea' and easy to use. The authors recommended that when discharging patients from an emergency department or hospital, the patient's physician should be contacted to discuss the possibility of discharging the patient with a home nebulizer.

In contrast to the above study, Butz et al reported a high rate of morbidity including frequent emergency department visits and hospitalizations among inner city children using home nebulizers.[29] It is important to note that only one out of seven children in this study were taking anti-inflammatory medication and the results most likely reflect poor overall asthma management.

In deciding whether or not to prescribe home nebulizers for exacerbations of either COPD or asthma, physicians must consider the possibility that patients may self-medicate to the point where they endanger their own health. In reporting the results of a questionnaire survey on some aspects of nebulizer use, nebulizer instructions and features relating to deteriorating asthma, Gregson and colleagues showed that although the majority (77–100%) of patients were aware of the '4-hour rule' for repeat bronchodilator use at home, there was considerable confusion about the acceptable time interval and what to do if there was inadequate relief of symptoms or improvement in peak expiratory flow rate (PEFR).[31] Only 32% of the adults with asthma (200 in the group) had a crisis plan for intervention. The authors concluded that every patient needs an action plan which clearly delineates which medications should be used during an exacerbation and how to use them. Clinical parameters should be clearly set as to when a patient needs to contact their physician for additional instructions or the need to proceed to the emergency department or hospital.

In summary, there is some evidence that the use of home nebulizers may decrease the number of emergency department visits or hospitalizations for selected patients with asthma or COPD. Additional cost savings may also be realized. It is important that the patients understand how to use the nebulizers and when to contact their physician when they are experiencing exacerbations so that significant morbidities can be prevented.

Effects on mucus secretion

Some uncontrolled studies have suggested that nebulizers can assist mucus clearance and symptomatically improve symptoms for selected patients.[32,33] There are no adequate studies to assess this effect of nebulizers and one should not recommend home nebulizer therapy for this indication alone.

Non-medical factors

As mentioned previously, it is possible that there are cost savings associated with home nebulizer use. Additionally, individual countries may vary with respect to Social Security benefits available to patients based on disease severity and home health needs. Ultimately, the decision as to whether or not to prescribe a home nebulizer should be based on the individual patient and their response to therapy.

Home nebulizers clearly have a role in optimizing care for some patients with COPD and asthma. Although the majority of patients can be effectively treated with MDIs and DPIs, there are some patients who will require home nebulizer therapy for the reasons discussed above. The next part of this chapter focuses on how to identify which patients will benefit from home nebulizers and how to initiate therapy.

Assessment of patients and initiation of therapy

The first step in assessing patients for home nebulizer therapy is to confirm the diagnosis of asthma or COPD with appropriate diagnostic evaluation. This should include formal pulmonary function tests and other tests as indicated based on the clinician's assessment of the patient. Conditions such as upper airway disease (vocal cord dysfunction), interstitial lung disease, congestive heart failure, and pulmonary vascular disease should be excluded. Diseases such as sinusitis or gastro-esophageal reflux that may complicate the management of COPD and asthma should be aggressively diagnosed and treated.

When the diagnosis of COPD or asthma is confirmed and the severity assessed, the physician should discuss the options with the patient to educate them as to what they may expect from different modalities of treatment. Handheld device technique must be repeatedly reviewed with the patients to ensure that they are in fact using their inhalers correctly and at the prescribed doses. Some patients may do better with DPIs rather than with MDIs and spacers. Additionally, other interventions such as pulmonary rehabilitation may be beneficial. There is emerging evidence that exercise capacity and quality of life can improve with pulmonary rehabilitation programs.[34] Patients may further benefit from smoking cessation programs, appropriate diet and attention to non-pharmacological interventions in their environment. Therefore, it is important to maximize all other therapeutic options prior to considering home nebulizer therapy.

At the current time, it is not possible to predict which patients will benefit from home nebulizer therapy. The majority of trials which report benefit have evaluated COPD patients with severe pulmonary function impairment (FEV_1 <30% predicted).[8–12] Patients with better lung function (mild to moderate disease) would probably not benefit from home nebulizers and there is no published experience to suggest otherwise. Patients with emphysema who do not demonstrate bronchodilator reversibility will not benefit from high-dose bronchodilator therapy and should not be considered for home nebulizers. Some patients with chronic severe asthma may develop relatively irreversible airflow obstruction, similar to COPD patients and should be considered for home nebulizer therapy. Patients with mild asthma and infrequent exacerbations should not be considered candidates for home nebulizer therapy.

The next step in determining which patients may benefit from home nebulizers is to perform a 'Domiciliary Nebulizer Trial or Inhaled therapy optimization protcol' as outlined in the ERS guidelines.[13] Previous studies have demonstrated that short-term laboratory studies using either single doses of bronchodilators or studying patients over several days do not necessarily correlate with which patients will benefit most from home nebulizer therapy. In a study of 20 patients (six with severe asthma, 14 with COPD) a double-blind laboratory assessment did not predict which patients were likely to respond to home nebulizer treatment.[8] Furthermore, adverse effects of treatment could not be predicted.

A study by Goldman and colleagues concluded that studying the improvement in PEFR and symptoms during a home trial of nebulized saline (1 week) and nebulized beta-agonist/ipratropium (1 week salbutamol and 1 week combination of salbutamol and ipratropium) was helpful in predicting which patients might benefit from home nebulizer therapy.[35] For the 98 patients that they studied (100 trials), they demonstrated an increase in

PEFR of 15% and improvement in symptoms (93% sensitivity and 87% negative predictive value) for 25 patients. They did note that no laboratory measurement predicted a positive trial. However, they suggested that patients who demonstrated a 15% increase in PEFR and subjective benefit could be candidates for home nebulizer therapy.

Inhaled therapy optimization trial

At the present time, there is no standard agreement as to the exact definition of a positive response to a trial of home nebulizer therapy. We recommend making a determination using the ERS guidelines which are summarized as follows.

First, the physician should determine which handheld device (MDI/spacer or DPI) can the patient best use. Once it is established that the patient is using the device correctly and taking their medications at the correct prescribed dosages, a 2-week baseline trial of collecting diary data and PEFR should begin. Patients should record their PEFR (best of three efforts) twice daily (am/pm) and when symptomatic. Patients should also record their use of rescue medication, symptoms, and exercise capacity. Ideally, FEV_1 and forced vital capacity should be obtained at baseline and after each treatment intervention.

Second, following the baseline period, a trial of increased bronchodilator therapy with PEFR and diary monitoring should be undertaken for at least another 2 weeks. Doses of salbutamol of 2.5–5 mg four times daily, ipratropium 250–500 μg four times daily, or the combination given via a nebulizer is recommended. As needed rescue medication should be continued.

A trial of long-acting beta-agonist or anticholinergic agent by handheld devices should also be considered for COPD patients prior to initiating nebulizer therapy. It is assumed that any severe asthma patient would be receiving a combination of high-dose inhaled corticosteroids and a long-acting beta-agonist as standard therapy prior to considering home nebulizer therapy. Objective monitoring should be continued during this 2-week period as well.

After completing the above trial with the establishment of baseline lung function and symptoms, a home nebulizer with appropriate medications can be prescribed. The patient should again be instructed to maintain PEFR and symptom diaries for comparison with the baseline period. Careful instructions as to how to use the nebulizer and administer the medications should be given as well as a written action plan which includes emergency instructions.

The ERS recommends assessing the response to treatment as shown in Box 5.1 and Table 5.1. The scheme should help physicians identify which

Box 5.1 Assessing the response to treatment (ERS guidelines).

Objective response

(compared with 2 weeks on usual therapy)

PEFR worse or unchanged or rise of 0–10%	Score 0
PEFR rise of 11–20%	Score 1
PEFR rise >20%	Score 2

Subjective response

(Ask the patient to respond to the following question: Compared with your previous treatment, how was your condition overall during this period of treatment?)

Worse	Score −1
Some or no definite change	Score 0
Definitely better	Score 1
Definitely much better	Score 2

PEFR, peak expiratory flow rate.

Table 5.1 Evaluation of outcomes (scores in Box 5.1).

Possible outcomes:	Suggested Action
Subjective response +1, +2 Objective response +1, +2	Consider continuing therapy long-term
Subjective response +1, +2 Objective response 0	Consider longer trial of therapy
Subjective response −1, 0 Objective response 0	Stop this treatment (and proceed to next step)
Subjective response −1, 0 Objective response +1, +2	Reconsider diagnosis and consider longer trial

patients will benefit from home nebulizer therapy. Periodic reassessment of the patients' condition and response to nebulizer therapy should be performed at reasonable intervals. Patient education is critical to optimizing this process.

Future directions

It is clear that much work needs to be done to define ultimately which patients with asthma and COPD will benefit from home nebulizer therapy. Physicians need to educate their patients about their disease and how to use the medications that are prescribed to them properly. The majority of patients should be able to use their inhalers with handheld devices. Patients who require nebulizers should be carefully selected and monitored such that they receive maximum benefit from their home nebulizers.

References

1. American Lung Association. http://www.lungusa.org
2. NPA (National Prescription Administration). http://www.npanet.com
3. IMS Provider Perspective. http://www.imshealth.com
4. Brocklebank D, Ram F, Wright J et al. Comparison of effectivenss of inhaler devices in asthma and chronic obstructive airways disease: a systemic review of the literature. *Health Technol Assess* 2001; **5**:1–149.
5. Cates CJ, Rowe BH. Holding chambers versus nebulizers for beta-agonist treatment of acute asthma. *Cochrane Database Syst Rev* 2000; CD000052.
6. Frei SP. Cost comparison of bronchodilator delivery methods in emergency department treatment of asthma. *J Emerg Med* 2000; **19**:323–6.
7. Karpel JP, Aldrich TK, Prezant DJ et al. Emergency treatment of acute asthma with albuterol metered-dose inhaler plus holding chamber. How often should treatments be administered? *Chest* 1997; **112**:348–56.
8. O'Driscoll BR, Kay EA, Weatherby H, Chetty MCP, Bernstein A. A long-term prospective assessment of home nebuliser treatment. *Respir Med* 1992; **86**:317–25.
9. Mossison JFJ, Jones PC, Muers MF. Assessing physiological benefit from domicilary nebulised bronchodilators in severe airflow limitation. *Eur Respir J* 1992; **5**:424–9.
10. O'Driscoll BR, Bernstein A. A long term study of symptoms, spirometry, and survival amongst home nebuliser uses. *Respir Med* 1996; **90**:561–6.
11. Gregson RK, Warner JO, Radford M. Assessment of the continued supervision and asthma management knowledge of patients possessing home nebulizers. *Respir Med* 1995; **7**:487–93.
12. Godden DJ, Robertson A, Currie N et al. Domiciliary nebuliser therapy – a valuable option in chronic asthma and chronic obstructive lung disease? *Scott Med J* 1998; **43**:48–51.
13. Boe J, Dennis JH, O'Driscoll BR. European Respiratory Society guidelines on the use of nebulisers. *Eur Respir J* 2001; **18**:228–42.
14. Nisar M, Walshaw MJ, Earis JE, Pearson MG, Calverley PMA. Assessment of reversibility of airway obstruction in patients with chronic obstructive airways disease. *Thorax* 1990; **45**:190–4.
15. Gross N, Petty TL, Freidman M et al. Dose response to ipratropium as a nebulised solution in patients with chronic obstructive pulmonary disease. *Am Rev Respir Dis* 1989; **139**:1188–91.

16. The Combivent Inhalation Study Group. Routine nebulized ipratropium and albuterol together are better than either alone in COPD. *Chest* 1997; **112**:1514–21.

17. Rodrigo GJ, Rodrigo C. The role of anticholinergics in acute asthma treatment: an evidence based evaluation. *Chest* 2002; **6**:1977–87.

18. Cates CJ, Adams N, Bestall J. Holding chambers versus nebulisers for inhaled steroids in chronic asthma. *Cochrane Database Syst Rev* 2001: DC001491.

19. Higgenbottam TW, Clark RA, Luksza AR et al. The role of nebulized budesonide in permitting a reduction in the dose of oral steroid in persistent severe asthma. *Eur J Clin Res* 1994; **5**:1–10.

20. Otulana BA, Varma N, Bullock A, Higenbottam T. High dose nebulized steroid in the treatment of chronic steroid-dependent asthma. *Respir Med* 1992; **86**:105–8.

21. Page CP, Morley J. Contrasting properties of albuterol stereoisomers. *J Allergy Clin Immunol* 1999; **2**:S31–S41.

22. Nelson HS. Clinical experience with levalbuterol. *J Allergy Clin Immunol* 1999; **2**:S77–S84.

23. Costello J. Prospects for improved therapy in chronic obstructive pulmonary disease by the use of levalbuterol. *J Allergy Clin Immunol* 1999; **2**:S61–S68.

24. Poole PI, Black PN. Mucolytic agents in chronic bronchitis and COPD. *Cochorane Database Syst Rev* 2000; CD001872.

25. Cross S. Asthma inhalation systems: the patient's viewpoint. *J Aerosol Med* 2001; **14**(Suppl 1):S3–S7.

26. Balzano G, Battiloro R, Biraghi M et al. Effectiveness and acceptability of a domiciliary multidrug inhalation treatment in elderly patients with chronic airflow obstruction: metered dose inhaler versus jet nebulizer. *J Aerosol Med* 2000; **13**:25–33.

27. Simpson AJ, Tweeddale PM, Crompton GK. Starting home nebulizer therapy: patients' expectations and subsequent outcome at 2 months. *Respir Med* 1998; **8**:1000–2.

28. White MV, Sander N. Asthma from the perspective of the patient. *J Allergy Clin Immunol* 1999; **104**:S47–S52.

29. Butz AM, Eggleston P, Huss K, Kolodner K, Rand C. Nebulizer use in inner-city children with asthma: morbidity, medications use, and asthma management practices. *Arch Pediatr Adolesc Med* 2000; **10**:984–90.

30. Yamamoto LG, Okamura D, Nagamine J et al. Dispensing home nebulizers for acute wheezing from the hospital is cost-effective. *Am J Emerg Med* 2000; **18**:164–7.

31. Gregson RK, Warner JO, Radford M. Assessment of the continued supervision and asthma management knowledge of patients possessing home nebulizers. *Respir Med* 1995; **7**:487–93.

32. Poole PJ, Brodie SM, Stewart JM, Black PN. The effects of nebulised isotonic saline and trebutaline on breathlessness in severe chronic obstructive pulmonary disease (COPD). *Aust NZ J Med* 1998; **28**:322–6.

33. Sutton PP, Gemmell HG, Innes N et al. The use of nebulised saline and nebulised terbutaline as an adjunct to chest physiotherapy. *Thorax* 1988; **43**:57–60.

34. Lacasse Y, Wong E, Guyatt GH et al. Meta-analysis of respiratory rehabilitation in chronic obstructive pulmonary disease. *Lancet* 1996; **348**:1115–19.

35. Goldman JM, Teale C, Muiers MF. Simplifying the assessment of patients with chronic airflow limitation for home nebulizer therapy. *Respir Med* 1992; **86**:33–8.

6. SPECIAL APPLICATIONS OF AEROSOL THERAPY

Torsten T Bauer and Patrice Diot

Introduction

Aerosol delivery to the lungs has become a well established therapy for chronic obstructive pulmonary disease (COPD) and asthma in the non-intubated patient. The drugs of choice are beta-2-adrenergic and anticholinergic drugs as well as inhaled corticosteroids. However, the applications in other fields or of other drugs is hampered by the sparse knowledge about the applicability of aerosol therapy. We have therefore included special applications of aerosol therapy in this chapter.

Aerosol therapy in the intensive care unit

In the intensive care unit (ICU) ventilator-supported patients often need numerous types of medications, both enteral or parenteral. In these patients aerosol therapy is particularly useful as an alternative route for drug delivery. Aerosols can be used to manage a large variety of pulmonary disorders in the ICU, but delivery of bronchodilators to patients with COPD is most common and best documented.[1] This group of agents will therefore be used initially to address the three major issues in delivery of aerosols to intubated patients: therapeutic response measurements, inhalation devices and dose finding studies. Thereafter, we will discuss other possible aerosol treatments in the ICU and special applications inside and outside the intensive care setting.

Therapeutic response measurements

Indications for bronchodilator therapy in intubated and mechanically ventilated patients are not well defined,[1,2] but may be regarded as similar to those in non-intubated subjects. Bronchospasm remains the most common indication for aerosol therapy in the ICU. However, bronchial obstruction may be missed in the mechanically ventilated patient, because communication is limited and auscultation altered. In general, all patients with a history of COPD should receive aerosolized bronchodilator therapy during mechanical ventilation but patients with pulmonary infection leading to or arising during ventilator support should also be treated with a bronchodilator, although scientific evidence is sparse.[3] In addition, the 'worsening' of the ventilatory situation with increasing ventilation pressures or increasing need for supplemental oxygen may indicate the presence of bronchospasm in mechanically ventilated patients. Arterial oxygenation, however, should not be used as the only treatment indicator or therapeutic response measurement, because most studies showed no change in oxygenation after application of bronchodilating aerosol therapy with one study even indicating a worsening.[4] In contrast, measurements of pulmonary mechanics are suitable for guiding therapy, because one rationale for aerosolized bronchodilator therapy in these patients is to reduce ventilation pressures and to decrease the risk of ventilator-induced lung injury. Dynamic pulmonary hyperinflation is common in patients with respiratory failure due to COPD and expiratory flow limitation and results in intrinsic positive end-expiratory pressure (PEEPi). Most studies used PEEPi, assessed by the interrupter technique (Figure 6.1)[5] and found a substantial reduction after administration of either anticholinergic or beta-2-adrenergic drugs. Other parameters such as total flow resistance (RT) or the 'interrupter' resistance (Rint) have been used (see equations in Figure 6.1). In a recent study, more elaborate methods for detection of flow limitation have been compared but no beta-adrenergic drug has been applied to verify their value for evaluating treatment efficacy.[6]

Nebulizers versus metered dose inhalers

There has been a substantial debate about the best way to deliver aerosols to the mechanically ventilated patient. The most prevalent indication will be obstructive flow limitation which can be treated with anticholinergic or beta-2-adrenergic drugs. Both types of medication are, with the exception of the long-acting tiotropium bromide, available as solutions and metered dose inhalers (MDI) and therefore suitable for application via nebulizers or MDI. Other substances like prostacyclin or surfactant are either not suitable for application via MDI or simply not available. The debate can therefore only be held in the field of bronchodilator therapy where Gay and colleagues, among the first to conduct a randomized study, studied 18 patients with sus-

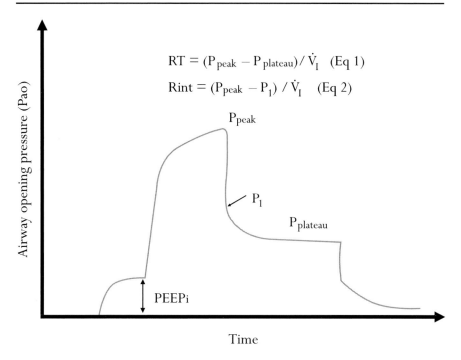

$$RT = (P_{peak} - P_{plateau})/\dot{V}_I \quad (Eq\ 1)$$

$$Rint = (P_{peak} - P_1)/\dot{V}_I \quad (Eq\ 2)$$

Figure 6.1 *Schematic illustration of airway opening pressure (Pao) using the interrupter technique. Pao rises from intrinsic end-expiratory pressure (PEEPi) to peak pressure (P_{peak}) and falls rapidly until P_1 followed by a slow decay until plateau pressure ($P_{plateau}$). Total flow resistance (RT) can be calculated according to equation 1 (Eq 1) using the immediately preceding flow (V_1). For the interrupter resistance (Rint) pressure (P_1) should be used instead of $P_{plateau}$ (Eq 2). (Adapted from Gottfried SB et al. J Appl Physiol 1985; 59:647–52.[5])*

pected airway obstruction (physician in charge had ordered bronchodilator aerosols). Patients were randomized to albuterol administered either by MDI or updraft small volume nebulizers. The nebulizer was placed close to the Y-junction between the ventilator tubing and the endotracheal tube, and the MDI was used during manual inflation of the lung with a postinspiratory pause. The dose aerosolized with the nebulizers (2.5 mg) was almost 10 times higher than with MDI (270 μg) but the authors did not find significant differences in airway mechanics between these two modes of aerosol preparation.[7] The authors concluded that aerosol delivery with MDI was equally effective as administration via nebulizer. Manthous and coworkers were the first to show that MDI administration can also be effective without manual inflation of the lung when a spacer is used. This spacer was connected to the Y-piece and actuated at end-expiration.[8] But non-valved spacers are also effective. This has been shown in a randomized comparison of MDI plus spacer with nebulizers for the efficacy of fenoterol and ipratropium.[9] However, ventilator settings varied in all studies and it was necessary to investigate ventilator settings for optimal drug delivery via MDI. This work was published in a series of papers[10–12] investigating the effect of an end-inspiratory pause (5 seconds versus none),[13] tidal volume (8 ml/kg body-weight versus 12 ml/kg bodyweight),[10] inspiratory flow pattern (pressure control and decelerating flow pattern versus volume control and square wave flow pattern),[11] and inspiratory flow rate (0.6 l/s versus 1.2 l/s). Although the sample size was small in all studies it became evident that no significant difference on the static or dynamic pressures between study groups could be observed and, even more important, a significant reduction in PEEPi up to 20% was observed in all patients. It is therefore reasonable to conclude that for the delivery of aerosolized bronchodilator therapy MDI has been shown to have similar efficacy to a nebulizer when an in-line chamber is used and basic rules are followed (Box 6.1).[14] Given the availability and easy use, the MDI could be considered the delivery device of choice. However, not all ventilation circuits are suitable for aerosol chamber

---

Box 6.1 Techniques for nebulizer and MDI use during mechanical ventilation.

Nebulizer
- Place drug and diluent in nebulizer, noting that nebulizer efficiency varies with brand
- Place the nebulizer in-line approximately 18 in from the circuit Y
- Ensure a 6–8 l/min gas flow to the nebulizer, continuously or intermittently
- Adjust tidal volume to 0.5 l; inspiratory flow to achieve Ti/Ttot >0.3
- Adjust minute volume if an external nebulizer gas flow is used
- Disable any continuous flow through the ventilator
- Assure nebulizer function throughout the treatment
- Remove the nebulizer from the circuit when the medication is spent
- Assure restitution of ventilator settings

MDI
- Adjust tidal volume to >0.5 l inspiratory flow
- Assure that patient's breath is synchronized with the ventilator
- Shake MDI and insert canister into chamber (inspiratory limb, no filter!)
- Synchronize attenuation with ventilator
- Allow exhalation
- Repeat in 20–30 seconds interval until dose is delivered

MDI, metered dose inhaler; Ti, time inspiratory; Ttot, total circuit time. (Adapted from Op't Holt TB. *AARC Times* 2000; **7**:18–24.[14])

insertion, because it requires a Y-connector. From the infection prevention point of view it also seems unwise to break the circuit four to six times daily to insert the chamber. A collapsible chamber that could remain within the ventilation tubing system with virtually no additional dead space had to be redesigned to meet new medical standards and will be available in the near future. The use of MDIs is regarded as more cost effective[15] and MDIs were cheaper than nebulizers in one cost comparison due to the lower preparation costs.[7] Nebulizers are potential reservoirs or vehicles for infectious micro-organisms. Routes of transmission may be from device to patient, from one patient to another, or from one body site to the lower respiratory tract of the same patient by hand or via the device.[16] Contaminated reservoirs of aerosol producing devices (e.g. nebulizers) may facilitate growth of hydrophilic bacteria that may be subsequently aerosolized during device use.[17] *Pseudomonas* spp., *Legionella* spp., or non-tuberculous mycobacteria can multiply to substantial concentrations in nebulizer fluid and increase the device user's risk of acquiring pneumonia.[16]

Dose finding studies

Manthous and coworkers were amongst the first to address this issue. They combined a randomized design (MDI versus nebulizer) with a dose–response study in 10 selected patients on mechanical ventilation (difference between P_{peak} and $P_{pause} > 15$ cmH$_2$O).[18] The results of this study were in contrast to previous findings, because, although albuterol was delivered in a high cumulative dose via MDI (9 mg, 100 puffs) no reduction of resistive pressures ($P_{peak} - P_{pause}$) was observed. In this study no manual inflation of the lung was used and the MDI was connected directly to the swivel adapter. The authors concluded that the poorly designed adapter was – at least in part – responsible for the deposition of the large majority of aerosol particles outside of the lung. A dose–response relationship could be established up to a cumulative dose of 7.5 mg with the nebulizer. A dose of 15 mg did not elicit further reduction of the resistive pressure and all patients experienced toxicity (dysrhythmias, nausea or tremor).[18] The introduction of spacers for aerosol delivery made it necessary to repeat this study with the new technology and lower doses. This work was carried out by Dhand and coworkers who first investigated the efficacy and safety of 900 mg albuterol (10 puffs)[19] and subsequently the dose–response relationship.[20] A cylindrical collapsible spacer chamber (Aerovent; Monahan Medical, Plattsburg, USA) was placed in the inspiratory limb of the ventilator circuit and actuated at approximately 20 s intervals just before the inspiratory flow generated by the ventilator. In these two studies, the efficacy was assessed in terms of changes in minimal and maximal inspiratory resistance (Rrs_{max}, Rrs_{min}) and PEEPi. The results of the dose–response study suggested that four puffs of albuterol (360 μg) administered with the above technique already produced significant bronchodilation in mechanically ventilated COPD patients with no further improvement after cumulative doses of 12 (1080 μg) and 28 puffs (2520 μg). A significant increase in heart rate was observed only after 28 puffs cumulative dose.[20] The response to bronchodilator therapy was observed for at least 60 min in this study but could be confirmed for up to four hours in a study by Duarte and coworkers.[21] Since that study also failed to demonstrate an additional benefit with a dose exceeding 400 μg of albuterol, we recommend a standard dose of 360–400 μg salbutamol (depending on the preparation available) four to six times daily. No studies are available to date to test the efficacy of newer long-acting beta-2-agonists such as salmeterol, which are readily available and are also delivered in standard canisters. However, there are no theoretical barriers to the use of such agents also in intensive care patients if the essential rules of administration of aerosols via MDI are followed.

Unfortunately there is no literature available investigating the efficacy of nebulizer or MDI therapy in patients with tracheostomy. However, as outlined above drug deposition outside the lung can be minimized by the correct use of nebulizers and MDI with spacers in mechanically ventilated patients and this experience should be transferable to patients with chronic respiratory failure and tracheostomy. If patients are breathing spontaneously, one might consider optimizing drug delivery by increasing tidal volume through a resuscitation bag connected to the chamber device. Efficacy may be further improved by applying an exhalation valve in case non-valved spacers are used. This is, however, based on clinical experience rather than published evidence and should be individualized for each patient.

Aerosolized antibiotics for the treatment and prevention of pulmonary infection

Topical antibiotics are usually delivered by nebulizers because the particle size is crucial to the deposition pattern.[22] An important limitation in many studies has been the inadequate characterization and control of variables affecting the efficiency of drug deposition, such as nebulizer design, operating conditions, particle size and patient's breathing pattern. Thus, the dose of antibiotics actually delivered to the lung was unknown. Inhalation antibiotic therapy has been investigated for both prophylactic and acute treatment of Gram-negative and, lately also, fungal pneumonia.[23] Several studies have shown that prophylactic inhaled antibiotics in patients are effective in reducing bacterial airway colonization with Gram-negative flora and decrease the incidence of pneumonia when used intermittently or for short periods.[24–27] In a recently study with pig models of pneumonia, nebulized amikacin yielded higher concentrations and killing rates in the lung compared to the parenteral route.[28] This may indicate a role for nebulized aminoglycosides as an additional therapy in pneumonic patients. However, the emergence of resistant bacteria has been a problem, and prolonged use has been associated with an unacceptably high rate of pneumonias caused by drug resistant bacteria. The use of aerosolized antibiotics should therefore be limited to well established bacterial pulmonary infections (e.g. cystic fibrosis, see Chapter 7).

Aerosolized pentamidine was a standard treatment for primary and secondary prevention of *Pneumocystis carinii* pneumonia in human immunodeficiency virus (HIV) patients until two randomized trials showed better outcomes using oral trimethoprim-sulfamethoxazole (co-trimoxazole).[29,30] This and the fact that severely immunocompromised patients are especially susceptible to contaminated aerosols led to a sparse use of inhaled pentamidine prophylaxis in these patients with the exception of those who do not tolerate prophylaxis with co-trimoxazole, dapsone/pyrimethamine or atovaquone.[31]

Aerosolized amphotericin B has been widely investigated for the prophylaxis of fungal infections in lung transplant recipients. Aerosolized amphotericin B lipid complex was administered in 355 cases in a study by Palmer and coworkers and there were no significant adverse events related to study medication in any patient, and 1-year survival for all enrolled patients was 78%.[32] Also non-liposomal amphotericin B seems to be well tolerated in nebulized quantities that result in sufficiently high intrabronchial fluid levels.[33] One trial also described a clinical benefit for such a prophylactic strategy. Monforte and associates applied aerosolized amphotericin B to 55 consecutive lung allograft recipients and found a significant reduction in *Aspergillus* infections (0.13; 95% confidence interval 0.02–0.69; $p < 0.05$).[34] However, this was not a randomized placebo-controlled trial which should be awaited, although data from animal studies are promising.

Pulmonary hypertension

Rationale for aerosol therapy

Pulmonary hypertension is defined by the World Health Organization to be present when the systolic pulmonary artery pressure is >40 mmHg and by the National Institutes of Health when the mean pulmonary artery pressure measured by catheterization is >25 mmHg at rest or >30 mmHg at exercise. The definition of primary pulmonary hypertension (PPH) excludes left-sided cardiac vascular diseases, myocardial disease, congenital heart disease, any previous or current clinically significant respiratory, connective tissue or chronic thromboembolic disease.[35] Portal hypertension, HIV infection, cocaine, fenfluramine and dexfenfluramine drugs can cause secondary pulmonary hypertension with clinical and histopathological patterns similar to PPH. PPH is a rare disease with an incidence of one to two cases per million in the general population, primarily affecting young women. It is linked with some genetic factors and generally associated with a poor prognosis. In the mid-1980s, the mean survival after diagnosis was 3 years, with 21% surviving for more than 5 years, and 10% for more than 10 years.[36] In pathophysiology the imbalance between prostacyclin and thromboxane metabolites plays a major role in the development of the disease which is characterized by vasoconstriction, vascular wall remodeling and thrombosis.[36] Prostacyclin is a powerful vasodilator of the systemic and pulmonary arterial and venous beds and also acts against pulmonary hypertension by inhibiting platelet aggregation and smooth muscle proliferation. Intravenous prostacyclin was introduced into therapy of PPH in the late 1980s[37] and the first randomized trial demonstrating benefits of long-term treatment by intravenous prostacyclin was published in 1990.[38] However, intravenous administration of prostacyclin has substantial disadvantages because it can induce vasodilatation in poorly ventilated lung regions leading to increased pulmonary shunting with a decrease in oxygenation. Further side effects include systemic hypotension, headache and flushing. Because of the instability of the drug and its short half-life continuous infusion and central venous catheter are required bearing the risk of infection.[38] This led other investigators to assess the effects of the aerosol route, with a first report by Walmrath and associates in 1993 in three ventilated patients with severe acute adult respiratory distress syndrome (ARDS).[39] The aerosol, characterized by a mass median aerodynamic diameter (MMAD) of 2.7 μm was nebulized into the inspiratory circuit of the ventilator in incremental doses ranging from 5 ng/kg per min for up to 30 min. A small but significant reduction in pulmonary artery pressure (PAP) was observed whereas cardiac output and capillary wedge pressure remained unchanged, suggesting a decrease in pulmonary vascular resistance. There was also an improvement in arterial oxygenation and a pronounced reduction in the shunt fraction. PAP and gas exchange returned to pretreatment values within 1 hour after this single aerosol withdrawal. There were no detectable side effects in the three patients described. An editorial in the same journal emphasized the similarity in the effects of nitric oxide and prostacyclin, and the potential of the presented data not only for prostacyclin but also for inhalation of nitric oxide donors (e.g. phosphodiesterase inhibitors).[40] This initial study was followed by a number of investigations in the field of aerosol therapy for pulmonary hypertension.

Iloprost aerosols in pulmonary hypertension

Iloprost is a stable prostacycline analog whose favorable effects administered as an aerosol to PPH patients were first reported in 1996.[41] It is a highly potent pulmonary vasodilator equally or even more effective on hemodynamics in some cases than nitric oxide.[42] Until the year 2002, two long-term uncontrolled studies reported contradictory data. Hoeper et al treated 24 patients with PPH and New York Heart Association (NYHA) functional class III and IV with six to eight inhalations of iloprost per day, up to a daily dose of 100 µg, over a 1-year period.[43] They concluded that aerosolized iloprost was a safe treatment with sustained effects on exercise capacity and pulmonary hemodynamics. In contrast, Machherndl et al concluded that inhaled iloprost at a daily dose of 100 µg/day in addition to conventional therapy was not efficient in severe pulmonary hypertension.[44] However, among the 12 studied patients, five suffered from thromboembolic pulmonary hypertension and six from Eisenmenger's syndrome. This discrepancy may therefore be attributable to the differences in the study populations, with a trend to a more pronounced effect in PPH. The Aerosolized Iloprost Randomized (AIR) study therefore represented a major step toward clarification of this problem.[45] This European multicenter placebo-controlled study was conducted on 203 patients (iloprost, 101 patients; placebo, 102 patients) with selected pulmonary arterial hypertension and chronic thromboembolic pulmonary hypertension with NYHA functional class III or IV despite conventional therapy. A maximum total dose of 5 µg of iloprost was inhaled by the patients using the Halolite

(MedicAid, UK) nebulizer six or nine times daily and treatment was assessed after 12 weeks based on improvement of NYHA class and a 6-min walk test. These combined endpoints were met by 16.8% of iloprost patients compared with 4.9% of placebo patients ($p = 0.007$). The results of this study are likely to establish aerosolized iloprost as a standard therapy for patients with severe primary pulmonary hypertension and selected forms of pulmonary arterial and chronic thromboembolic pulmonary hypertension. Ultrasonic nebulization should be preferred over jet nebulization, because a randomized comparison showed higher efficiency and shorter inhalation times with an ultrasonic device.[46] However, whether inhalation therapy with iloprost will be effective in decreasing mortality awaits further investigation.

Phosphodiesterase inhibitors and other agents

A total of 11 isoenzymes of phosphodiesterase (PDE) have been described in mammals. Inhibition of PDE-3 and PDE-4 primarily increases cyclic adenosine monophosphate (cAMP) which also mediates prostacyclin effects. Inhibition of PDE-5 increases not only the intracellular concentration of cyclic guanidine monophosphate (cGMP), which mediates the vasodilatory effect of nitric oxide, but also cAMP.[42] Synthetic inhibitors of phosphodiesterases are under development to treat vascular disorders and some have been studied in PPH as aerosols, alone or in combination with iloprost. The PDE-5/6 inhibitor sildenafil has recently been shown to induce selective pulmonary vasodilatation in a randomized comparison of patients with lung fibrosis and secondary pulmonary hypertension. In contrast to prostacyclin, sildenafil did not increase ventilation–perfusion mismatching.[47] A study in a sheep model also confirmed that nebulized sildenafil is a selective pulmonary vasodilator that can increase the vasodilating effect of inhaled nitric oxide on the pulmonary vessels.[48] Inhaled zaprinast, which is an inhibitor of guanosine-$3',5'$-cyclic monophosphate (cGMP)-selective phosphodiesterase, selectively dilates the pulmonary circulation and potentiates and prolongs the pulmonary vasodilating effects of nitric oxide in lambs with experimental pulmonary hypertension.[49] The demonstration of synergistic effects of phosphodiesterase inhibitors coadministered by oral or aerosol route with inhaled prostacyclin or iloprost is also promising but there are no reports on humans. Other substances are currently under evaluation for aerosolized therapy of pulmonary hypertension.[42] Among those are compounds that are formed by reacting nitric oxide with various nucleophiles (NONOates) which release nitric oxide spontaneously and induce vasodilatation (e.g. dimethylaminoethyl-putreanine, diethylentriamine). This mechanism seems promising in various animal models to reduce pulmonary hypertension without reducing systemic arterial pressure and without systemic toxicity. However, at present, all agents are far from clinical application.

Lung transplantation

Aerosolized cyclosporine A

The introduction of cyclosporine A in the treatment of lung allograft recipients is probably one of the major reasons for prolonged survival of these patients. Cyclosporine A has a narrow therapeutic index when administered orally and the efficacy of aerosolized cyclosporine A to prevent acute pulmonary rejection was first demonstrated in a canine model.[50] Experimental data in rat models with unilateral orthoptic lung transplanation showed that aerosolized cyclosporine A prevents acute rejection in a dose-dependent fashion.[51]

Because cyclosporine A is insoluble in water, ethanol was used as the solvent in the first studies (CSA-ethanol). Muggenberg et al labeled CSA-ethanol with [99 mTc] sulfur colloid and demonstrated by gamma camera techniques in healthy beagle dogs that the aerosol could be produced by a jet nebulizer and deposited in the lungs.[52] In five lung transplanted patients with acute persistent rejection and bronchiolitis obliterans, O'Riordan et al measured lung deposition of CSA-ethanol aerosols from a 250 mg cyclosporine A nebulizer charge between 20 mg and 53 mg.[53] Deposition in the graft correlated with regional ventilation and with perfusion. Keenan et al demonstrated the clinical efficacy of aerosolized CSA-ethanol to control refractory chronic rejection in 18 patients with chronic rejection receiving aerosolized cyclosporine A (300 mg) 3 days per week after a period of 10 consecutive days when compared to 23 control patients. Histologic score of rejection and pulmonary function tests improved in 14 of the 16 evaluable patients in the group treated by aerosolized cyclosporine A. Two patients were unable to tolerate the treatment and withdrew from the study but there was no renal or hepatic toxicity. Cough, which is the most frequent side effect led to the replacement of ethanol by propylene glycol which is better tolerated. The efficacy of aerosolized cyclosporine A dissolved in propylene glycol was first assessed in treatment of acute rejection after lung transplantation in nine patients.[55] A dose of 300 mg was administered three times a week and the follow-up ranged between 12 and 200 days. Eight of the nine patients had histological improvement and mean forced expiratory volume in one second (FEV_1) of the population increased significantly. Cyclosporine A aerosol deposition in the graft was measured by gamma camera techniques in seven patients. The deposited mass in the transplant ranged between 5.6 mg and 29.7 mg per lung. There was a strong correlation between the deposition of the drug in the transplant and the improvement of FEV_1. However, nebulized cyclosporine A is not a standard therapy and the improvement over systemic therapy awaits further research. Newer immunosuppressant agents with fewer systemic side effects may also solve most of the problems associated with systemic immunosuppression with cyclosporine A.

Palliative care

Pain, cough, breathlessness, tenacious secretions and stridor are frequent and difficult-to-treat symptoms in palliative care. Nebulization is unlikely to have a place in the management of pain,[56] but tenacious secretions and stridor have been at least anecdotally treated with various agents such as saline, budesonide and ipratropium. However, controlled studies are lacking. Nebulized lidocaine (lignocaine) has been extensively studied to reduce the dose of topical anesthetics for bronchoscopy and as a suppressant of coughing after bronchoscopy. It has also been proven to be effective in severe glucocorticoid-dependent asthma, allowing in some cases reduction of oral glucocorticoid therapy. The potential of nebulized lidocaine to treat intractable cough has only been reported in a single and uncontrolled study with four patients in addition to anecdotal reports.[57]

Dyspnea is a subjective feeling that is difficult for the physician to quantify since it reflects personal perception and certain external features may have influence.[58] It is also difficult to treat because there is no correlation between the extent of disease and the severity of dyspnea. Dyspnea has been studied on a visual analogue scale, but lidocaine at 100 mg and 200 mg was not more efficient than saline in cancer patients.[59] Conclusions about the effects of nebulized opioids are also difficult to draw because there is no standard treatment protocol, and treatment is decided on a case-by-case basis. Orally or intravenously administered morphine has been proposed as a treatment for dyspnea in the terminally ill patient. It provides relief but has side effects.[58] This is the reason why inhalation has been proposed as an alternative method of administration and in some hospital departments it has been accepted as common practice. The mode of action of inhaled morphine is still unclear, but there are at least two hypotheses: that there is a central action of opiates similar in type to pain inhibition[60] and/or that morphine acts on peripheral pulmonary receptors.[58] Although one uncontrolled study conducted in 17 patients with nebulized morphine at doses of 20 mg every 4 hours during 48 hours gave promising results,[61] in a placebo-controlled, double-blind randomized study conducted in 17 patients, nebulized morphine did not prove to have a specific effect on dyspnea.[62] These conflicting data should not discourage randomized trials involving well defined populations with end-stage disease, because nebulized opioids may have an important place in palliative care.

References

1. Dhand R, Tobin MJ. Inhaled bronchodilator therapy in mechanically ventilated patients. *Am J Respir Crit Care Med* 1997; **156**:3–10.
2. Cakar N. Inhalation therapy during mechanical ventilation. *Intensive Care Med* 1999; **25**:233–5.
3. Bauer TT, Roussos C, Torres A. Aerosol therapy in intubated and mechanically ventilated patients in the intensive care unit. *Eur Respir Rev* 2000; **10**:536–40.
4. Bernasconi M, Brandolese R, Poggi R et al. Dose-response effects and time course of effects of inhaled fenoterol on respiratory mechanics and arterial oxygen tension in mechanically ventilated patients with chronic airflow obstruction. *Intensive Care Med* 1990; **16**:108–14.
5. Gottfried SB, Higgs BD, Rossi A et al. Interrupter technique for measurement of respiratory mechanics in anesthetized humans. *J Appl Physiol* 1985; **59**:647–52.
6. Lourens MS, Berg BV, Hoogsteden HC, Bogaard JM. Detection of flow limitation in mechanically ventilated patients. *Intensive Care Med* 2001; **27**:1312–20.
7. Gay PC, Patel HG, Nelson SB et al. Metered dose inhalers for bronchodilator delivery in intubated, mechanically ventilated patients. *Chest* 1991; **99**:66–71.
8. Manthous CA, Chatila W, Schmidt GA, Hall JB. Treatment of bronchospasm by metered-dose inhaler albuterol in mechanically ventilated patients. *Chest* 1995; **107**:210–13.
9. Guerin C, Chevre A, Dessirier P et al. Inhaled fenoterol-ipratropium bromide in mechanically ventilated patients with chronic obstructive pulmonary disease. *Am J Respir Crit Care Med* 1999; **159**:1036–42.
10. Mouloudi E, Katsanoulas K, Anastasaki M et al. Bronchodilator delivery by metered-dose inhaler in mechanically ventilated COPD patients: influence of tidal volume. *Intensive Care Med* 1999; **25**:1215–21.

11. Mouloudi E, Prinianakis G, Kondili E, Georgopoulos D. Bronchodilator delivered by metered-dose inhaler in mechanically ventilated COPD patients. Influence of flow pattern. *Eur Respir J* 2000; **16**:263–8.

12. Mouloudi E, Prinianakis G, Kondili E, Georgopoulos D. Effect of inspiratory flow rate on b_2-agonist induced bronchodilatation in mechanically ventilated COPD patients. *Intensive Care Med* 2000; **27**:42–6.

13. Mouloudi E, Katsanoulas K, Anastasaki M et al. Bronchodilator delivery by metered-dose inhaler in mechanically ventilated COPD patients: influence of the end-inspiratory pause. *Eur Respir J* 1998; **12**:165–9.

14. Op't Holt TB. Aerosol therapy during mechanical ventilation. *AARC Times* 2000; **7**:18–24.

15. Bowton DL, Goldsmith WM, Haponik EF. Substitution of metered-dose inhalers for hand-held nebulizers: success and cost savings in a large acute-care hospital. *Chest* 1999; **101**:305–8.

16. Centers for Disease Control and Prevention. Guidelines for prevention of nosocomial pneumonia. *MMWR* 1997; **46**:1–79.

17. Craven DE, Lichtenberg DA, Goularte TA et al. Contaminated medication nebulizers in mechanical ventilator circuits. *Am J Med* 1984; **77**:834–8.

18. Manthous CA, Hall JB, Schmidt GA, Wood LDH. Metered-dose inhaler versus nebulized albuterol in mechanically ventilated patients. *Am Rev Respir Dis* 1993; **148**:1567–70.

19. Dhand R, Jubran A, Tobin MJ. Bronchodilator delivery by metered-dose inhaler in ventilator-supported patients. *Am J Respir Crit Care Med* 1995; **151**:1827–33.

20. Dhand R, Duarte AG, Jubran A et al. Dose-response to bronchodilator delivered by metered-dose inhaler in ventilator-supported patients. *Am J Respir Crit Care Med* 1996; **154**:388–93.

21. Duarte AG, Momii K, Bidani A. Bronchodilator therapy with metered-dose inhaler and spacer versus nebulizer in mechanically ventilated patients: comparison of magnitude and duration of response. *Respir Care* 2000; **45**:817–23.

22. Rosenfeld M, Cohen M, Ramsey B. Aerosolized antibiotics for bacterial lower airway infections: principles, efficacy, and pitfalls. *Clin Pulm Med* 1997; **4**:101–12.

23. Lode H, Höffken G, Kemmerich B, Schaberg T. Systemic and endotracheal antibiotic prophylaxis of nosocomial pneumonia in the ICU. *Intensive Care Med* 1992; **18**:S24–S27.

24. Klastersky J, Huysmans E, Weerts D et al. Endotracheally administered gentamicin for the prevention of infections of the respiratory tract in patients with tracheostomy: a double-blind study. *Chest* 1974; **65**:650–4.

25. Levine BA, Petroff PA, Slade L, Pruitt BA. Prospective trials of dexamethasone and aerosolized gentamicin in the treatment of inhalation injury in the burned patient. *J Trauma* 1978; **18**:188–93.

26. Greenfield S, Teres D, Bushnell LS et al. Prevention of Gram-negative bacillary pneumonia using aerosol polymyxin as prophylaxis. I. Effect on the colonization pattern of the upper respiratory tract of seriously ill patients. *J Clin Invest* 1973; **52**:2935–40.

27. Klick JM, Du Moulin GC, Hedley-White J et al. Prevention of Gram-negative bacillary pneumonia using polymyxin aerosol as prophylaxis. II. Effect on the incidence of pneumonia in seriously ill patients. *J Clin Invest* 1975; **55**:514–19.

28. Goldstein I, Wallet F, Nicolas-Robin A et al. Lung deposition and efficiency of nebulized amikacin during *Escherichia coli* pneumonia in ventilated piglets. *Am J Respir Crit Care Med* 2002; **166**:1375–81.

29. Schneider MM, Hoepelman Al, Eeftinck Schattenkerk JK et al. A controlled trial of aerosolized pentamidine or trimethoprim-sulfamethoxazole as primary prophylaxis against *Pneumocystis carinii* pneumonia in patients with human immunodeficiency virus infection. The Dutch AIDS Treatment Group. *N Engl J Med* 1992; **327**:1837–41.

30. Hardy WD, Feinberg J, Finkelstein DM et al. A controlled trial of trimethoprim-sulfamethoxazole or aerosolized pentamidine for secondary prophylaxis of *Pneumocystis carinii* pneumonia in patients with the acquired immunodeficiency syndrome. AIDS Clinical Trials Group Protocol 021. *N Engl J Med* 1992; **327**:1842–8.

31. Miller R, Hermant C, Escamilla R, Benfield T. Nebulizer use in patients with human immunodeficiency virus infection and acquired immunodeficiency syndrome. *Eur Respir Rev* 2000; **10**:523–6.

32. Palmer SM, Drew RH, Whitehouse JD et al. Safety of aerosolized amphotericin B lipid complex in lung transplant recipients. *Transplantation* 2001; **72**:545–8.

33. Marra F, Partovi N, Wasan KM et al. Amphotericin B disposition after aerosol inhalation in lung transplant recipients. *Ann Pharmacother* 2002; **36**:46–51.

34. Monforte V, Roman A, Gavalda J et al. Nebulized amphotericin B prophylaxis for *Aspergillus* infection in lung transplantation: study of risk factors. *J Heart Lung Transplant* 2001; **20**:1274–81.

35. Rubin LJ. Primary pulmonary hypertension. *N Engl J Med* 1997; **336**:111–17.

36. Fuster V, Steele PM, Edwards WD et al. Primary pulmonary hypertension: natural history and the importance of thrombosis. *Circulation* 1984; **70**:580–7.

37. Higenbottam T. The place of prostacyclin in the clinical management of primary pulmonary hypertension. *Am Rev Respir Dis* 1987; **136**:782–5.

38. Rubin LJ, Mendoza J, Hood M et al. Treatment of primary pulmonary hypertension with continuous intravenous prostacyclin (epoprostenol). Results of a randomized trial. *Ann Intern Med* 1990; **112**:485–91.

39. Walmrath D, Schneider T, Pilch J et al. Aerosolised prostacyclin in adults respiratory distress syndrome. *Lancet* 1993; **342**:961–2.

40. Royston D. Inhalational agents for pulmonary hypertension. *Lancet* 1993; **342**:941–2.

41. Olschewski H, Walmrath D, Schermuly R et al. Aerosolized prostacyclin and iloprost in severe pulmonary hypertension. *Ann Intern Med* 1996; **124**:820–4.

42. Hoeper MM, Galie N, Simonneau G, Rubin LJ. New treatments for pulmonary arterial hypertension. *Am J Respir Crit Care Med* 2002; **165**:1209–16.

43. Hoeper MM, Schwarze M, Ehlerding S et al. Long-term treatment of primary pulmonary hypertension with aerosolized iloprost, a prostacyclin analogue. *N Engl J Med* 2000; **342**:1866–70.

44. Machherndl S, Kneussl M, Baumgartner H et al. Long-term treatment of pulmonary hypertension with aerosolized iloprost. *Eur Respir J* 2001; **17**:8–13.

45. Olschewski H, Simonneau G, Galie N et al. Inhaled iloprost for severe pulmonary hypertension. *N Engl J Med* 2002; **347**:322–9.

46. Gessler T, Schmehl T, Hoeper MM et al. Ultrasonic versus jet nebulization of iloprost in severe pulmonary hypertension. *Eur Respir J* 2001; **17**:14–19.

47. Ghofrani HA, Wiedemann R, Rose F et al. Sildenafil for treatment of lung fibrosis and pulmonary hypertension: a randomised controlled trial. *Lancet* 2002; **360**:895–900.

48. Ichinose F, Erana-Garcia J, Hromi J et al. Nebulized sildenafil is a selective pulmonary vasodilator in lambs with acute pulmonary hypertension. *Crit Care Med* 2001; **29**:1000–5.

49. Ichinose F, Adrie C, Hurford WE et al. Selective pulmonary vasodilation induced by aerosolized zaprinast. *Anesthesiology* 1998; **88**:410–16.

50. Dowling RD, Zenati M, Burckart GJ et al. Aerosolized cyclosporine as single-agent immunotherapy in canine lung allografts. *Surgery* 1990; **108**:198–205.

51. Mitruka SN, Pham SM, Zeevi A et al. Aerosol cyclosporine prevents acute allograft rejection in experimental lung transplantation. *J Thorac Cardiovasc Surg* 1998; **115**:28–37.

52. Muggenberg BA, Hoover MD, Griffith BP. Administration of cyclosporine by inhalation: a feasibility study in beagle dogs. *Aerosol Med* 1990; **3**:1–13.

53. O'Riordan TG, Iacono A, Keenan RJ et al. Delivery and distribution of aerosolized cyclosporine in lung allograft recipients. *Am J Respir Crit Care Med* 1995; **151**:516–21.

54. Keenan RJ, Iacono A, Dauber JH et al. Treatment of refractory acute allograft rejection with aerosolized cyclosporine in lung transplant recipients. *J Thorac Cardiovasc Surg* 1997; **113**:335–41.

55. Iacono AT, Smaldone GC, Keenan RJ et al. Dose-related reversal of acute lung rejection by aerosolized cyclosporine. *Am J Respir Crit Care Med* 1997; **155**:1690–8.

56. Ahmedzai S, Davis C. Nebulised drugs in palliative care. *Thorax* 1997; **52**:S75–S77.

57. Howard P, Cayton RM, Brennan SR, Anderson PB. Lignocaine aerosol and persistent cough. *Br J Dis Chest* 1977; **71**:19–24.

58. Chandler S. Nebulized opioids to treat dyspnea. *Am J Hosp Palliat Care* 1999; **16**:418–22.

59. Wilcock A, Corcoran R, Tattersfield AE. Safety and efficacy of nebulized lignocaine in patients with cancer and breathlessness. *Palliat Med* 1994; **8**:35–8.

60. Woodcock AA, Gross ER, Gellert A et al. Effects of dihydrocodeine, alcohol, and caffeine on breathlessness and exercise tolerance in patients with chronic obstructive lung disease and normal blood gases. *N Engl J Med* 1981; **305**:1611–16.

61. Zeppetella G. Nebulized morphine in the palliation of dyspnoea. *Palliat Med* 1997; **11**:267–75.

62. Noseda A, Carpiaux JP, Markstein C et al. Disabling dyspnoea in patients with advanced disease: lack of effect of nebulized morphine. *Eur Respir J* 1997; **10**:1079–83.

7. NEBULIZED ANTIBIOTICS IN CYSTIC FIBROSIS AND NON-CF BRONCHIECTASIS IN CHILDREN AND ADULTS

A Kevin Webb, Mary E Dodd and Andrew Bush

Introduction

Survival for patients with cystic fibrosis (CF) now extends into the fourth decade of life. Morbidity and mortality for this lethal disease are almost entirely related to progressive pulmonary sepsis.[1,2] It is the aggressive and informed use of oral, inhaled and intravenous antibiotics against the organisms which infect the CF lung, which have transformed this lethal disease from one leading to death in childhood to survival into adulthood.[3,4] The care of CF patients is complex and the judicious use of antibiotics for these patients is best delivered by a multidisciplinary team in a CF center.[5]

Nebulized antibiotics (using penicillin) were first described for the treatment of lung disease (pneumonia) in the mid-1940s.[6] Over two decades ago, a randomized controlled trial using nebulized carbenicillin and gentamicin demonstrated a reduction in hospitalization and an improvement in pulmonary function in adult patients with CF.[7] There have been multiple publications, guidelines and consensus documents evaluating the indications and benefits of nebulized antibiotics in CF.[8–10]

This chapter focuses specifically on the current usage and clinical indications of inhaled antibiotics for children and adults with CF. The results from well conducted studies are now being published but significant questions still need to be answered with further research and trials. We also review how the information derived from the extensive use of nebulized antibiotics in CF has been applied to the treatment of non-CF bronchiectasis.

Microbiology of cystic fibrosis

In order to understand the use of antibiotics and, in particular, nebulized antibiotics in the treatment of CF, it is important to have some knowledge of the unique microbiology of the CF lung.

The basic defect in CF lies on the long arm of chromosome 7 that results in impermeability of the chloride channel in the epithelial cells lining the bronchial tree. The normal protein for the chloride channel is termed the cystic fibrosis transmembrane conductance regulator (CFTR). How defective CFTR renders the airways of patients with CF susceptible to bacterial infection in early childhood is poorly understood. However, some of the recognized pathological consequences are an alteration in fluid transport across the airways, inefficient mucociliary clearance of infected secretions and reduced activity of local host defense mechanisms.

In early childhood, the airways of patients with CF are infected with *Staphylococcus aureus*. Four decades ago this bacterial pathogen was responsible for death in childhood, a situation which was improved by the introduction of prophylactic oral anti-staphylococcal antibiotics. As survival into adulthood improves, *Pseudomonas aeruginosa* is becoming the predominant pathogen infecting over 80% of the adult CF lungs. CFTR appears to be an epithelial cell receptor for clearance of *P. aeruginosa* from the lung.[11] Defective CFTR function possibly promotes adherence and binding of this pathogen to damaged airway receptors.[12] Initial acquisition of *P. aeruginosa* is usually from the environment. In the early stages of acquisition the *P. aeruginosa* strains have a relatively benign phenotype, are sensitive to antibiotics, are few in number and have a non-mucoid appearance.

Recently, the genome for *P. aeruginosa* has been cloned leading to greater understanding of its genetic versatility.[13] The large genome of *P. aeruginosa* enables it to thrive in and adapt to different environments, in particular, the CF lung. It has intrinsic antibiotic resistance due to its lower outer membrane permeability with an active efflux system for antibiotics.[14] It secretes several virulence factors including toxins, lipases and proteases. Alginate biosynthesis is regulated by specific loci on the *P. aeruginosa* genome; these gene promoters (algD and algC) present in non-mucoid strains are switched on to produce alginate (biofilms) in response to critical environmental signals in the CF lung.[15]

Once chronic infection has become established the environment of the CF lung appears to rapidly promote a more virulent phenotype (Table 7.1). The evolution of *P. aeruginosa* from a relatively benign to a more virulent

Table 7.1 Characteristics of *Pseudomonas aeruginosa* in the CF lung: early infection versus chronic infection.

Early	Chronic
Non-mucoid phenotype	Mucoid phenotype with biofilm
Low bacterial density	High bacterial density
Antibiotic sensitive	Some antibiotic resistance
Smooth lipopolysaccharide	Rough lipopolysaccharide
Less inflamed airways	Inflamed airways

CF, cystic fibrosis.

pathogen during the progression from early to chronic infection presents a window of opportunity for eradicating this bacterial pathogen.

The pathology of chronic endobronchial infection is characterized by large numbers of mucoid *P. aeruginosa* producing a dense neutrophil inflammatory response (Figure 7.1). This illustrates why it is impossible to eradicate chronic *P. aeruginosa* infection. Neither the antibiotics nor the neutrophils can penetrate the inflammatory bacterial mass (Figure 7.2), and subsequently the neutrophils degranulate releasing potent enzymes, in particular, neutrophil elastase which destroys surrounding lung tissue.

Chronic infection with *P. aeruginosa* has profound clinical consequences. It is correlated with an accelerated decline in pulmonary function, worsening nutrition, reduced growth velocity in children and a poorer prognosis compared to the non-infected patient.[2,16,17] Patients chronically infected with *P. aeruginosa* have a mean survival to 28 years compared to a mean survival to 39 years in non-infected patients.[18] Aggressive use of antibiotics and control of infection are therefore crucial to delay the progression of lung disease. Delivery by the inhaled route affords many advantages compared to the systemic and oral route.

The use of nebulized antibiotics in patients with cystic fibrosis

Studies have shown that regular nebulized antibiotics decrease hospital admissions and improve patients' quality of life.[7,19] Large doses can be

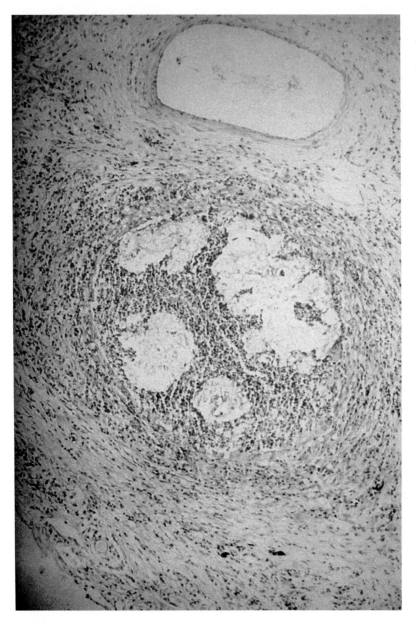

Figure 7.1 Small airways surrounded by a dense inflammatory infiltrate of neutrophils. (H and E stain; courtesy of Professor J Govan.)

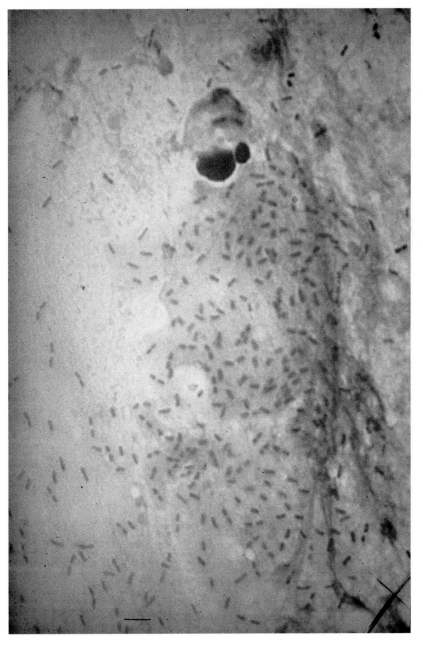

Figure 7.2 Neutrophils trying to and failing to penetrate alginate surrounding Pseudomonas aeruginosa. Correspondingly, antibiotic penetration is decreased. (H and E stain; courtesy of Professor J Govan.)

Box 7.1 Indications for use of nebulized antibiotics in patients with CF.

Eradication at time of first infection with *Pseudomonas aeruginosa*

Chronic infection with *Pseudomonas aeruginosa*

Severe sinus disease

Infection with MRSA

Colonization/infection with *Aspergillus fumigatus*

CF, cystic fibrosis; MRSA, methicillin-resistant *Staphylococcus aureus*.

---

inhaled from which some drug will reach the small airways producing drug concentrations in the bactericidal range and peak serum concentrations that are safe in young children and adults.[20] They can be used lifelong on a daily basis in the home environment. Nebulized antibiotics may decrease the requirement for intravenous antibiotics, and they do not have the same number of side effects which are associated with intravenous antibiotics. A meta-analysis of published trials of inhaled antibiotics demonstrated that the benefits (which included a reduced pseudomonal load and improved pulmonary function) significantly outweighed any risk.[21] Although lifelong treatment mainly for prevention of disease progression is being introduced it may have no immediate discernible benefit as perceived by the patient.

There are recognized clinical indications for using nebulized antibiotics for the treatment of patients with CF (Box 7.1).

Nebulized antibiotics used for the prevention and eradication of early infection with *Pseudomonas aeruginosa*

Recent research using bronchoalveolar lavage (BAL) as a diagnostic tool has established that infection and inflammation commence in infancy and early childhood in patients with CF.[22] During these early years, the patients are often clinically well and may be asymptomatic. In addition, *P. aeruginosa* has not yet acquired its virulent characteristics. The bacteria are present in small numbers, are non-mucoid and antibiotic sensitive, and endobronchial inflammation is not established. It takes approximately 12 months from initial isolation of *P. aeruginosa* for infection to become chronic.[23] This time period is now recognized as a window of opportunity to introduce inhaled antibiotics, eradicate *P. aeruginosa*, delay disease progression and potentially improve survival.

Published studies have shown that nebulized antibiotics can eradicate *P. aeruginosa* in children and adults at time of first identification.[24–31] The results of these studies are presented in Table 7.2. Overall, they demonstrate that an eradication policy with nebulized antibiotics is effective for 80–90% of patients initially infected with *P. aeruginosa*. Further review of these studies shows that chronic infection can be delayed for up to 3 years with preservation of pulmonary function.[27]

Although published studies have clearly established that it is imperative to institute inhaled antibiotics at time of first isolation of *P. aeruginosa* uncertainty remains as to which is the best treatment protocol. In the published studies different antibiotics with different doses for different lengths of time were used. Inhaled drugs were not compared with each other but were combined on some occasions with oral antibiotics and in some studies outcome was compared with historical controls. This therapeutic uncertainty is reflected in the considerable variability in the individual prescription of nebulized antibiotics by experienced CF physicians working in CF centers.[32] There is a need for a prospective, large, multicenter controlled trial to evaluate the efficacy and long-term clinical benefit of inhaled antibiotics in preventing early infection with *P. aeruginosa*. Such a study could be undertaken in Europe or North America.

Nebulized antibiotics used for the treatment of chronic colonization with *Pseudomonas aeruginosa* in patients with cystic fibrosis

The initial paper of Hodson et al described the clinical benefit of inhaled antibiotics for patients chronically infected with *P. aeruginosa*.[7] Further studies have been undertaken.[33–37] Essentially, these studies showed improvement and maintenance of pulmonary function, reduction in hospital admissions, improved weight gain and enhanced patient wellbeing. The nebulized antibiotics used in the studies were ceftazidime, gentamicin, carbenicillin, colistin, cefaloridine and tobramycin. The design for the studies varied (parallel or crossover), the patient numbers were small and treatment length was from months to years. As a consequence it has been difficult to decide which is the best treatment modality.

In the United Kingdom (UK) and Denmark, colistin has been the inhaled drug of choice for treating chronic infection with *P. aeruginosa*; until recently this was the only antibiotic licensed for nebulization in the UK. Unfortunately, despite the length of usage, there are no published randomized controlled trials using colistin showing a definite benefit in the long term for this indication. Also, unlike eradication treatment, the indications for commencing nebulized antibiotics in chronically infected patients are

Table 7.2 Review of studies of outcome of treatment for eradication of *Pseudomonas aeruginosa* using nebulized antibiotics.

Study design and reference	Level of evidence*	N	Drug regimen	Observation period (months)	Outcome (eradication vs non-eradication)
Descriptive[24]	3	7	Colistin 0.5 MU twice daily	11	3/7 patients eradicated PA
RCT[25]	1b	26	Cases: colistin 1 MU twice daily + ciprofloxacin Controls: no treatment	27	12/14 treated patients eradicated PA in treated group
Case–control (historical controls)[26]	2b	16	Cases: colistin 1 MU twice daily + ciprofloxacin + tobramycin 100 mg twice daily Controls: iv antibiotics	27	5/8 treated patients eradicated PA No data
Case–control (historical controls)[27]	2b	91	Cases: colistin 1 MU twice daily + ciprofloxacin Controls: standard treatment (not ciprofloxacin + colistin)	44	41/48 treated patients eradicated PA 24/43 non-treated patients eradicated PA
RCT[28]	1b	22	Cases: tobramycin 80 mg twice daily Controls: placebo	12	8/9 treated patients eradicated PA (2 withdrew) 1/5 non-treated patients eradicated PA (6 withdrew)
Case–control[29]	2b	28	Cases: continuous gentamicin 80–120 mg twice daily Controls: intermittent gentamicin	36	12/12 treated patients eradicated PA 5/16 control patients eradicated PA
Descriptive[30]	3	15	Tobramycin 80 mg twice daily for 12 months	36	14/15 patients eradicated PA at one year. 14/15 still free of PA at 2 years
Descriptive[31]	3	27	Colistin 1 MU twice daily + ciprofloxacin for 3 weeks	60	20/27 patients eradicated PA

* Petrie GJ et al on behalf of the Scottish Intercollegiate Guidelines Network. Clinical guidelines: criteria for appraisal for national use. Edinburgh: Royal College of Physicians, 1995. RCT, randomized controlled trial; MU, million units; PA, *Pseudomonas aeruginosa*.

not clear cut. They are usually commenced on an individual basis in patients who have declining respiratory function despite repeated course of intravenous antibiotics.

Two landmark studies enrolling large numbers of patients inhaling high-dose preservative-free tobramycin (TOBI; Chiron Corporation, Annandale, NJ, USA) have studied and defined the benefits and risks for patients with CF chronically infected with *P. aeruginosa*.[38,39] The first study, published in 1993, was a randomized crossover study, which evaluated the safety and efficacy of TOBI. Seventy-one patients received 600 mg of TOBI or physiological saline at one time. Group 1 received 600 mg of TOBI for 28 days followed by physiological saline for two 28-day periods. Group 2 received placebo for 28 days followed by TOBI for two 28-day periods. The drug dose was chosen to achieve a sputum concentration of tobramycin which was 10-fold greater than the minimum inhibitory concentration (MIC) for *P. aeruginosa*. Levels achieved with inhalation were higher than those achieved with intravenous administration. The drug has a low absorption rate into the systemic circulation with a median (peak) serum concentration of 0.98 mg/l at 1 hour after inhalation.[40] Renal function and ototoxicity were monitored. In the first 28-day period of active drug treatment there was almost a 10% improvement in forced expiratory volume in one second (FEV_1) predicted and a decrease in density of *P. aeruginosa* in sputum by a factor of 100. There was no increase in nephrotoxicity or ototoxicity. The increase in number of tobramycin-resistant bacteria was similar for both the active and the placebo arm of the study.

In the second study, published in 1999 (which was double-blind and placebo-controlled), TOBI was inhaled in alternating monthly cycles of antibiotic and saline versus continuous placebo for a period of 6 months. Five hundred and twenty patients participated in the study. The concept of using alternating cycles of active drug was to diminish the development of persistent TOBI resistance and allow susceptible pathogens to repopulate the airways during the 'drug holiday'. In this extended study, the pulmonary function improved by 10% at week 20 as compared with week 0. Sputum density of *P. aeruginosa* decreased but there was an increase in the MIC of the drug against *P. aeruginosa* in the active group. Hospital admissions were decreased by 26% when compared to the placebo group and the requirement for intravenous antibiotics was decreased in the active group when compared to placebo.

This study was extended for a further 18 months and 242 patients received TOBI on an open cyclical basis.[41] The improvement in pulmonary function was maintained for the whole group with a mean FEV_1 of 4.7% above the baseline.

When these data were further analyzed for subgroup benefit, the most marked benefit was in the adolescent population with a 14.3% improvement in FEV_1 compared with baseline.[42] Adolescence is a vulnerable period for young people with CF. Self-care often declines and associated loss of lung function can be irreversible. It is recognized that a 10% decline in lung function doubles the risk of patient death.[2] These results highlight an additional indication for nebulized antibiotics be given to adolescents who are deteriorating.

A major concern in these studies was the decreased antibiotic susceptibility of *P. aeruginosa* to TOBI but the authors concluded that the benefits of improved lung function and weight gain over time outweighed the risk of increased antibiotic resistance. A limited retrospective study demonstrated that patients receiving TOBI had an improved Global Rating for Health Related Quality of Life.[19]

There is no evidence for an increased benefit of combining nebulized and intravenous antibiotics.[43]

Recently, a multicenter randomized controlled trial has compared TOBI (300 mg twice daily) with colistin 1 MU twice daily for 1 month in 115 patients with CF chronically infected with *P. aeruginosa*.[44] The mean difference in change for FEV_1 % predicted between the two groups was 6.33% in favor of TOBI. However, the standard dose for adults receiving colistin is 2 MU twice daily. Also, clinical use of TOBI usually incorporates 1 month on and 1 month off the drug. Comparisons were made at the end of 1 month rather than 2 months. These differences from usual clinical practice for TOBI and colistin somewhat invalidates the conclusions of the study.

Other indications for the use of nebulized antibiotics in CF

Sinus disease

The epithelial cells which line both the sinuses and the bronchi in patients with CF express the same basic defective function of CFTR. The sinuses are also chronically infected with similar pathogens (in particular, *P. aeruginosa*) that infect the lung. The sinuses can infect a transplanted lung following transplantation. Nebulized antibiotics delivered with a face mask can be used to try to sterilize the airways prior to transplantation and are routinely used to keep the new lungs free of infection following the transplantation.[45] There are no trials evaluating the value of this clinical practice.

Unusual pathogens

Methicillin-resistant *Staphylococcus aureus* (MRSA): There are increasing reports of MRSA infection in CF.[46–48] The impact of infection with MRSA upon disease progression is uncertain. One study in adults has suggested the organism does not alter disease progression[46] but a study in children suggested MRSA had an adverse effect upon growth and was associated with a requirement for more intravenous antibiotics and worse findings on chest radiographs than controls.[47]

However, acquisition of MRSA does result in further segregation for infected patients. Since these patients spend a considerable amount of time in hospital they feel increasingly isolated and it is worth attempting to eradicate the organism. Nebulized vancomycin at a dose of 5 mg/kg three times daily made up with saline has been used as an adjunct to intravenous and oral therapy with some success (reference 48 and personal practice).

Aspergillus fumigatus

Aspergillus fumigatus is frequently found in the sputum of patients with CF. Despite an enormous number of publications debating whether it is a commensal related to repeated antibiotic treatment, an allergen causing allergic bronchopulmonary aspergillosis, an infecting organism[49] or all of these, uncertainty remains as to the best course of management. Transplant physicians prefer the fungus to be eliminated prior to transplantation. Nebulized amphotericin has been used on an individual basis to eliminate *Aspergillus fumigatus* from sputum.[50]

Burkholderia cepacia

Because of the multiple antibiotic resistance of the *Burkholderia cepacia* complex pathogens there is no evidence that nebulized antibiotics have a definitive role in management. Clearly, nebulized antibiotics can be used for concurrent chronic *P. aeruginosa* infection.

Unusual indications

It has been recognized recently that low doses of gentamicin will improve chloride channel impermeability (a CFTR function) in those patients with codon stop mutations.[51] A recent study showed improved chloride transport as evaluated by measuring changes in nasal potential difference after local application of gentamicin.[52]

Nebulized antibiotics for non-CF bronchiectasis

The incidence and prevalence of non-CF bronchiectasis is unknown. In a recent study no cause was identified in 53% of patients.[53] However, in the same study the following common causes were identified: post-infective (29%), an immune defect (8%), and allergic bronchopulmonary aspergillosis (7%). Unusual causes included primary ciliary dyskinesia (PCD), aspiration, Young's syndrome, rheumatoid arthritis, ulcerative colitis and panbronchiolitis. PCD is increasingly being identified in adults and children as the second most common inherited lung disease resulting in severe bronchiectasis and these patients need considerable clinical input.[54]

Non-CF bronchiectasis shows enormous variability in disease severity and progression. The spectrum of disease includes patients who may require hospitalization, regular intravenous antibiotics and daily physiotherapy, or be totally asymptomatic. The majority of these patients, unlike their CF counterparts, survive into the fifth and sixth decade of life. These patients (children and adults) are usually seen in a general respiratory clinic and do not receive the same level or intensity of care provided by a multidisciplinary CF team. However, slowly, some of the knowledge acquired from CF care is being applied to non-CF bronchiectasis. It is now appreciated that patients with bronchiectasis who are infected with *P. aeruginosa* have greater sputum production, worse lung function and an accelerated decline in pulmonary function.[55,56]

The heterogeneous nature of non-CF bronchiectasis is the main reason for limited guidelines regarding the use of nebulized drugs, in particular, nebulized antibiotics in non-CF bronchiectasis.[57]

Long-term oral antibiotics are prescribed for bronchiectatic patients infected with *S. aureus*, *Pneumococcus* and *Haemophilus* influenzae. However, nebulized and intravenous antibiotics are the optimum treatment for bronchiectactic patients chronically infected with *P. aeruginosa*. Although no controlled trials have been published, an eradication regimen for *P. aeruginosa* similar to that used for patients with CF should be instituted at time of first isolation. *P. aeruginosa* infecting non-CF bronchiectatic patients does not usually have the same virulence characteristics as the pathogen which infects patients with CF. CFTR functions normally in non-CF bronchiectasis and adherence of *P. aeruginosa* to bronchial mucosa may be less and consequently more easily eradicated with nebulized antibiotics.

A recent placebo-controlled, double-blind randomized study has evaluated the microbiological efficacy of TOBI 300 mg administered twice daily for 4 weeks to 74 non-CF bronchiectatic patients infected with *P. aeruginosa*.[58] The main outcome at week 6 was eradication of *P. aeruginosa* in 35% of the treated group. Additional positive findings were a reduction in *P. aeruginosa* density in the sputum compared to no change in the placebo group. Sixty-eight percent of the patients in the active group, compared to 35% in the placebo group, had an improved medical condition. On the downside, there was no improvement in pulmonary function and tobramycin resistance developed in 11% of the treated patients. An older study showed that inhaled gentamicin compared with placebo reduced airway neutrophil activity and mucus secretion in non-CF bronchiectasis.[59]

Safety of nebulized antibiotics

Antibiotic resistance

The two most commonly nebulized antibiotics are colistin and more recently TOBI. The early *P. aeruginosa* eradication trials have utilized colistin (usually with ciprofloxacin) and its therapeutic benefit has stood the test of time. Temporary or chronic resistance of *P. aeruginosa* to colistin is very unusual and partly explains its popular use in Europe and the UK. The trials of TOBI for patients with CF chronically infected with *P. aeruginosa* have shown considerable therapeutic benefit.[38,39] The extended trials have shown an increased resistance to TOBI. The maintained clinical benefit may be explained by the high levels of TOBI in the sputum. However, it is important to ensure that this increased resistance of *P. aeruginosa* to TOBI continues to be monitored longitudinally. Tobramycin is probably the most frequently used intravenous antibiotic in tandem with a beta-lactam and increased aminoglycoside resistance would pose a real threat to the efficacy of intravenous antibiotic therapy. Although high doses of nebulized antibiotics have greater sputum penetration it has been suggested that sublethal doses of antibiotics may also diminish the virulence and pathogenicity of *P. aeruginosa*.[60]

Bronchoconstriction

Studies have now unequivocally established that bronchoconstriction occurs with inhalation of antibiotics in both children and adults (Table 7.3). Various

Table 7.3 Bronchoconstriction (mean fall in FEV$_1$) and nebulized antibiotics.

Drug	% fall		Reference
Colistin	7.2–5.5		Dodd et al[63]
Colistin	5.9		Cunningham et al[61]
Tobramycin	3.5–5.6		Nikolaizik et al[64]
TOBI	Not significant		Ramsey et al[39]
TOBI	4		Nikolaizik et al[65]
	LR*	HR*	
Tobramycin	12	17	Alothman et al[66]
TOBI	4	16	

* Low risk and high risk of bronchospasm.
FEV$_1$, forced expiratory volume in one second.

mechanisms have been studied and suggested which include the tonicity, the pH, the preservative, the drug itself and the hyperreactivity of the patient's airways.

Bronchoconstriction occurs with nebulized colistin in both children[61] and adults[62] with CF and with solutions of different osmolalities.[63] Bronchoconstriction also occurs with the use of nebulized tobramycin but it is uncertain whether the bronchoconstriction is due to the preservative phenol, the antioxidant sodium metabisulfite or the higher osmolality of the solution.[64] In a recent study, bronchial reactions to different formulations of high-dose tobramycin were studied.[65] It was found that there was a similar fall in lung function immediately or 5 min after usage with all preparations including preservative (phenol)-free TOBI. A further study suggests that heightened airway reactivity in children with CF places them at risk of bronchospasm whatever the composition of the inhaled therapy.[66]

On the basis of these results it is recommended that before prescription every patient should be administered a hospital-supervised dose and spirometric tests performed before and after inhalation at intervals up to 30 min.[8] For the majority of patients maximum constriction occurs immediately after the challenge.[62] The test should be performed when the patient is clinically stable. Nebulized antibiotics are usually prescribed life-long and the repeated effect of long-term bronchoconstriction is unknown. If nebulized antibiotics are recommended to ensure improved disease control, it is important to protect against bronchoconstriction. In one study salbutamol was shown to be more effective than sodium cromogly-cate, possibly through its bronchodilator activity in addition to inhibition of mast cell degeneration.[67]

Patient allergy

Although severe allergy (anaphylaxis) is well recognized with the use of intravenous antibiotics this does not occur with inhaled antibiotics. Itchy cutaneous rashes on the arms and face are uncommon.

Ototoxicity and nephrotoxicity

There is no evidence of ototoxicity or nephrotoxicity from two large multi-center studies using inhaled antibiotics[38,39] although a smaller study of the use of long-term nebulized gentamicin found increased urinary N-acetyl-beta-D-glucosamidase activity had a positive correlation with cumulative doses of gentamicin posing a risk of renal toxicity.[68]

Pregnancy

Inhaled antibiotics should be prescribed with caution in pregnancy but based on the current available evidence are not contraindicated.

Environmental safety

Concern has been expressed that medical personnel are at risk from the pollution in the atmosphere by nebulized antibiotics. There are reports of staff experiencing bronchoconstriction and skin rashes. It has also been suggested that pollution of the hospital and home environment will lead to the establishment of resistant organisms, particularly in intensive care units where patients may receive nebulized antibiotics following transplantation. Although there is no evidence to support this, it is generally recommended that the nebulizer is fitted with a high efficiency breathing filter on the expiratory port to prevent any environ-mental contamination.[8]

Nebulized antibiotics: practical issues

Cross infection

Nebulizers may act as a source of bacterial contamination with both
B. cepacia and P. aeruginosa.[69] It is recommended that nebulizers are washed
and thoroughly dried after every use and compressors are not shared
between patients. As patients with CF grow older and aggressive antibiotic
therapy is maintained drug resistance is increasing and cross infection
which has long been recognized with B. cepacia is also occurring with
multiresistant P. aeruginosa.[70] It is advisable for patients to nebulize antibiotics in a separate area.[50]

Delivery

Effective therapy is determined by an efficient delivery system and patient
characteristics. The nebulizer compressor system, the characteristics of the
drug particle size, deposition pattern, dose and pharmacokinetics, the age
of the patient, degree of airways narrowing, breathing patterns and adherence to treatment are all factors which influence the efficacy of the therapy.
Drug delivery devices are continually being refined and innovations being
introduced to meet patient requirements and control for the varying factors.
Adaptive aerosol delivery delivers the drug during the first half of inspiration, matches the patient's breathing pattern, eliminates waste and provides
patient feedback to deliver the same dose with every treatment. A recent
study has shown that patients prefer this device to the conventional nebulizer compressor system, the quality of inhalation is superior and patients
are more compliant.[71] Currently, inhaled antibiotics can only be delivered
by the nebulized route, which is time consuming and burdensome for the
patients. A preliminary trial of an inhaler device to deliver colistin showed
increased coughing as an adverse effect.[72] Refinements to that mode of
delivery are being developed.

However, even with a variety of different nebulizer devices available, it
has been shown from measuring concentration in sputum, urine and distribution within the lung, that adequate therapeutic levels of drugs can be
achieved.[73–75]

Children versus adults

Although the clinical indications for introducing nebulized antibiotics will be
the same for infants, children and adults it is important not to extrapolate

Table 7.4 Factors influencing efficacy of nebulized antibiotics in children and adults.

Children	Adults
Less cooperative	Cooperative
More adherent	Less adherent
Smaller bronchial surface area	Large bronchial surface area
Large variability in lung deposition of nebulized drug	Less variability of lung deposition of nebulized drug
Low inspiratory flow rate	High inspiratory flow rate
Greater small airways penetration	Lesser small airways penetration (damaged)
More suitable for P. aeruginosa eradication	Majority chronically infected with P. aeruginosa

and apply the results of a study from one patient age group to another. It has been suggested that the aerosol dosage deposited in children is lower and with greater variability than in adults.[76] Younger patients have a reduced bronchial surface area but there may be greater penetration of drug into the small airways, inspiratory flow may be less in infants and children[77,78,79] and they may be less cooperative with treatment (Table 7.4). However, young children and adolescents are probably the main group to be targeted for introducing nebulized antibiotics at time of first infection with P. aeruginosa when airways are less damaged. By adulthood over 80% of patients are chronically infected with P. aeruginosa.

Increasing disease severity adversely influences lung deposition of nebulized antibiotic. Peripheral deposition is inversely correlated with FEV_1 due to mucous plugging and inflammation in the small airways.[79,80]

Conclusion

Nebulized antibiotics are very effective treatment for children and adults with CF who are infected with P. aeruginosa. In addition, they have the potential to improve quality of life and survival. There is considerable variation in usage of nebulized antibiotics between CF centers and it is an area of continuing research (Box 7.2).

Box 7.2 Further research potential: time of first acquisition of *Pseudomonas aeruginosa*.

Which is the best nebulized antibiotic?

What dosage to prescribe?

Which is the optimum eradication time?

How long should antibiotics be continued after eradication?

How to treat eradication failures?

Cost-benefit studies for nebulized antibiotics

References

1. Kerem E, Corey M, Gold R, Levison H. Pulmonary function and clinical course in patients with cystic fibrosis after pulmonary colonisation with *Pseudomonas aeruginosa*. *J Pediatr* 1990; **116**:714–19.

2. Kerem E, Reisman J, Corey M et al. Prediction of mortality in patients with cystic fibrosis. *New Engl J Med* 1992; **326**:1187–91.

3. Dodge JA, Morrison S, Lewis PA et al. Incidence population and survival of cystic fibrosis patients in the UK, 1968–95. *Arch Dis Child* 1997; **77**:493–6.

4. Cystic Fibrosis Foundation. Patient Registry 1999, Annual Report. Bethesda, MD: Cystic Fibrosis Foundation, 2000.

5. Mahadeva R, Webb AK, Westerbeek RC et al. Management in pediatric and adult cystic fibrosis centres improves clinical outcome; a cross sectional study. *BMJ* 1998; **316**:1771–5.

6. Bryson V, Sansome E, Laskines S. Aerosolisation of penicillin solutions. *Science* 1944; **100**:33–5.

7. Hodson M, Penketh ARL, Batten J. Aerosol carbenicillin and gentamicin treatment of *Pseudomonas aeruginosa* infection in patients with cystic fibrosis. *Lancet* 1981; **ii**:1137–9.

8. Webb AK, Dodd ME. Nebulised antibiotics for adults with cystic fibrosis. *Thorax* 1997; Supp 2:S69–S71.

9. Conway S. Evidence for using nebulised antibiotics in cystic fibrosis. *Arch Dis Child* 1999; **80**:307–9.

10. Saiman L. Consensus Conference. Use of aerosolised antibiotics in patients with cystic fibrosis. *Chest* 1999; **116**:775–87.

11. Pier GB, Grout M, Zaidi TS. Cystic fibrosis transmembrane conductance regulator is an epithelial cell receptor for clearance of *Pseudomonas aeruginosa* from the lung. *Proc Natl Acad Sci USA* 1997; **94**:12088–93.

12. Scheid P, Kempster L, Griesenbach U et al. Inflammation in cystic fibrosis airways: relationship to increased bacterial adherence. *Eur Respir J* 2001; **17**:27–35.

13. Stover CK, Pham XO, Erwin AL, Mizoguchi SD et al. Complete genome sequence of *Pseudomonas aeruginosa* PAO1, an opportunistic pathogen. *Nature* 2000; **406**:959–64.

14. Hancock RE. Resistance mechanisms in *Pseudomonas aeruginosa* and other nonfermentative gram negative bacteria. *Clin Infect Dis* 1998; **27**:S93–S99.

15. Davies DG, Chakrabarty AM, Geesey GG. Exopolysaccharide production in biofilms: substratum activation of alginate gene expression by *Pseudomonas aeruginosa*. *App Environ Microbiol* 1993; **59**:1181–6.

16. Kosorok MR, Zeng L, West SE et al. Acceleration of lung disease in children with cystic fibrosis after *Pseudomonas aeruginosa* acquisition. *Pediatr Pulmonol* 2001; **32**:277–87.

17. Pammucku A, Bush A, Buchdahl R. Effects of *Pseudomonas aeruginosa* colonisation on lung function and anthropometric variables in children with cystic fibrosis. *Pediatr Pulmonol* 1995; **19**:1–15.

18. Fitzsimmons S. The Cystic Fibrosis Foundation, Patient Registry Report 1996. *Pediatrics* 1997; **100**:11–19.

19. Quittner AL, Buu A. Effects of tobramycin solution for inhalation on Global Ratings of Quality of Life in patients with cystic fibrosis and *Pseudomonas aeruginosa* infection. *Pediatr Pulmonol* 2002; **3**:269–76.

20. Rosenfeld M, Gibson R, McNamara S et al. Serum and lower respiratory tract concentrations after tobramycin inhalation in young children with cystic fibrosis. *J Pediatr* 2001; **139**:572–7.

21. Mukhopadhyay S, Singh M, Cater JI et al. Nebulised antipseudomonal antibiotic therapy in cystic fibrosis: a meta-analysis of benefits and risks. *Thorax* 1996; **51**:364–8.

22. Dakin CJ, Numa AH, Wang H et al. Inflammation infection, and pulmonary function in infants and young children with cystic fibrosis. *Am J Respir Care Med* 2002; **165**:904–10.

23. Johansen HK, Hoiby N. Seasonal onset of initial colonisation and chronic infection with *Pseudomonas aeruginosa* in patients with cystic fibrosis in Denmark. *Thorax* 1992; **47**:109–11.

24. Littlewood JM, Miller MG, Ghonheim AT, Ramsden CH. Nebulised colomycin for early pseudomonas colonisation in cystic fibrosis. (Letter). *Lancet* 1985; **(i)**:865.

25. Valerius NH, Koch C, Hoiby N. Prevention of chronic *Pseudomonas aeruginosa* colonisation in cystic fibrosis by early treatment. *Lancet* 1991; **338**:725–6.

26. Vazquez C, Municio M, Corera M et al. Early treatment of *Pseudomonas aeruginosa* colonisation in cystic fibrosis. *Acta Pediatr* 1993; **82**:308–9.

27. Frederiksen B, Koch C, Hoiby N. Antibiotic treatment of initial colonisation with *Pseudomonas aeruginosa* postpones chronic infection and prevents deterioration of pulmonary function in cystic fibrosis. *Pediatr Pulmonol* 1997; **23**:330–5.

28. Wiesemann HG, Steinkamp G, Ratjen F et al. Placebo-controlled, double blind, randomised study of aerosolised tobramycin for early treatment of *Pseudomonas aeruginosa* colonisation in cystic fibrosis. *Pediatr Pulmonol* 1998; **25**:88–92.

29. Heinzl B, Eber E, Oberwaldner B, Haas G, Zach MS. Effects of inhaled gentamicin prophylaxis on acquisition of *Pseudomonas aeruginosa* in children with cystic fibrosis: a pilot study. *Pediatr Pulmonol* 2002; **33**:32–7.

30. Ratjen F, Doring G, Nikolaizik WH. Effect of inhaled tobramycin on early *Pseudomonas aeruginosa* colonisation in patients with cystic fibrosis. *Lancet* 2001; **358**:983–4.

31. Taccetti G, Repetto T, Procopio E et al. Early *Pseudomonas aeruginosa* colonisation in cystic fibrosis patients. *Lancet* 2001; **359**:625–6.

32. Taylor R, Hodson M. Cystic fibrosis: antibiotic prescribing practices in the United Kingdom. *Eur Respir Med J* 1993; **7**:535–40.

33. Nolan G, McIvor P, Levison H et al. Antibiotic prophylaxis in cystic fibrosis: inhaled cephaloridine as an adjunct to cloxacillin. *J Pediatr* 1982; **4**:626–30.

34. Kun P, Landau LI, Phelan PD. Nebulised gentamicin in children and adolescents with cystic fibrosis. *Aust Paediatr J* 1984; **20**:43–5.

35. Jensen T, Pedersen SS, Garnes S, Heilmann C et al. Colistin inhalation therapy in cystic fibrosis patients with chronic *Pseudomnas aeruginosa* lung infection. *J Antimicrob Chemother* 1987; **19**:831–8.

36. Stead RJ, Hodson ME, Batten JC. Inhaled ceftazidime compared with gentamicin and carbenicillin in older patients with cystic fibrosis infected with *Pseudomonas aeruginosa*. *Br J Dis Chest* 1987; **81**:272–9.

37. Macluskey IB, Gold R, Corey M, Levison H. Long-term effects of inhaled tobramycin in patients with cystic fibrosis colonised with *Pseudomonas aeruginosa*. *Pediatr Pulmonol* 1989; **7**:42–8.

38. Ramsey BW, Dorkin HL, Eisenberg JD et al. Efficacy of aerosolised tobramycin in patients with cystic fibrosis. *N Engl J Med* 1993; **328**:1740–6.

39. Ramsey BW, Pepe MS, Quan JM et al. Intermittent administration of inhaled tobramycin in patients with cystic fibrosis. *New Engl J Med* 1999; **340**:23–30.

40. Lamb HM, Goa KL. Management of patients with cystic fibrosis. Defining the role of inhaled tobramycin. *Dis Manage Health Outcomes* 1999; **6**:93–108.

41. Moss RB. Administration of aerosolized antibiotics in cystic fibrosis patients. *Chest* 2001; **120**:107S–113S.

42. Moss RB. Long-term benefits of inhaled tobramycin in adolescent patients with cystic fibrosis. *Chest* 2002; **121**:55–63.

43. Schaad UB, Wedgwood-Krucko J, Suter S et al. Efficacy of inhaled amikacin as adjunct to intravenous combination therapy (ceftazidime and amikacin) in cystic fibrosis. *J Pediatr* 1987; **111**:599–605.

44. Hodson M, Gallagher CG, Govan JRW. Randomised UK/Eire clinical trial of the efficacy and safety of tobramycin 300/5 ml nebuliser solution or nebulised colistin in CF patients. *Eur Respir J* 2002; **20**:658–64.

45. Madden BP, Kamalvand K, Chan CM et al. The medical management of patients with cystic fibrosis following heart-lung transplantation. *Eur Respir J* 1993; **6**:965–70.

46. Thomas SR, Gyi KM, Gaya H, Hodson ME. Methicillin-resistant *Staphylococcus aureus*: impact at a national cystic fibrosis centre. *J Hosp Infec* 1998; **40**:203–9.

47. Miall LS, McGinley NT, Brownlee KG, Conway SP. Methicillin resistant *Staphylococcus aureus* (MRSA) infection in cystic fibrosis. *Arch Dis Child* 2001; **84**:160–2.

48. Maiz L, Canton R, Mir N, Baquero F, Escobar H. Aerosolized vancomycin for the treatment of methicillin resistant *Staphylococcus aureus* infection in cystic fibrosis. *Pediatr Pulmonol* 1998; **26**:287–9.

49. Denning DW, Van Wye JE, Lewiston NJ, Stevens DA. Adjunctive therapy of allergic bronchopulmonary aspergillosis with itraconazole. *Chest* 1991; **100**:813–19.

50. Cystic Fibrosis Trust. Antibiotic treatment for cystic fibrosis. Bromley, Kent: Cystic Fibrosis Trust, 2002.

51. Howard M, Frizell RA, Bedwell DM. Aminoglycosides antibiotics restore CFTR function by overcoming premature stop mutations. *Nat Med* 1996; **2**:467–9.

52. Wilchanski M, Famini C, Blau A et al. A pilot study of the effect of gentamicin on nasal potential difference measurements in cystic fibrosis patients carrying stop mutations. *Am J Respir Crit Care Med* 2000; **161**:860–5.

53. Pasteur MC, Helliwell SM, Houghton SJ et al. An investigation into causative factors in patients with bronchiectasis. *Am J Respir Crit Care Med* 2000; **162**:1277–84.

54. Meeks M, Bush A. Primary ciliary dyskinesia: state of the art. *Pediatr Pulmonol* 2000; **29**:307–16.

55. Ho P, Chan K, Ip M et al. The effect of *Pseudomonas aeruginosa* infection on clinical parameters in steady-state bronchiectasis. *Chest* 1998; **114**:1594–8.

56. Evans S, Turner SM, Bosch BJ, Hardy CC, Woodhead MA. Lung function in bronchiectasis: the influence of *Pseudomonas aeruginosa*. *Eur Respir J* 1996; **9**:1601–4.

57. Currie DC. Nebulisers for bronchiectasis. *Thorax* 1997; **52**:S72–S74.

58. Barker A, Couch L, Fiel S et al. Tobramycin solution for inhalation reduces sputum *Pseudomonas aeruginosa* density in bronchiectasis. *Am J Respir Crit Care Med* 2000; **162**:481–5.

59. Lin H-C, Chenh H-F, Wang C-H et al. Inhaled gentamicin reduces airway neutrophil activity and mucus secretion in bronchiectasis. *Am J Respir Crit Care Med* 1997; **155**:2024–9.

60. Geers TJ, Cooke RE. The effect of sublethal levels of antibiotics on the pathogenicity of *Pseudomonas aeruginosa* from tracheal tissue. *J Antimicrob Chem* 1987; **19**:569–78.

61. Cunningham S, Prasad A, Collyer L et al. Bronchoconstriction following nebulised colistin in cystic fibrosis. *Arch Dis Child* 2000; **84**:432–3.

62. Maddison J, Dodd M, Webb AK. Nebulised colistin causes chest tightness in adults with cystic fibrosis. *Respir Med* 1994; **88**:145–7.

63. Dodd ME, Maddison J, Abbott J, Webb AK. The effect of tonicity of nebulised colistin on chest tightness and lung function in adults with cystic fibrosis. *Thorax* 1997; **52**:656–8.

64. Nikolaizik WH, Jenni- Galovic S, Schoni M. Bronchial constriction after nebulised tobramycin preparations and saline in patients with cystic fibrosis. *Eur J Pediatr* 1995; **155**:608–11.

65. Nikolaizik WH, Trociewicz K, Ratjen F. Bronchial reactions to the inhalation of high dose tobramycin in cystic fibrosis. *Eur Respir J* 2002; **20**:122–6.

66. Alothman GA, Alsadi MM, Ho BL et al. Evaluation of bronchial constriction in children with cystic fibrosis after inhaling two different preparations of tobramycin. *Chest* 2002; **122**:930–4.

67. Chua HL, Walker SL, LeSouef PN, Sly PD. Comparison of efficacy of salbutamol and sodium cromoglygate in the prevention of ticarcillin-induced bronchoconstriction. *Pediatr Pulmonol* 1993; **16**:311–15.

68. Ring E, Eber E, Erwa W, Zach MS. Urinary N-acetyl-beta-D-glucosaminidase activity in patients with cystic fibrosis on long term gentamicin inhalation. *Arch Dis Child* 1998; **78**:540–3.

69. Hutchinson GR, Parker S, Pryor JA et al. Home-nebulizers: a potential primary source of *Burkholderia cepacia* and other colistin-resistant, gram-negative bacteria in patients with cystic fibrosis. *J Clin Microbiol* 1996; **34**:584–7.

70. Jones AM, Govan JR, Doherty C et al. Spread of a multiresistant strain of *Pseudomonas aeruginosa* in adult cystic fibrosis clinic. *Lancet* 2001; **358**:557–8.

135

71. Marsden RJ, Conway SP, Dodd ME. A multi-centre, randomised study comparing the Halolite adaptive aerosol delivery (AAD) system with a high output nebuliser system in patients with cystic fibrosis. *Pediatr Pulmonol* 2002; Suppl 24:A414.

72. LeBrunn PPH, deBoer AH, Frijlink HW, Heijerman HGM. Inhalation of colistin dry powder. Design and evaluation of a new dosage form. Proceedings of 24th European CF Conference, Vienna, 2001:S2.3.

73. Eisenberg J, Pepe M, Williams-Warren J et al. A comparison of peak sputum tobramycin concentration in patients with cystic fibrosis using jet and ultrasonic nebuliser systems. *Chest* 1997; **111**:955–62.

74. Dequin PF, Faurisson F, Lemarie E et al. Urinary excretion reflects lung deposition of aminogycoside aerosols in cystic fibrosis. *Eur Respir J* 2001; **18**:316–22.

75. Le Conte P, Potel G, Peltier P et al. Lung distribution and pharmacokinetics of aerosolised tobramycin. *Am Rev Respir Dis* 1993; **147**:1279–82.

76. Everard ML. Aerosol delivery in infants and young children. *J Aerosol Med* 1996; **9**:71–7.

77. Mallol J, Rattray S, Walker G et al. Aerosol deposition in infants with cystic fibrosis. *Pediatr Pulmonol* 1996; **21**:276–81.

78. Alderson PO, Secker-Walker RH, Strominger DB et al. Pulmonary deposition of aerosols in children with cystic fibrosis. *J Pediatr* 1974; **84**:479–84.

79. Chua HL, Collis GG, Newbury AM et al. The influence of age on aerosol deposition in children with cystic fibrosis. *Eur Respir J* 1994; **7**:2185–91.

80. Mukhopadhyay S, Staddon GE, Eastman C et al. The quantitative distribution of nebulised antibiotic in the lung in cystic fibrosis. *Respir Med* 1994; **88**:203–11.

8. Nebulizers in Cystic Fibrosis and non-CF Bronchiectasis in Children and Adults: Therapies other than Antibiotics

Andrew Bush, Ranjan Suri and A Kevin Webb

Introduction

Patients with cystic fibrosis (CF) and bronchiectasis have to perform daily time-consuming therapies such as chest physiotherapy, and often follow an exercise program. Thus the additional burden of nebulized therapy should only be imposed if:

1. The patient really needs that additional therapy and benefits from it.
2. The therapy can only be given by the nebulized route, and not, for example, with inhalers or dry powder devices.

Patients frequently mix medications in the same nebulizer, to cut down on the time of treatment. This may be deleterious, because interactions may inactivate both components of the mixture, or have unknown effects on the aerosol properties.[1] It is vital to give careful instructions as to what can and cannot be mixed. Furthermore, single dose nebulizers are frequently re-used.[1] The effect of this practice on nebulizer performance has been assessed in two studies.[1,2] When properly maintained, there is no deterioration in performance, but unwashed units containing tobramycin had impaired performance after 40 runs (evidence level 2b).[2]

Drug deposition is reduced by any cause of airway obstruction including CF;[3] it may be possible to influence deposition favorably by imposing low inspiratory flows, altering posture or adding an expiratory resistance during treatment. One in vivo study comparing standard nebulization with a pressure support device demonstrated that the pressure support device improved total lung aerosol deposition without increasing particle impaction in the

137

airways.[4] When considering the relevance of published data to individual patients, it should be remembered that it may not be appropriate to use different nebulizers interchangeably,[5–7] although, in fact, differences between nebulizers demonstrated in the laboratory may not translate into clinically relevant effects.[7] It is also wrong to extrapolate results between groups of patients with different degrees of airway obstruction or patients of different ages.[8,9] (Evidence level 2b.) In one study,[9] 12 infants were compared with eight older children. When inhaling by the nasal route, infant lung deposition of an aerosol was lower in sleeping infants (median 1.3%, range 0.3–1.6%) compared with the older children (median 2.7%, range 1.6–6.4%). Note how small the percentage of the total dose was deposited in the airway in either age group even in the context of a clinical trial; how much less is deposited in real life can only be a subject of speculation. This is particularly relevant to the use of recombinant human deoxyribonuclease (rhDNase) in infants (see below). In the older children there was no difference between orally and nasally inspired drug deposition; obviously this could not be determined in the obligate nose breathing infant.

Even at best, currently available nebulizers must be considered to be inefficient devices in CF.[10,11] In general, beta-2-agonists (if indicated, see below) are given before physiotherapy, and all other nebulized medications after airway clearance, to try to ensure maximal access to the inflamed airway.

Infection control is a major issue in CF, and concerns have been expressed that improperly maintained nebulizers may actually act as a constant source of reinfection. In one study, *Burkholderia cepacia* was isolated from three of 35 home nebulizers;[12] only one of the three patients had one of the two strains present in the nebulizer also present in the sputum. Four of 35 nebulizers were contaminated with *Stenotrophomonas maltophilia*. None of the 34 patients with *Pseudomonas aeruginosa* in their sputum had this organism isolated from the nebulizer. Sixty-nine percent of the nebulizers were contaminated, and up to 16 environmental, colomycin-resistant strains were found. The major site of contamination was beneath the chamber atomizer. Those who on questionnaire were identified as following recommended practices for good nebulizer hygiene, in particularly drying the equipment properly, had minimal or no contamination. Another study reported the isolation of *Staphylococcus aureus* from 55% of returned nebulizers, and *P. aeruginosa* from 35%.[1] The clinical significance of these findings is unknown, but it probably underscores the need to give repeated instruction in nebulizer hygiene, and the undesirability of sharing nebulizers between patients with CF.

This chapter will also cover such studies as there are in non-CF bronchiectasis; due to the paucity of clinical trials in this field, there will be no separate section on this topic; references pertain to CF unless otherwise stated. Nebulized antibiotics are covered in Chapter 7.

Mucolytics

Hypertonic saline

Sputum induction with hypertonic saline is a well established clinical and research procedure. There have been several short-term studies looking at safety and efficacy in CF. In a dose finding study, mucociliary clearance (MCC) was measured using a radioaerosol/gamma camera technique in 10 patients with CF.[13] There was a stepwise increase in MCC up to 6% hypertonic saline, with no further improvement with 12%. However, the salty taste of 12% hypertonic saline was unacceptable to some patients. In a comparative study, 6% hypertonic saline was equally efficacious as mannitol in improving MCC, but both resulted in bronchoconstriction (fall in forced expiratory volume in one second (FEV_1) with hypertonic saline $5.8 \pm 1.2\%$, mannitol $7.3 + 1.2\%$).[14] Addition of amiloride to the hypertonic saline did not improve MCC.[15] In a systematic study of 23 CF patients,[16] 10% hypertonic saline result was shown to cause bronchoconstriction, but in 15 subjects there was also subsequent bronchodilation, similar to the paradoxical bronchodilation seen after exercise in some patients with CF.[17] Efficacy studies of hypertonic saline have focused on changes in lung function and changes in the weight of expectorated sputum. However, sputum induction and enhanced sputum clearance may not be the same procedure. A short-term study has demonstrated increases in pulmonary function with hypertonic saline similar to those obtained with rhDNase in Phase II studies.[18–20] FEV_1 increased by $15 \pm 16\%$ from the baseline after 2 weeks, compared with $2.8 \pm 13\%$ using normal saline, $p <0.02$. The wide scatter emphasizes that there are important individual differences in response with this as with other treatments in CF. Another short-term study demonstrated an increased weight of sputum expectorated with 6% compared with 0.9% (normal) saline, with patients preferring the 6% solution;[21] no changes in lung function were shown. The longest and largest trial of 7% hypertonic

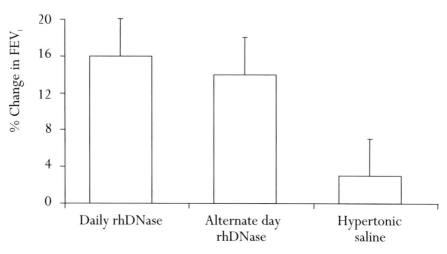

Figure 8.1 *Percentage change in FEV₁ following 12 weeks treatment. There was no significant difference between the responses for daily and alternate day rhDNase, both of which significantly improved lung function compared with baseline, but hypertonic saline resulted in no improvement in lung function over a 12-week period. FEV₁, forced expiratory volume in one second. (Adapted from Suri R et al. Lancet 2001; 358:1316–21[22] with permission from Elsevier.)*

saline, in which 48 children were randomly allocated in a crossover design to either 7% hypertonic saline, daily rhDNase or alternate day rhDNase for 12 weeks, showed that for the group, there was no significant change over baseline hypertonic saline (change in FEV₁ 3 ± SD 21%) when was administered by a jet nebulizer twice daily (Figure 8.1).[22] The study was powered to have a more than 90% chance of detecting a change of 100 ml in FEV₁ significant at the 5% level. Looking at individual patients, 35% did have an improvement in FEV₁ of at least 10% with hypertonic saline, including some children who did not improve with rhDNase (Figure 8.2).[22,23] It is possible that the use of an ultrasonic nebulizer might have resulted in greater improvements in lung function, but the widespread use of these devices on a domiciliary basis is unlikely to be practical due to cost; furthermore, since the data on other CF medications are mainly of only using jet nebulizers, it would mean the expense of providing two different devices to the patient, and the investment of time to clean and dry two devices. In terms of safety, in this trial, patients already taking short acting beta-2-agonists were allowed to take them prior to nebulizing hypertonic saline, and only three were

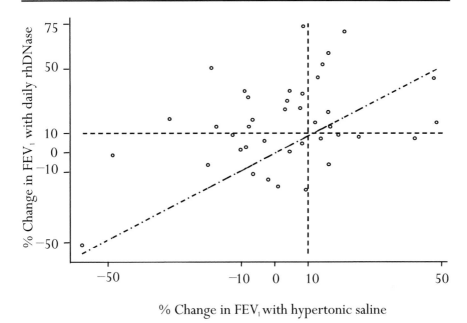

Figure 8.2 *Individual patients' responses to daily rhDNase and hypertonic saline. Each point represents a single patient. There are marked individual differences in response both to rhDNase and hypertonic saline. FEV₁, forced expiratory volume in one second. (Data from Suri R et al. Lancet 2001; 358:1316–21[22] with permission from Elsevier and Suri R. MD Thesis, University of Manchester.[23])*

unable to use the medication.[24] Benefit at 6 weeks was less than at 12 weeks, so a 12-week trial on an individual basis was recommended (Figure 8.3). There is an Australian trial of hypertonic saline which has yet to report (personal communication); the results will certainly be interesting in the further evaluation of the role of this medication. A much smaller short-term study concluded that efficacy for 5.85% hypertonic saline and rhDNase was similar,[25] but examination of the individual data reveals that there was marked individual differences in response, as found by ourselves (see above), with some responding better to rhDNase, and some to hypertonic saline.

In addition to the effects on airway reactivity, concerns about the effects of hypertonic saline on airway defenses and its possible proinflammatory potential have been raised. Although the tonicity of CF airway surface liquid is a matter of ongoing controversy, it is clear that there are a number of salt-sensitive peptides (beta-defensins, other cationic peptides and components of the innate airway mucosal defense systems[26]) whose antibacterial properties might be impaired by rendering the epithelial lining fluid hypernatremic.[26,27]

(a)

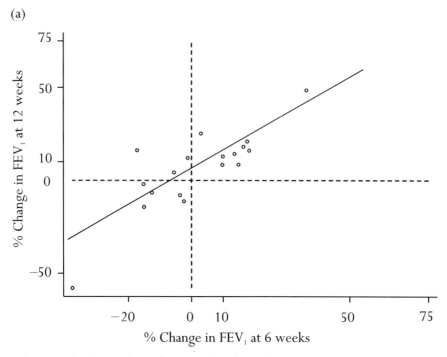

Figure 8.3 *(a) Correlation between 6-week and 12-week FEV₁ responses to hypertonic saline (p <0.001). Note that although response at 6 weeks is strongly predictive of response at 12 weeks, there are individuals who took 12 weeks to respond.*

Although conceivably this may be a factor in very young children with no lower airway bacterial infection (and no study has evaluated this), it seems unlikely to be important in older children and adults with established neutrophilic airway inflammation. Repetitive induction of sputum with hypertonic saline has been reported to cause increased airway neutrophilia,[28,29] which is intrinsically undesirable in CF; however, in the large hypertonic saline study reported above,[22] hypertonic saline did not result in any short- or long-term increase in sputum interleukin (IL)-8, myeloperoxidase or neutrophil elastase, and no change in sputum culture results. Furthermore, there were no correlations between changes in lung function and changes in inflammatory markers.[30] This suggests that there is no clinically significant proinflammatory effect of hypertonic saline over at least a 12-week period.

We conclude that the use of hypertonic saline as an adjunct to physiotherapy should be evaluated on an individual basis (level 1b). It is probable that patients who respond to both will prefer to use rhDNase because of the

(b)

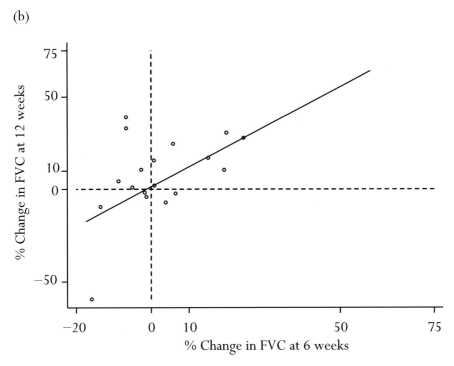

Figure 8.3 (Continued) *(b) Correlation between 6-week and 12-week FVC responses to hypertonic saline (p = 0.02). Note that although response at 6 weeks is strongly predictive of response at 12 weeks, there are individuals who took 12 weeks to respond. FEV_1, forced expiratory volume in one second; FVC, forced vital capacity. (Data from Suri R. MD Thesis, University of Manchester.[23])*

short nebulization time, but rhDNase therapeutic failures should certainly be considered for a trial of hypertonic saline.

RhDNase

Studies in older children and adults

The largest randomized controlled clinical trial ever performed in CF demonstrated improvement in lung function and reduction in infective exacerbations sustained over 6 months in patients with moderately severe CF.[31] For the rhDNase-treated group, mean improvement in FEV_1 was just under 7%; one third had an improvement of more than 10%. The reduction in antibiotic use was statistically significant but clinically trivial (<2 days in 6 months). This trial and a retrospective audit[32] demonstrated marked individual variation in response, with some individuals showing no benefit or even harmful effects. Benefit was also seen in two trials of severely ill

143

patients with CF.[33,34] The long-term benefits are controversial; open studies have demonstrated sustained benefits out to 22 months.[35] There have been concerns that rhDNase may mask underlying deterioration, and be merely a cosmetic therapy – these concerns have arisen as a result of the apparent deterioration below baseline on stopping treatment after 22 months. The usual dose is 2.5 mg once daily; anecdotally, some patients may benefit from higher doses. As yet, no effect on mortality has been demonstrated, partly due to the current flat survival curves.[36,37] The possible effects of rhDNase on sputum inflammatory markers will be discussed below. RhDNase is expensive, but a trial is justified in individual CF patients who meet the following criteria (level 1b):

- age 5 years and over
- fixed airflow obstruction, with spirometry below the normal range
- chronic sputum production
- adherent to conventional treatment
- ready and willing to take on an additional treatment burden.

Detailed protocols for $n = 1$ trials for rhDNase have been devised.[38] Obviously it is vital not to confuse spontaneous fluctuations in disease severity with treatment effects. The most rigorous protocol involves three periods of 4 weeks each. Each of these periods involves 2 weeks of rhDNase and 2 weeks of saline, with measurement of exercise, oximetry and spirometry. FEV_1 was the best discriminator: half the group studied showed a beneficial response to rhDNase. Although this is a demanding protocol, it is statistically rigorous. It could be criticized for being unblended, but in practice it is very difficult in real life to find a true matched placebo. Although it would seem from the plateau of lung function after 10–14 days which was reported in the Phase II studies to assume that a 2-week trial is adequate, data validating this are sparse. In two separate studies, we have shown that 6-week response is strongly predictive of 12-week response (Figure 8.4),[23] and 12-week is strongly predictive of 9-month response (Figure 8.5).[10] Note that in one of the studies in severely ill CF patients, responses took 3 months to reach a peak.[33] Studies have assessed the use of different nebulizers for rhDNase. Shah et al compared the Hudson Nebulizer (Hudson, Irvine, CA, USA) and Pulmo-Aide compressor (Devilbiss, Somerset, Philadelphia, PA, USA) to the Sidestream nebulizer driven by the CR-50 compressor (both Profile Respiratory Systems, Sussex, UK).[39] The Sidestream/CR-50 combination was quicker and more efficient in vitro, but

(a)

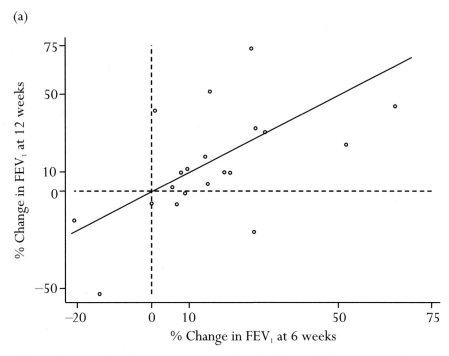

Figure 8.4 *(a) Correlation between 6-week and 12-week FEV_1 responses to daily rhDNase ($p = 0.008$). Note that the response at 6 weeks is strongly predictive of response at 12 weeks, and there are no individuals who took 12 weeks to respond.*

this was less significant in vivo. The authors point out that clinically there is little to choose between the systems. A similar conclusion was reached by Fiel et al in a three-way comparison between the Marquest Acorn 11 (Marquest Medical Inc, Eaglewood, CO, USA) and the Hudson T Up-draft (Hudson, Irvine, CA, USA) driven by the DeVilbiss Pulmo-Aide compressor, and the Pari LC Jet Plus nebulizer with the Pari inhaler boy compressor (Pari-Werk, Starnberg, Germany).[40] Geller et al studied patients with early lung disease, using the Medic-Aid Durable Sidestream nebulizer powered by the MobilAire Compressor with the Hudson T Up-draft driven by the DeVilbiss Pulmo-Aide compressor.[41] The Medic-Aid system tended to produce greater improvement in lung function, but all changes were small in this very well group of patients, and any significance of these findings is likely to be minimal.[36] Overall, it would seem that most properly maintained jet nebulizers and compressors can be used interchangeably for rhDNase therapy. Age is another factor: Diot et al found that there was greater lung deposition in older people with more severe lung disease.[8]

(b)

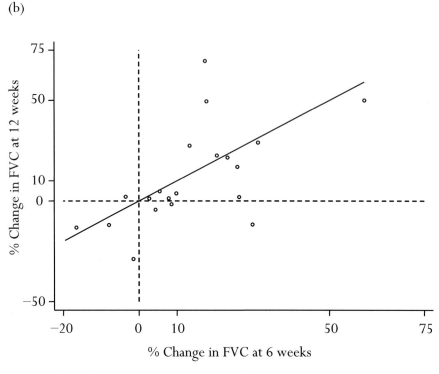

Figure 8.4 (Continued) *(b) Correlation between 6-week and 12-week FVC responses to daily rhDNase (p = 0.005). Note that the response at 6 weeks is strongly predictive of response at 12 weeks, and there are no individuals who took 12 weeks to respond. FEV$_1$, forced expiratory volume in one second; FVC, forced vital capacity. (Data from Suri R. MD Thesis, University of Manchester.[23])*

Although there was an inverse correlation ($r = -0.61$, $p = 0.015$) between lung deposition and FEV$_1$, there was no correlation between clinical response and lung deposition.

Other important practical aspects of therapy include not mixing rhDNase with any other medication (level 2b); having at least a 30-min rest (preferably up to 2 hours) between rhDNase and the next session of physiotherapy or any other nebulized treatment (level 4).[42] Patients vary in how best they fit the timing into their schedule; commonly it is administered as soon as the patient has come home from school or work. The use of short course rhDNase as an adjunct to intravenous antibiotics for a pulmonary exacerbation conveys no additional benefit (level 1b).[43] RhDNase does not appear to be effective in most cases of non-CF bronchiectasis (level 1b).[44]

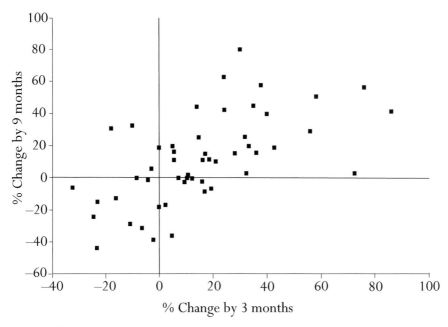

Figure 8.5 *Correlation between 12-week and 9-month FEV$_1$ responses to daily rhDNase (n = 51, p <0.001). Note that the response at 12 weeks is strongly predictive of response at 1 year, and there are no individuals who took 12 weeks to respond. FEV$_1$, forced expiratory volume in one second. (Data from Davies J.* Pediatr Pulmonol *1997; 23:243–8.[32])*

Comparison of rhDNase with hypertonic saline

A recent study compared daily rhDNase with alternate day rhDNase and 7% saline[22] (the hypertonic saline data are discussed above). Both treatments improved lung function compared with baseline (see Figure 8.1) (increase in FEV$_1$ 16% (SD 25%) daily rhDNase vs 14% (SD 22%) alternate day). There was no significant difference between daily and alternate day rhDNase treatment (2% FEV$_1$ 95% confidence intervals –4–9%). The study was inadequately powered to assess cost saving, but there was a trend for overall cost of treatment to be less in the alternate day limb of the study.[45]

A safety issue with regard to rhDNase therapy is the possible risk of increase in free inflammatory markers in the airway lumen. DNA is a strongly cationic compound, and binds chemokines, immobilizing them and thus making them inactive in sputum.[46] There have been concerns that breaking down DNA may result in the release of neutrophil chemoattractants such as free and total IL-8, with consequent worsening of airway inflammation.[46,47] An initial report was reassuring,[48] although it was difficult

147

to assess the evidence in detail from the information provided. An in vitro study documented the increased release of free IL-8 (the likely active compound) when bovine DNase was mixed with CF sputum.[47] In another relatively short-term study although no change in IL-8 was shown, sputum human neutrophil elastase and human leukocyte cathepsin G did increase, reverting to baseline when rhDNase was stopped.[49] The clinical relevance of this observation could not be shown. However, in the rhDNase: hypertonic saline study reported above,[22] there was no change over baseline for free and total IL-8, neutrophil elastrase or myeloperoxide with 12 weeks of treatment with daily or alternate day rhDNase.[30] There was no correlation between the changes in any of the inflammatory markers and changes in lung function. This study probably gives the most reassuring evidence to date of an absence of a clinically important in vivo proinflammatory effect of rhDNase.

From the above, it is clear that rhDNase has become an established treatment in patients with both moderate[31] and severe[33,34] CF lung disease. There are clearly marked and unpredictable individual differences in response, with only some patients gaining benefit,[32,50] and some actually getting worse,[32] despite feeling better (level 1b).

RhDNase in early CF lung disease
The above data have led to the study of rhDNase in early stage CF lung disease, and in very young children who would not conventionally be prescribed this medication. It is well known that there is evidence of inflammation and increase in DNA in lavage fluid in so-called early lung disease[51–53] and recent research has shown that lung function is impaired very early, even in a group of babies which appear to be free of any respiratory disease.[54] The theoretical basis is sound; as always the issues are safety and efficacy. The monitoring of efficacy in patients with mild or no clinically apparent CF lung disease is not straightforward. In patients with moderate or severe CF lung disease, lung function improvements have been well documented.[31,33,34] The issues in children and well patients have been reviewed recently.[36] Mortality is the endpoint which most concerns patients' families at diagnosis[55] but current survival curves are too flat[37] to make this a useful endpoint; a study to show a change would need to last decades, with thousands of children enrolled. The most common surrogate is lung function, in particular, FEV_1. Even in advanced disease, lung function is only as accurate as tossing a coin to determine mortality.[56] In young children, a significant change in FEV_1 is 190 ml or 8% of baseline,[57] a change unlikely to be

148

achieved in young children in a study of rhDNase in early stage lung disease. The use of flow at low lung volumes is even more fraught with difficulty; variability may be as much as 20–30%.[58] Although there are data documenting improvements in the short term in these parameters,[41] the long-term clinical significance of these changes is difficult to assess.[36] The use of infective exacerbations as an endpoint is dogged by difficulties in definition.[59]

The safety record of rhDNase in older children and adults is impressive, even in the very sick.[33,34] What is unknown in infants and young children is the potential effect on in particular alveolar development (the first 2 years of life in particular). CF infants and young children are in the main well, with the likelihood of many years of life ahead of them, and therefore have much more to lose than adults with severe lung disease, in whom the intense infection and inflammation are far more likely to wreak severe damage than any medication. We know that medications such as triamcinolone have the potential in animals to impair secondary septation and alveolar development,[60,61] and it would be wrong to assume that other agents do not have the potential to damage the growing lung. The risk–benefit balance, in a really well child, may be tilted unacceptably to the risk end.

Among early clinical work was a bronchoscopic study in which 65 infants aged 3 months to 5 years, and 33 children between the ages of 5 and 10 years were enrolled.[62] They all had a single nebulized dose of rhDNase and then underwent bronchoalveolar lavage. There was huge variation in lavage DNase activity, unrelated to patient age, weight or height, or whether the patient used a mask or a mouthpiece. This highlights the difficulty in getting consistent and adequate drug deposition in well young children, which were discussed above.[8,10] These children then went on to have 2 weeks of rhDNase treatment, without adverse effects. This was a short-term study, albeit an important one. There are clearly major problems in this sort of trial work in very young children.

However, the recent publication of an impressive clinical trial has challenged us to consider the use of nebulized rhDNase in early disease.[63] The trial is by any standards a highly impressive piece of work. It was a 2-year study, which was completed by 410 children, and showed reduced time to first exacerbation (but did not comment on total exacerbations; it is unclear if these were reduced) and maintained lung function in the treatment group, compared with placebo.[63] (Treatment benefit for FEV_1 3.2 + 1.2%, $p = 0.006$; for forced vital capacity (FVC) $0.7 \pm 1.0\%$, p = not significant.) Criticisms of what is by any standards a herculean task may seem churlish, but the following points must be considered.[64] First, it is unclear that all the children were truly early

149

stage, in that more than one third had digital clubbing, and calculation from their own data show that some would have had an FEV_1 as low as 66%, FVC as low as 79% and a Brasfield score as low as 18, assuming their group statistics are normally distributed and correctly calculated. Using the same calculations and the same assumptions, some children would not have met the entry criteria (FVC >85%). It is unclear why there was an early and non-sustained peak in lung function in the rhDNase group. Second, some minor technical points include the use of 1983 normal ranges for lung function, when there are more modern data;[65] the study, as the authors state, was underpowered to detect a rate of change in lung function. The lack of individual data, or an attempt to correlate response with initial lung function, is a weakness; if all those with FEV_1 <80% responded, and those with better lung function did not, this tells us little more than previous studies.[31,33,34] Finally, unpublished follow-up data from the large Phase III study showed that when the placebo patients received active medication (after a delay of 6 months necessitated by the trial), their response in terms of both lung function and infective exacerbation was as least as good as the trial patients.[31] This implies the delay did not prejudice their response, and is an argument against an imperative for early treatment.

A novel approach to the problem of endpoints in this age group is the use of high resolution computerized tomography (CT) scanning, with modern techniques to reduce radiation exposure. Pathological changes on CT scanning have been shown to correlate with lung function, although disappointingly, not with sputum inflammatory markers.[66] In a study of 12 children with CF aged less than 5 years, high resolution CT was performed before and after 100 days therapy with rhDNase or placebo.[67] High resolution CT but not chest radiograph scores improved significantly (-1.0 ± 0.53 vs 0.58 ± 0.24, $p = 0.02$) in the rhDNase group compared with placebo.[67] This exciting study suggests that at least early structural changes may be partially reversed by rhDNase. There are important ethical implications inherent in the widespread use of high resolution CT in CF children who have a good long-term prognosis, and the study was of course too small to be the basis of any general recommendations. Nonetheless, the results are potentially extremely interesting.

Overall, based on the current evidence, rhDNase cannot be recommended for all CF infants at the time of diagnosis. The data would certainly support its use on an $n = 1$ trial basis in young children who are doing badly. Monitoring of response in the individual is essential, but difficult in practice, and the best means is not clear. We need better ways to detect deterioration, and monitor therapeutic response early, so that subgroups who are

150

doing badly can be targeted early. Finally, given the equivalence of daily and alternate day rhDNase, future studies in early stage disease should probably employ the latter strategy.

There have been anecdotal reports of the use of nebulized rhDNase in other, non-CF lung disease, including airway mucus impaction causing acute[68] and chronic[69] atelectasis, primary ciliary dyskinesia,[70,71] premature neonates,[72] and severe bronchiolitis.[73] Treatment under these circumstances should be considered to be experimental, but worth attempting if conventional treatment is failing (level 4).

In conclusion, rhDNase is an effective mucolytic in half to two thirds of CF patients. There is compelling evidence that it need only be given on alternate days. It should not be administered to people with early stage disease, particularly young children, outside the context of a controlled trial.

Other mucolytics

We found no evidence in the published literature to support the use of any other agent as a mucolytic in CF or bronchiectasis. There have been three trials of N-acetylcysteine as a mucolytic,[74–76] none of which have shown any benefit. A recent systematic review confirmed the lack of benefit for either nebulized or oral N-acetylcysteine.[77] The continued popularity of this medication remains a source of wonder. The possibility that there may be particular individuals who benefit from other mucolytics cannot be excluded from published data, and careful $n = 1$ trials may occasionally be warranted. N-acetylcysteine cannot be recommended generally as a treatment for CF lung disease (level 1a).

There is interest in using Nacystelyn, a salt derivative of N-acety cysteine, administered via a metered dose inhaler (MDI) and spacer as a mucolytic.[78] In a pilot acute study, there was evidence of improved rheological characteristics of mucus, but no change in lung function with this medication. There was some wheezing with the higher doses. More data are needed before its place (if any) in therapy can be assessed.

Summary

The only two nebulized mucolytics for which any proof of efficacy are available are rhDNase and hypertonic saline. It is clear that there is marked and unpredictable response to both. It is recommended that patients with CF are evaluated individually and sequentially for response, using FEV_1 as the endpoint. There is still a need for new, and also more effective mucolytics, because some patients respond neither to rhDNase nor hypertonic saline. It may be that inhaled mannitol will fulfill that role, although trials to assess it have yet to be conducted.

Bronchodilators

Bronchial hyperreactivity is common in CF, but is variable between patients and over time with the same patient. Bronchodilators (either beta-2-agonists or anticholinergics) may be given before nebulized antibiotics (above) or particularly in patients with prominent wheeze. Trials of bronchodilators by any route should be monitored with pulmonary function measurements, since paradoxical bronchoconstriction has been described (level 2b).[79] In CF and primary ciliary dyskinesia, exercise may improve airway obstruction more than bronchodilators,[17,80] and may be a preferable strategy (level 2a) not least for the potential favorable effects on CF bone disease (level 1b).[81,82] Since there is good evidence in the context of asthma (level 1a)[83] that for all but the severest attacks of wheezing, inhaled beta-2-agonist via an MDI and spacer is at least as effective as the same drug given by nebulizer provided comparable doses are used,[84,85] nebulized beta-2-agonist is rarely indicated for most CF patients, except possibly at the time of acute chest exacerbations. There is little evidence of long-term efficacy of bronchodilators in CF;[86] however, some patients will wish to use nebulized rather than inhaled bronchodilators for the possible effect of humidified inspirate on airway secretions (level 4).

In acute infective CF exacerbations, there is evidence that intravenous bronchodilator may be more efficacious than nebulized (level 1b)[87] Twenty-three adult patients received either intravenous or nebulized terbutaline. The intravenous group improved more rapidly, and, on day 10, FEV_1 and FVC were similar to best values during the previous year, whereas in the nebulized group, there were still decrements in these parameters.

A study of bronchodilator responsiveness in 24 patients with bronchiectasis demonstrated that nearly half responded to one or both of fenoterol and ipratropium bromide.[88] There was a non-significant trend for nebulized ipratropium, but not fenoterol, to give better bronchodilatation than the same medication via an MDI and spacer. It is unclear from the paper whether this merely reflects a dose effect. We recommend that a trial of nebulized bronchodilators is warranted in non-CF bronchiectasis (level 2b).

Steroids and chromones

Evidence from a randomized controlled clinical trial has shown improved pulmonary function in CF patients infected with *P. aeruginosa* treated with oral prednisolone in doses of both 1 mg/kg and 2 mg/kg, given on alternate days, but at the cost of unacceptable side effects (level 1b).[89] Attempts to obtain the benefits of inhaled steroids without the adverse effects have produced variable results,[90,91] and there is an ongoing trial in the United Kingdom looking at inhaled steroid withdrawal in CF (CF WISE study). There are no trials of nebulized steroids in CF or bronchiectasis, and they cannot be recommended for routine use. By analogy with studies in severe asthma,[92] a trial of nebulized budesonide may rarely be considered in the CF patient with severe and refractory wheeze, but only after high-dose inhaled corticosteroid and long-acting beta-2-agonists have failed (level 4). A single randomized crossover trial of nebulized sodium cromoglycate in CF complicated by bronchial hyperreactivity but not asthma showed no benefit.[93] This medication cannot be recommended routinely in CF (level 1b).

Other treatments

Nebulized amiloride showed promise as a long-term therapy in an initial trial,[94] but this was not subsequently confirmed in large randomized trials.[95,96] Amiloride was also not a useful adjunct in the treatment of acute exacerbations.[97] At the present time amiloride cannot be recommended as a routine treatment for CF (level 1b). There is some evidence that the combination of amiloride and tobramycin may be effective in the treatment of multiresistant organisms, including *B. cepacia* (level 3).[98] Various forms of *Aspergillus* lung disease including allergic bronchopulmonary aspergillosis (ABPA) and chronic sputum colonization are not uncommon in CF. There are anecdotal reports of the use of nebulized amphotericin and liposomal amphotericin in the prophylaxis and occasionally treatment of *Aspergillus* lung disease in the context of systemic immunosuppression.[99] There are only isolated reports of this treatment in the context of CF.[100] It might be reasonable to consider nebulized amphotericin in the context of failure of conventional treatment, for example prednisolone for ABPA or persistent chronic infection associated with symptoms and not responding to oral itraconazole (level 4). As with nebulized antibiotics, bronchospasm may occur (level 2b),[101] which may be less with the more expensive liposomal preparation.[102]

Nebulized heparin has been used in one short-term, pilot study in six adult patients chronically infected with *B. cepacia*.[103] There were no changes in lung function; sputum was subjectively easier to expectorate, and there were reductions in serum and sputum IL-6 and IL-8. Sputum volume was unchanged. There were no complications, and specifically no evidence of bleeding. In the absence of further trials, however, nebulized heparin therapy can only be recommended on an experimental basis (level 4).

Future roles: innovative therapies

New therapies, currently at an experimental stage, such as α-antitrypsin and secretory leukoprotease inhibitor are given nebulized. Their place in routine therapy is yet to be established.

Although many trials of gene therapy have used direct endobronchial administration of vector, this is not likely to be practical in the long term, and it is likely that nebulized gene therapy will be preferred. Studies have already shown the practicality of using nebulized delivery of liposomes[104, 105] and recombinant adenoviruses.[106] A detailed discussion is beyond the scope of this chapter, but has been reviewed recently.[107] Finally, newer mucolytics such as actin-resistant DNase,[108] gelsolin[109, 110] which break down actin filaments as well as DNA in the sputum, thus giving more potential benefit on the rheological properties of mucus, are likely to be tested in the future.

Summary

Many valuable medications for CF can only be given nebulized. If every medication that *could* be given nebulized was given by this route, treatment time would escalate dramatically, and adherence to treatment likely to plummet. The use of a nebulizer should always be a last resort in CF, and only continued if there is clear evidence of benefit. We still use nebulizers inconsistently throughout Europe;[111] the challenge for all CF centers is now to achieve a rational and evidence-based consensus.[10]

Appendix The criteria for the gradings of evidence used in this paper

Levels of evidence

Level	Type of evidence[112]
I a	Evidence obtained from meta-analysis of randomized controlled trials
I b	Evidence from at least one randomized controlled trial
2a	Evidence obtained from at least one well designed study without randomization
2b	Evidence obtained from at least one other type of well designed, quasi-experimental study
3	Evidence obtained from well designed non-experimental descriptive studies, such as comparative studies, correlation studies and case-controlled studies
4	Evidence obtained from expert committee reports or opinions and/or clinical experience of respected authorities

Grading of recommendations

Grade	Type of recommendation[113]
A (levels I a, I b)	Requires at least one randomized controlled trial as part of the body of literature of overall good quality and consistency addressing the specific recommendation
B (levels 2a, 2b, 3)	Requires availability of well conducted clinical studies but no randomized clinical trials on the topic of recommendation
C (level 4)	Requires evidence from expert committee reports or opinions and/or clinical experience of respected authorities. Indicated absence of directly applicable studies of good quality

References

1. Rosenfeld M, Emerson J, Astley S et al. Home nebulizer use among patients with cystic fibrosis. *J Pediatr* 1998; **132**:125–31.
2. Standaert TA, Morlin GL, Williams-Warren J et al. Effects of repetitive use and cleaning techniques of disposable jet nebulizers on aerosol generation. *Chest* 1998; **114**:577–86.
3. Mukhopadhya S, Staddon GE, Eastman C et al. The quantitative distribution of nebulized antibiotics in the lung in cystic fibrosis. *Respir Med* 1994; **88**:203–11.

4. Fauroux B, Itti E, Pigeot J et al. Optimization of aerosol deposition by pressure support in children with cystic fibrosis: an experimental and clinical study. *Am J Respir Crit Care Med* 2000; **162**:2265–71.

5. Faurisson F, Dessanges JF, Grimfeld A et al. Performances and ergonomics of nebulizers in cystic fibrosis. *Rev Mal Respir* 1996; **13**:155–62.

6. Coates AL, McNeish CF, Meisner D et al. The choice of jet nebulizer, nebulizing flow, and addition of albuterol affects the output of tobramycin aerosols. *Chest* 1997; **111**:1206–12.

7. Faurisson F, Dessanges JF, Grimfeld A et al. Nebulizer performance: AFLM study. *Respiration* 1995; **62**(Suppl 1):13–18.

8. Diot P, Palmer LB, Smaldone A et al. RhDNase 1 aerosol deposition and related factors in cystic fibrosis. *Am J Respir Crit Care Med* 1997; **156**:1662–8.

9. Chua HL, Collis GG, Newbury AM et al. The influence of age on aerosol deposition in children with cystic fibrosis. *Eur Respir J* 1994; **7**:2185–91.

10. Bush A, Bisgaard H, Geddes D, Lannefors L. Nebulizers in cystic fibrosis. *Eur Respir Rev* 2000; **10**:552–7.

11. Hung JCC, Hambleton G, Super M. Evaluation of two commercial jet nebulisers and three compressors for the nebulisation of antibiotics. *Arch Dis Child* 1994; **71**:335–8.

12. Hutchinson GR, Parker S, Pryor JA et al. Home use nebulizers: a potential primary source of *Burkholderia cepacia* and other colistin-resistant, gram-negative bacteria in patients with cystic fbrosis. *J Clin Microbiol* 1996; **34**:584–7.

13. Robinson M, Hemming AL, Regnis JA et al. Effect of increasing doses of hypertonic saline on mucociliary clearance in patients with cystic fibrosis. *Thorax* 1997; **52**:900–3.

14. Robinson M, Daviskas E, Eberl S et al. The effect of inhaled mannitol on bronchial mucus clearance in cystic fibrosis patients: a pilot study. *Eur Respir J* 1999; **14**:678–85.

15. Robinson M, Regnis JA, Bailey DL et al. Effect of hypertonic saline, amiloride, and cough on mucociliary clearance in patients with cystic fibrosis. *Am J Respir Crit Care Med* 1996; **153**:1503–9.

16. Rodwell LT, Anderson SD. Airway responsiveness to hyperosmolar saline challenge in cystic fibrosis: a pilot study. *Pediatr Pulmonol* 1996; **21**:282–9.

17. McFarlane PI, Heaf D. Changes in air flow obstruction and oxygen saturation in response to exercise and bronchodilators in cystic fibrosis. *Pediatr Pulmonol* 1990; **8**:4–11.

18. Ranasinha C, Assoufi B, Shak S et al. Efficacy and safety of short-term administration of aerosolised recombuinant human Dnase 1 in adults with stable cystic fibrosis. *Lancet* 1993; **342**:199–202.

19. Ramsey B, Astley SJ, Aitken KL et al. Efficacy and safety of short term administration of aerosolized recombinant human deoxyribonuclease in patients with cystic fibrosis (CF). *Am Rev Respir Dis* 1993; **148**:145–51.

20. Eng PA, Morton J, Douglas JA et al. Short term efficacy of ultrasonically nebulised hypertonic saline in cystic fibrosis. *Pediatr Pulmonol* 1996; **21**:77–83.

21. Riedler J, Reade T, Button B, Robertson CF. Inhaled hypertonic saline increases sputum expectoration in cystic fibrosis. *J Pediatr Child Health* 1996; **32**:48–50.

22. Suri R, Metcalfe C, Lees B et al. Comparison of hypertonic saline and alternate-day or daily recombinant human deoxyribonuclease in children with cystic fibrosis: a randomised trial. *Lancet* 2001; **358**:1316–21.

23. Suri R. A cross-over comparative study of hypertonic saline, alternate day and daily rhDNase in children with cystic fibrosis. MD Thesis, University of Manchester, Manchester, 2001.

24. Suri R, Wallis C, Bush A. Tolerability of nebulised hypertonic saline in children with cystic fibrosis. *Pediatr Pulmonol* 2000; Suppl 20:306.

25. Ballman M, von der Hardt H. Hypertonic saline and recombinant human Dnase: a randomized cross-over pilot study in patients with cystic fibrosis. *J Cystic Fibrosis* 2002; **1**:35–7.

26. Travis SM, Conway B-AD, Zabner J et al. Activity of abundant antimicrobials of the human airway. *Am J Cell Mol Biol* 1999; **20**:872–9.

27. Smith JJ, Travis SM, Greenberg EP, Welsh MJ. Cystic fibrosis airway epithelia fail to kill bacteria because of abnormal airway surface fluid. *Cell* 1996; **85**:229–36.

28. Nightingale JA, Rogers DF, Barnes PJ. Effect of repeated sputum induction on cell counts in normal volunteers. *Thorax* 1998; **53**:87–90.

29. Holz O, Richter K, Jones RA et al. Changes in sputum composition between two inductions performed on consecutive days. *Thorax* 1998; **53**:83–6.

30. Suri R, Marshall LJ, Wallis C et al. Effects of rhDNase and hypertonic saline on airway inflammation in children with cystic fibrosis. *Am J Respir Crit Care Med* 2002; **166**:352–5.

31. Fuchs HJ, Borowitz DS, Christiansen DH et al. Effect of aerosolized recombinant human DNase on exacerbations of respiratory symptoms and on pulmonary function in patients with cystic fibrosis. *N Engl J Med* 1994; **331**:637–42.

32. Davies J, Trindade M-T, Wallis C et al. Retrospective review of the effects of rhDNase in children with cystic fibrosis. *Pediatr Pulmonol* 1997; **23**:243–8.

33. Shah PI, Bush A, Canny GJ et al. Recombinant human DNase 1 in cystic fibrosis patients with severe pulmonary disease: a short-term, double blind study followed by six months open label treatment. *Eur Respir J* 1995; **8**:954–8.

34. McCoy C, Hamilton S, Johnson C. Effects of 12-week administration of dornase alfa in patients with advanced cystic fibrosis lung disease. *Chest* 1996; **110**:889–95.

35. Shah P, Scott SF, Fuchs HJ, Geddes DM, Hodson ME. Medium term treatment of stable stage cystic fibrosis with recombinant DNase 1. *Thorax* 1995; **50**:333–8.

36. Bush A. Early treatment with dornase alfa in cystic fibrosis: what are the issues? *Pediatr Pulmonol* 1998; **25**:79–82.

37. Elborn JS, Shale DJ, Britton JR. Cystic fibrosis: current survival and population estimates to the year 2000. *Thorax* 1991; **46**:881–5.

38. Bollert FG, Paton JY, Marshall TG et al. Recombinant Dnase in cystic fibrosis: a protocol for targeted introduction through n-of-1 trials. Scottish Cystic Fibrosis Group. *Eur Respir J* 1999; **13**:107–13.

39. Shah PL, Scott SF, Geddes DM et al. An evaluation of two aerosol delivery systems for rhDNase. *Eur Respir J* 1997; **10**:1261–6.

40. Fiel SB, Fuchs HJ, Johnson C, Gonda I, Clark AR. Comparison of three jet nebulizer aerosol delivery systems used to administer recombinant human DNase 1 to patients with cystic fibrosis. The Pulmozyme rhDNase Study Group. *Chest* 1995; **108**:153–6.

41. Geller DE, Eigen H, Fiel SB et al. Effect of smaller droplet size of dornase alfa on lung function in mild cystic fibrosis. *Pediatr Pulmonol* 1998; **25**:83–7.

42. Conway SP, Watson A. Nebulised bronchodilators, corticosteroids, and rhDNase in adult patients with cystic fibrosis. *Thorax* 1997; **52**(Suppl 2):S64–S68.

43. Wilmott RW, Amin RS, Colin AA et al. Aerosolized recombinant DNase in hospitalized cystic fibrosis patients with acute pulmonary exacerbations. *Am J Respir Crit Care Med* 1996; **153**:1914–17.

44. Wills PJ, Wodehouse T, Corkery K et al. Short-term recombinant human DNase in bronchiectasis: effect on clinical status and in vitro sputum transportability. *Am J Respir Crit Care Med* 1996; **154**:413–17.

45. Suri R, Grieve R, Normand C et al. Effects of hypertonic saline, alternate day and daily rhDNase on healthcare use, costs and outcomes in children with cystic fibrosis. *Thorax* 2002; **57**:841–6.

46. Allen J, Harborne N, Rau DC, Gould H. Participation of core histone 'tails' in the stabilization of the chromatin solenoid. *J Cell Biol* 1982; **93**:285–97.

47. Perks B, Shute JK. DNA and actin bind and inhibit interleukin-8 function in cystic fibrosis sputa: in vitro effect of mucolytics. *Am J Respir Crit Care Med* 2000; **162**:1767–72.

48. Costello CM, O'Connor CM, Finlay GA et al. Effect of nebulised recombinant DNase on neutrophil elastase load in cystic fibrosis. *Thorax* 1996; **51**:619–23.

49. Rochat RT, Patore FD, Schlegel-Haueter SE et al. Aerosolized rhDNase in cystic fibrosis: effect on leucocyte proteases in sputum. *Eur Respir J* 1996; **9**:2200–6.

50. Davis PB. Evolution of therapy for cystic fibrosis. *New Engl J Med* 1994; **331**:672–3.

51. Khan TZ, Wagener JS, Boat T et al. Early pulmonary inflammation in infants with cystic fibrosis. *Am J Respir Crit Care Med* 1995; **151**:1075–82.

52. Kirchner KK, Wagener JS, Khan TZ, Copenhaver SC, Accurso F. Increased DNA levels in bronchoalveolar lavage fluid obtained from infants with cystic fibrosis. *Am J Respir Crit Care Med* 1996; **154**:1426–9.

53. Birrer P, McElvaney NG, Rudeberg C et al. Protease-antiprotease imbalance in the lungs of children with cystic fibrosis. *Am J Respir Crit Care Med* 1994; **150**:207–13.

54. Ranganathan S, Dezateux C, Bush A et al. Airway function in infants newly diagnosed with cystic fibrosis [research letter]. *Lancet* 2001; **358**:1964–5.

55. Jedlicka-Kohler I, Gotz M, Eichler I. Parents' recollection of the initial of the initial communication of the diagnosis of cystic fibrosis. *Pediatrics* 1996; **97**:204–9.

56. Kerem E, Reisman J, Corey M, Canny GJ, Levison H. Prediction of mortality in cystic fibrosis. *N Engl J Med* 1992; **326**:1187–91.

57. Strachan DP. Repeatability of ventilatory function measurements in a population of 7 year old children. *Thorax* 1989; **44**:474–9.

58. Nickerson BG, Lemen RJ, Gerdes CB et al. Within-subject variability and percent change for significance of spirometry in normal subjects and in patients with cystic fibrosis. *Am Rev Respir Dis* 1980; **122**:855–9.

59. Dakin C, Henry RL, Field P, Morton J. Defining an exacerbation of pulmonary disease in cystic fibrosis. *Pediatr Pulmonol* 2001; **31**:436–42.

60. Thibeault DW, Heimes B, Rezaiekhaligh M, Mabry S. Chronic modification of lung and heart development in glucocorticoid treated newborn rats exposed to hyperoxia or room air. *Pediatr Pulmonol* 1993; **16**:81–8.

61. Tschanz SA, Damke BM, Burri PH. Influence of postnatally administered glucocorticoids on rat lung growth. *Biol Neonate* 1995; **68**:229–45.

62. Wagener JS, Rock MJ, McCubbun MM et al. Aerosol delivery and safety of human recombinant deoxyribonuclease in young children with cystic fibrosis: a bronchoscopic study. *J Pediatr* 1998; **133**:486–91.

63. Quan JM, Tiddens AWM, Sy JP et al. A two year randomized, placebo-controlled trial of dornase alfa in young patients with cystic fibrosis with mild lung function abnormalities. *J Pediatr* 2001; **139**:813–20.

64. Bush A. Early use of dornase alpha in cystic fibrosis: Con. *J Cystic Fibrosis* 2002; 1(Suppl 11):S26.

65. Rosenthal M, Bain SH, Cramer D et al. Lung function in white children aged 4–19 years: I-spirometry. *Thorax* 1993; **48**:794–802.

66. Dakin CJ, Pereira JK, Henry RL, Wang H, Morton JR. Relationship between sputum inflammatory markers, lung function, and lung pathology on high-resolution computed tomography in children with cystic fibrosis. *Pediatr Pulmonol* 2002; **33**:475–82.

67. Nasr SZ, Kuhns LR, Brown RW et al. Use of computed tomography and chest x-rays in evaluating efficacy of aerosolized recombinant human Dnase in cystic fibrosis patients younger than age 5 years: a preliminary study. *Pediatr Pulmonol* 2001; **31**:377–82.

68. Greally P. Human recombinant DNase for mucus plugging in status asthmaticus. *Lancet* 1995; **346**:1423–4.

69. Gershan WM, Rusakow LS, Chetty A. Resolution of chronic atelectasis in a child with asthma after aerosolized recombinant human DNase. *Pediatr Pulmonol* 1994; **18**:268–9.

70. Ten Berge M, Brinkhorst G, Kroon A, De Jongste JC. DNase treatment in primary ciliary dyskinesia – assessment by nocturnal pulse oximetry. *Pediatr Pulmonol* 1999; **27**:59–61.

71. Desai M, Weller PH, Spencer DA. Clinical benefit from nebulized human recombinant DNase in Kartagener's syndrome. *Pediatr Pulmonol* 1995; **20**:307–8.

72. El Hassan NO, Huysman MWA, Merkus PJFM, Chess PR, de Jongste JC. Rescue use of DNase in critical lung atelectasis and mucus retention in premature neonates. *Pediatrics* 2001; **108**:468–71.

73. Merkus PJFM, de Hoog M, Gent van R, de Jongste JC. DNase treatment for atelectasis in infants with severe RSV bronchiolitis. *Eur Respir J* 2001; **18**:734–7.

74. Denton R, Kwart H, Litt M. N-acetylcysteine in cystic fibrosis. *Am Rev Respir Dis* 1967; **95**:643–51.

75. Howatt WF, DeMuth GR. A double-blind study of the use of acetylcysteine in patients with cystic fibrosis. *Univ Mich Med Center J* 1966; **32**:82–5.

76. Romano L, Calvi A, Gaiero A. Mid-term response to treatment with rhDNase can not be anticipated from the basis of sputum production. *Pediatr Pulmonol* 1995; Suppl 12:237.

77. Duijvestijn YC, Brand PL. Systematic review of N-acetylcysteine in cystic fibrosis. *Acta Paediatrica* 1999; **88**:38–41.

78. App EM, Baran D, Dab I et al. Dose-finding and 24-h monitoring for efficacy and safety of aerosolized Nacestelyn in cystic fibrosis. *Eur Respir J* 2002; **19**:294–302.

79. Zach MS, Oberwaldner B, Forche G, Polgar G. Bronchodilators increase airway instability in cystic fibrosis. *Am Rev Respir Dis* 1985; **131**:537–43.

80. Philips GE, Thomas S, Heather S, Bush A. Airway response of children with primary ciliary dyskinesia to exercise and β-2 agonist challenge. *Eur Respir J* 1998; **11**:1389–91.

81. Duncan CS, Blimkie CJ, Cowell CT et al. Bone mineral density in adolescent female athletes: relationship to exercise type and muscle strength. *Med Sports Exer* 2002; **34**:286–94.

82. MacKelvie KJ, McKay HA, Petit MA et al. Bone mineral response to a 7-month randomized controlled, school based jumping intervention in 121 prepubertal boys: associations with ethnicity and body mass index. *J Bone Min Res* 2002; **17**:834–44.

83. Cates CJ, Rowe BH, Bara A. Holding chambers versus nebulisers for beta-agonist treatment of acute asthma. In: the *Cochrane Library*, Issue 3, 2002. Oxford: Update Software.

84. Parkin PC, Saunders NR, Diamond SA, Winders PM, Macartur C. Randomised trial spacer v nebuliser for acute asthma. *Arch Dis Child* 1995; **72**:239–40.

85. Kerem E, Levison H, Schuh S et al. Efficacy of albuterol administered by nebulizer versus spacer device in children with acute asthma. *J Pediatr* 1993; **123**:313–17.

86. Orenstein DM. Long-term inhaled bronchodilator therapy in cystic fibrosis. *Chest* 1991; **99**:1061.

87. Finnegan MJ, Hughes DV, Hodson ME. Comparison of nebulized and intravenous terbutaline during exacerbations of pulmonary infection in patients with cystic fibrosis. *Eur Respir J* 1992; **5**:1089–91.

88. Hassan JA, Saadiah S, Roslan H, Zainudin BM. Bronchodilator response to inhaled beta-2 agonist and anticholinergic drugs in patients with bronchiectasis. *Respirology* 1999; **4**:423–6.

89. Eigen H, Rosenstein B, Fitxsimmons S, Schidlow D. A multi-center study of alternate day prednisolone therapy in patients with cystic fibrosis. *J Pediatr* 1995; **126**:515–23.

90. Balfour-Lynn IM, Klein NJ, Dinwiddie R. Randomised controlled trial of inhaled corticosteroids (fluticasone propionate) in cystic fibrosis. *Arch Dis Child* 1997; **77**:124–30.

91. Bisgaard H, Pedersen SS, Nielsen KG et al. Controlled trial of inhaled budesonide in patients with cystic fibrosis and chronic bronchopulmonary *Pseudomonas aeruginosa* infection. *Am J Respir Crit Care Med* 1997; **156**:1190–6.

92. Llangovan P, Pedersen S, Godfrey S et al. Treatment of severe steroid dependent preschool asthma with nebulised budesonide suspension. *Arch Dis Child* 1993; **68**:356–9.

93. Sivan Y, Arce P, Eigen H, Nickerson BG, Newth CJ. A double-blind, randomized study of sodium cromoglycate versus placebo in patients with cystic fibrosis and bronchial hyperreactivity. *J Allergy Clin Immunol* 1990; **85**:649–54.

94. Knowles MR, Church NL, Waltner WE et al. A pilot study of aerosolised amiloride for the treatment of lung disease in cystic fibrosis. *N Engl J Med* 1990; **322**:1189–94.

95. Graham A, Hasani A, Alton EWFW et al. No added benefit from nebulized amiloride in patients with cystic fibrosis. *Eur Respir J* 1993; **6**:1243–8.

96. Pons G, Marchand MC, d'Athis P et al. French multicenter randomized double-blind placebo-controlled trial on nebulized amiloride in cystic fibrosis patients. The Amiloride-AFLM Collaborative Study Group. *Pediatr Pulmonol* 2000; **30**:25–31.

97. Bowler IM, Kelman B, Worthington D et al. Nebulised amiloride in respiratory exacerbations of cystic fibrosis: a randomised controlled trial. *Arch Dis Child* 1995; **73**:427–30.

98. Cohn RC, Rudzienski L. Further observations on amiloride-tobramycin synergy in cystic fibrosis [abstract]. *Pediatr Pulmonol* 1991; Suppl 6:279.

99. Schwartz S, Behre G, Heinemann V et al. Aerosolized amphotericin B inhalations as prophylaxis of inhaled aspergillus infections during prolonged neutropenia: results of a prospective randomized multicenter trial. *Blood* 1999; **93**:3654–61.

100. Brown K, Rosenthal M, Bush A. Fatal invasive aspergillosis in an adolescent with cystic fibrosis. *Pediatr Pulmonol* 1999; **27**:130–3.

101. DuBois J, Bartter T, Gryn J, Pratter MR. The physiological effects of inhaled amphotericin B. *Chest* 1995; **108**:750–3.

102. Purcell IF, Corris PA. Use of nebulised liposomal amphotericin B in the treatment of aspergillus fumigatus empyema. *Thorax* 1995; **50**:1321–3.

103. Ledson M, Gallagher M, Hart CA, Walshaw M. Nebulized heparin in *Burkholderia cepacia* colonized adult cystic fibrosis patients. *Eur Respir J* 2001; **17**:36–8.

104. Eastman SJ, Tousignant JD, Lukason MJ et al. Aerosolization of cationic lipid:pDNA complexes – in vitro optimization of nebuliser parameters for human clinical studies. *Hum Gene Ther* 1998; **9**:43–52.

105. Schreier H, Gagna L, Conary JT, Laurian G. Simulated lung transfection by nebulization of liposome cDNA complexes using a cascade impactor seeded with 2-CFSME-cells. *J Aerosol Med* 1998; **11**:1–13.

106. Joseph PM, O'Sullivan BP, Lapey A et al. Aerosol and lobar administration of a recombinant adenovirus to individuals with cystic fibrosis. 1. Methods, safety and clinical implications. *Hum Gene Ther* 2001; **12**:1369–82.

107. Flotte TR, Laube BL. Gene therapy in cystic fibrosis. *Chest* 2001; **120**(Suppl 3):124S–131S.

108. Zahm JM, Debordeaux C, Maurer C et al. Improved activity of an actin-resistant DNase 1 variant on the cystic fibrosis airway secretions. *Am J Respir Crit Care Med* 2001; **163**:1153–7.

109. Vasconcellos CA, Allen PG, Wohl ME et al. Reduction in viscosity of cystic fibrosis sputum in vitro by gelsolin. *Science* 1994; **263**:969–71.

110. Davoodian K, Ritchings BW, Ramphal R, Bubb MR. Gelsolin activates Dnase1 in vitro and cystic fibrosis sputum. *Biochemistry* 1997; **36**:9637–41.

111. Borsje P, de Jongste JC, Mouton JW, Tiddens HA. Aerosol therapy in cystic fibrosis: a survey of 54 CF centers. *Pediatr Pulmonol* 2000; **30**:368–76.

112. Petrie GJ, Barnwell E, Grimshaw J, on behalf of the Scottish Intercollegiate Guidelines Network. *Clinical guidelines: criteria for appraisal for national use.* Edinburgh: Royal College of Physicians, 1966.

113. Agency for Health Care Policy and Research. *Acute pain management, operative or medical procedures and trauma 92–0032. Clinical practice guideline.* Rockville, MD: Agency for Healthcare Policy and Research Publications, 1992.

9. DIAGNOSTIC USES OF NEBULIZERS

Chris Stenton and John Dennis

Introduction

The administration of an aerosol via a nebulizer is an important step in a number of diagnostic procedures. These include the measurement of airway responsiveness, inhalation challenge testing with allergens and occupational agents, bronchodilator reversibility testing, sputum induction, and the administration of radioisotopes. The performance of the nebulizer is most critical in the measurement of airway responsiveness as this requires precise quantification of the effect of the inhaled agent, and discussion of this forms the main part of this chapter. The issues of nebulizer output, aerosol particle size distribution, variability of nebulizer output, and the influence of breathing patterns are similar so far as other forms of inhalation challenge and reversibility testing are concerned. With sputum induction and radioisotope administration the response to the nebulized agent is not quantified directly but the performance of the nebulizer remains important for the standardization of the tests.

Airway responsiveness

Airway responsiveness is the term used to describe the tendency of the airways to narrow in response to a variety of constrictor stimuli.[1] These can be naturally occurring such as exercise, cold air, smoke or dust, or they can be pharmacological agonists such as methacholine or histamine. Some degree of airway responsiveness can be quantified in most individuals but it is markedly increased in asthma, and airway hyperresponsiveness can be considered a fundamental characteristic of that condition. Its measurement has proved very useful in diagnosing asthma clinically and in investigating the condition epidemiologically.

Airway responsiveness is akin to many other physiological characteristics in being unimodally distributed in the population (Figure 9.1). Subjects with

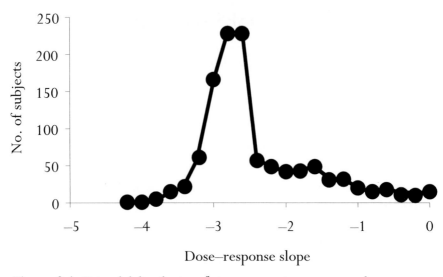

Figure 9.1 *Unimodal distribution of airway responsiveness measured as dose–response slope from a population study of 600 20–45-year-old subjects. (Adapted from Barraclough R et al.* Eur Respir J *2002; **20**:826–33[2] with permission from European Respiratory Society Journals Limited.)*

asthma are at one end of the responsiveness spectrum but there is no clear distinction between the range of asthma and the normal range. Nevertheless, broad categories can be identified in which there is either a high or a low probability that the individual has asthma (Figure 9.2).[2–4] The measurements can therefore be very useful in assessing individuals whose disease presents with atypical symptoms such as cough, or those with some other condition such as hyperventilation that is masquerading as asthma. A number of other diseases including smoking-induced chronic obstructive pulmonary disease (COPD) can increase airway responsiveness[5] and so the predictive value of the test for asthma depends on the clinical context in which it is used. Almost all individuals with currently active asthma have increased airway responsiveness and a clearly negative test is very useful in excluding the diagnosis.

One setting in which the measurement is particularly useful is in the diagnosis of occupational asthma.[6] In this condition the affected individual is often intermittently exposed to the asthmagenic agent, and the severity of the asthma together with the degree of airway responsiveness increases and decreases with exposure. Serial measurements confirming a work-related pattern can help establish the diagnosis (Figure 9.3).[7,8]

Epidemiological surveys suggest that there has been a marked increase in asthma prevalence over the past few decades[9] and quantifying the

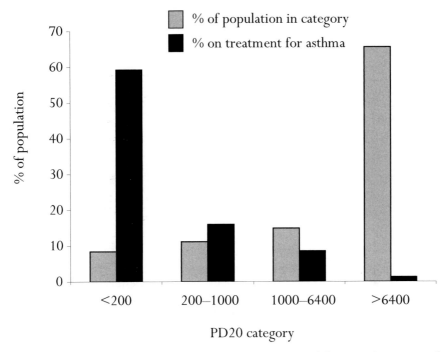

Figure 9.2 *Relationship between airway responsiveness and diagnosis/treatment of asthma.[2] At one end of the spectrum 8% of the population have PD20 FEV₁ <200 μg and 60% of these are on treatment for asthma. At the other end, 65% of the population have PD20 >6400 μg and approximately 1% are on treatment for asthma. FEV₁, forced expiratory volume in one second; PD20, provoking dose calculated to cause a 20% fall in FEV₁.*

precise extent of the disease is of considerable current importance. Epidemiological measures of asthma such as symptom frequency and severity or use of medication can be influenced by subjective changes in awareness or changes in diagnostic criteria. Airway responsiveness measurements alone are able to provide relevant objective information about the disease prevalence. The European Community Respiratory Health Study (ECRHS) is one major asthma study that has quantified airway responsiveness in 36 centers in 16 countries and has demonstrated that geographic differences in asthma symptom prevalence are accompanied by differences in airway responsiveness.[10] Other investigators have shown that marked increases in asthma symptoms in the late 1990s were not accompanied by increases in airway responsiveness and were likely to have been a consequence of changes in diagnostic awareness.[2] However, the conclusions of these and many other multicenter or longitudinal studies

165

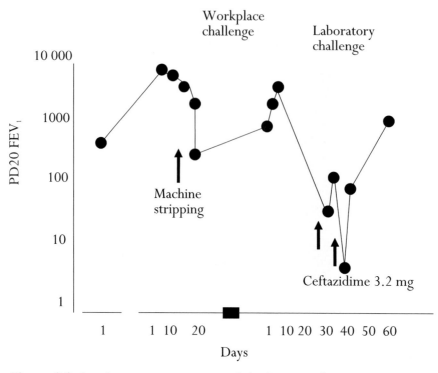

Figure 9.3 *Serial airway responsiveness and the diagnosis of occupational asthma. Initial PD20 measurement with the subject at work was 800 μg. There was an improvement associated with a period off work followed by a further fall when machinery was stripped. The subject was off work again and then underwent a series of inhalation challenge tests. These were associated with further improvements and worsening of airway responsiveness (increases and decreases in PD20). FEV₁, forced expiratory volume in one second; PD20, provoking dose calculated to cause a 20% fall in FEV₁. (Adapted from Stenton SC et al.* Eur Respir J *1995; 8:1421–3[8] with permission from European Respiratory Society Journals Limited.)*

depend on the careful standardization of the techniques and this has been a matter of considerable debate, if not controversy.[10–13]

Airway responsiveness is usually measured by quantifying the response to a bronchoconstrictor agent delivered to the airways from a jet nebulizer.[1,14] Increasing doses of the bronchoconstrictor are inhaled at 5 min intervals, and ventilatory function (forced expiratory volume in one second (FEV_1)) is measured after each dose, and expressed as a percentage of the starting value. The test continues until FEV_1 has fallen by 20% or until a predetermined maximum dose of bronchoconstrictor has been administered. Within that framework, there is huge diversity in the way the tests are carried out. Both methacholine and histamine are used as bronchoconstrictors although methacholine is generally preferred because it causes fewer side effects. The bronchoconstrictor is sometimes administered by the *tidal breathing method* which involves continuous inhalation of each dose of aerosol over 2 min. Alternatively, the *dosimeter method* delivers aerosol boluses during the initial part of a series of inspiratory maneuvers with the timing and dose controlled by a breath-actuated dosimeter. Several commercial and purpose built dosimeters with differing operating characteristics are available, there is a wide choice of nebulizers, and there is variation in the dosage and administration schedule for the bronchoconstrictor.

The response to the bronchoconstrictor is normally measured as the FEV_1. A variable number of FEV_1 measurements can be made after each dose and because making forced expiratory maneuvers partially antagonizes the effect of bronchoconstrictor agents this influences the outcome.[3] The test result is usually quantified as the PD20, the provoking dose of agonist calculated by linear interpolation from a dose–response plot to cause exactly a 20% fall in FEV_1 (Figure 9.4). If a tidal breathing method is used the dose delivered to the airways is not known and the PC20, the

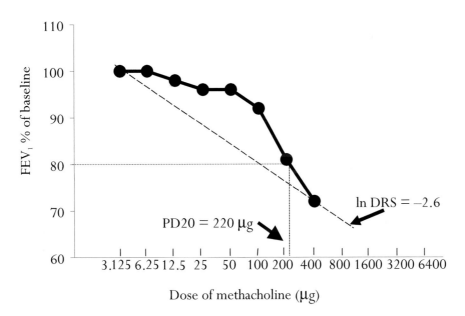

Figure 9.4 *Measurement of airway responsiveness.*[2–6] *Methacholine is administered by nebulizer in doubling doses at 5 min intervals until there is a 20% fall in FEV_1. The test result is quantified either as PD20, the dose of methacholine calculated by interpolation to cause exactly 20% fall in FEV_1, or dose–response slope (DRS).*

provoking concentration, is calculated. Most normal subjects do not experience a 20% fall in FEV_1 and PD20 or PC20 cannot be calculated. In epidemiological studies it is common to measure the dose–response slope, i.e. the slope of a line connecting the baseline value with the final FEV_1 as this can be quantified in all subjects.[2] Other summary measures are sometimes used.[10]

The technique used in the challenge test can influence airway responsiveness measurements either by affecting their absolute magnitude or their repeatability. Often the influences are subtle, and challenge techniques that appear superficially similar can conceal important differences. This can lead to difficulties when comparing measurements between laboratories, and in the interpretation of multicenter or longitudinal studies. Recent guidelines[1,14] should lead to some uniformity but at present airway responsiveness measurements remain poorly standardized in comparison with other tests of lung function.

Nebulizers and airway responsiveness measurements

Airway responsiveness measurements are at best repeatable in the same individual within one and a half doubling doses, i.e. an initial PD20 of 200 μg can vary from 75 μg to 600 μg when repeated. Often the repeatability is less than this.[15] Dosimeters allow greater control over the dose of agonist and are associated with more repeatable measurements than the tidal breathing method, although the method used to measure the bronchoconstrictor response probably contributes more to that than the method of drug delivery.[15] It is not known to what extent the residual variability of airway responsiveness measurements reflects a biological phenomenon or is due to variation in the nature of the aerosol delivered to the airways. However, for optimum precision it is important to understand and control the administration of the aerosol as closely as possible.[16]

Nebulizer output

The mass output of a nebulizer is the chief determinant of the amount of agonist delivered to the lungs, and of its biological effect.[17] It is related to nebulizer type, pressure and flow rate of the driving gas, the type of inhalation maneuver, and the extent of air entrainment in breath-enhanced devices. It is important for the accuracy of airway responsiveness measurements that this is quantified and controlled as much as possible. Nebulizers should be calibrated before use and if this is carried out incorrectly there will be an effect on the airway responsiveness measurement in direct proportion to the calibration error.[1]

Quantifying the output of nebulizers is not straightforward and has the potential to introduce considerable error into airway responsiveness measurements. For many years, nebulizers were calibrated from their weight loss during use but this caused problems with accuracy as the weight lost during normal use is usually only a very small proportion of the overall weight. A 25 g nebulizer delivering 50 μl loses only 0.0005% of its weight per activation. Longer periods of nebulization were often used for calibration but they did not mimic clinical use because the nebulizer cooled with repeated use, output was reduced by 25–40% over 10 min, and there was a calibration error of similar magnitude.[18] Variations in weight calibration techniques have led to differences in estimated nebulizer output of the order of 20–40%.[18]

More fundamentally, it is now recognized that calibrating jet nebulizers by weight loss overestimates their aerosol output by failing to take into account the evaporation that occurs during use.[19] The latter is irrelevant so far as delivery of agonist is concerned but it contributes significantly to the weight loss. It is also responsible for cooling of the nebulizer and concentration of the solution in the reservoir.[18] Weight loss overestimates the true aerosol output of most commonly used nebulizers by approximately 40–60%.[20] The Wright nebulizer (Roxon Medi-Tech, Montreal, PQ, Canada) which is commonly used with the tidal breathing method derives a particularly high proportion of its output from evaporation and its effective output can be overestimated several fold.[19] Evaporation would matter little if the aerosol fraction was a constant proportion of the total nebulizer output, but there is evidence that it is influenced by both nebulizer type and batch.[19–21] A 30% difference in the aerosol fractions of two batches of nebulizers manufactured for use with the Mefar dosimeter (Mefar, Bresica, Italy) was found in one study,[21] and in the ECRHS the aerosol fraction differed between centers over the range of 40–52%.[11] Thus even with careful calibration by weight one center was unknowingly administering 30% more methacholine with each dose than another.

It is now recommended that nebulizers are calibrated by ion or radioactive tracer methods.[19,22,23] The aerosol is entrained and impacted onto a filter, the solute is desorbed from the filter, and the ion content is assayed against standard solutions or the radioactivity counted. This eliminates the systematic calibration errors associated with the measurement of output by weight loss.

When a dosimeter is used to control the activation of a nebulizer this needs to be calibrated separately but there is evidence that this is not always carried out. In the ECRHS study it was found that the majority of dosimeters were operating outside the manufacturer's specified range of driving pressures (180 kP ± 5%), and sometimes markedly so. Driving pressures of 70–245 kP were found in 15 dosimeters[24] and this is likely to have had a substantial effect on the airway responsiveness measurements as aerosol output is closely related to the driving pressure and flow. Other modifications were observed such as replacement of the compressor with an external compressed air source and this is likely to have increased the output by increasing the proportion of time the nebulizer was driven at peak pressure.[24,25]

Calibration errors of the order of 50–100% probably matter little for clinical diagnostic purposes as the range of airway responsiveness over which asthma is probable is separated from the range over which asthma is unlikely by an indeterminate zone of at least two doubling doses.[26] Calibration errors alone are unlikely to be sufficient to make a clear change to an individual's diagnostic category but they are important in epidemiological investigations in which a small population shift in airway responsiveness distribution can assume significance. This was illustrated in a 2-year survey of shipyard workers in which the nebulizers for the second year were incorrectly calibrated[3] resulting in an unexpected difference in the population distribution of airway responsiveness between the 2 years. The error was identified when the nebulizers were recalibrated at the end of the study and when the airway responsiveness measurements were recalculated the difference between the 2 years disappeared.[27] A similar effect was seen in the ECRHS in which correction for the greater than anticipated nebulizer output resulted in a 13% reduction in the number of subjects with a PD20 of less than 2 mg.[11] A longitudinal study of asthma in children which showed a 1.5–2-fold increase in the prevalence of airway hyperresponsiveness over a 10-year period used a DeVilbiss 40 nebulizer for the first survey and a DeVilbiss 45 (DeVilbiss Health Care Inc, Somerset, PA, USA) for the second.[28] It was later shown that although the two nebulizers had a similar output quantified by weight loss, the DeVilbiss 45 had almost twice the aerosol output of the DeVilbiss 40 and this might have accounted for the observed changes in airway responsiveness distribution.[29]

Variability of nebulizer output

The outputs of commercially available nebulizers vary considerably not only between nebulizer type but between and within batches of the same nebulizer.[24,33] Typically the coefficient of variation from one measurement to another is in the region of 10% whether measured by weight loss or by aerosol output.[11,19,21,31] Coefficients of variation of up to 38% have been calculated[32] indicating that output can vary by approximately 80% from one measurement to another, sufficient to have a substantial influence on the repeatability of airway responsiveness measurements. Some nebulizers have less inherent variability than others. The reusable DeVilbiss 646 (Somerset, PA, USA) which is commonly used with inhalation dosimeters appears to have a particularly variable output,[1,33] possibly related to the consistency with which its components can be reassembled in identical positions after cleaning. It has been suggested that glueing the nebulizer together after calibration might improve its performance.[1] The vent on the DeVilbiss 646 allows entrainment of air and increases output but this makes it more variable and it is recommended that the vent is closed during challenge testing.[34] Improved engineering might lead to a reduction in the variability of some high specification nebulizers though variability is likely to change little for the majority of 'disposable' nebulizers used for inhalation challenge studies.

Particle size distribution

The particle size distribution of an aerosol influences the overall amount entering the lung and the pattern of deposition, and is an important determinant of its biological effect. Particles of >10 μm are largely deposited in the mouth, central airway deposition is maximal at 6–7 μm, and peripheral airway deposition is maximal at 2–3 μm.[35,36] Commercially available nebulizers show a wide variation in their particle size distribution with mean values ranging from <1 μm to >10 μm.[36,37] The total amount of aerosol entering the lung is likely to vary by about 40% over this range and deposition in the peripheral airways will vary several fold.[38] This is likely to have a significant effect on airway responsiveness measurements. The air flow rate through the nebulizer further influences particle size distribution as smaller particles are produced at higher driving pressures and flows.[39]

Although the amount of aerosol entering the lung clearly influences the response, the evidence that the site of deposition within the lung is important is much less consistent. Ruffin and colleagues showed that a maneuver designed to deposit histamine centrally in the airways was associated with an increase in PD20 of approximately 3.5 doubling doses.[40] On the other hand, Ryan and colleagues showed that there was no difference in PD20 when the same dose of aerosol was delivered as 3.6 μm particles rather than 1.3 μm particles.[17] The optimum particle size distribution for inhalation challenge studies is thus not known.

Like total output, the particle size distribution of nebulizers shows some variability from measurement to measurement. Standaert and colleagues showed coefficients of variation for the mass mean diameter of five nebulizers of 3–20% with coefficients for the respirable fraction (<5 μm) ranging from 4% to 24%.[31] The effective dose of bronchoconstrictor delivered to the lung with the poorest performing nebulizer could vary over almost a four-fold range introducing significant variability into the measurement of airway responsiveness. The effect might be even more marked if the site of deposition within the lung is a significant determinant of the response.

Once generated, aerosols can decrease markedly in size because of evaporation, or they can slowly increase in size if they are hypertonic and absorb fluid from the surrounding air.[41] A 1 μm water droplet, for example, evaporates within 0.5 s at room temperature even under saturated conditions because of internal pressures caused by surface tension. The particle size distribution of an aerosol is thus affected by the temperature, air flow rate, degree of humidification of the driving air,[42–44] and the distance traveled along tubing, etc.[31] The cooling effect of continuous nebulization and a decrease in the relative humidity of air from >90% to 13% each cause approximately a 40% decrease in aerosol droplet size,[45,46] and traveling along a 1.5 m length of tubing can cause a 12% decrease.[31] Evaporation can also increase the solute concentration in the remaining aerosol to more than 10 times that of the initial nebulizer reservoir solution.[45] These dynamic changes create difficulties in accurately characterizing particle size distribution at the point of impaction in the airways where they have their biological effect though the significance of this is not known. The high flow rates of conventional cascade impactors which are used to measure particle size distribution are likely to lead to significant evaporation which is not found at the lower flow rates achieved during normal nebulizer use. This might lead to inappropriately low particle size measurements.[47] Low flow cascade impaction might provide a more clinically representative measurement though this has not yet been used to fully investigate nebulizer outputs.[28,48–49]

Breathing pattern

The deposition of aerosols in the lungs increases with breathing rate and volume up to a minute volume of 10–15 l/min and falls off above that level.[49] However, if the rate of inspiration is greater than the rate of gas flow through a nebulizer then air will be entrained and the aerosol will be diluted,

172

and in practice slower inspiratory maneuvers can result in a several fold greater inhaled dose than more rapid inspiration.[17] Slow inspiration also reduces inertial impaction in the upper airways and leads to more peripheral aerosol deposition,[17] and together these effects can have a substantial effect on airway responsiveness measurements. Ryan and colleagues,[17] for example, demonstrated that that PC20 histamine was 3.3-fold lower with an 8 s inspiratory maneuver compared with a 2 s maneuver. Intake of air via the nose has a diluting effect on aerosol inhaled via the mouth and nose clips are often used although there is no evidence of their effectiveness. Substantial differences have been noted in minute ventilation during inhalation challenge tests both between and within individuals[50] and careful control of the inspiratory flow rate appears to increase the repeatability of airway responsiveness measurements probably by reducing the variability of the inhaled dose of agonist.[51] Other aspects of breathing pattern can influence measurements with both the dosimeter and the tidal breathing techniques.[17,51] In one study increasing the duration of the pause between inspiration and expiration from 5 s to 15 s reduced the coefficient of variability of aerosol deposition from 104% to 5%.[52] Under normal operating conditions the breathing pattern is more carefully regulated with the dosimeter technique than with tidal breathing and this might contribute to its greater repeatability.

Changes with duration of nebulization

It has been recognized for some time that the weight loss of nebulizers is greatest during the early phase of nebulization[52,53] and that this is a consequence of the cooling which takes place due to evaporation.[18] This is a potential source of error if nebulizers are calibrated by weight loss over a period longer than that used during the challenge test.[18,54] Cooling reduces the evaporative weight loss but has little effect on the aerosol output.[19] Decreased evaporation from the nebulizer has the secondary effect of decreasing particle size distribution by increasing evaporation from the aerosol into the drier surrounding air.[50]

A further consequence of progressive evaporation from the reservoir during nebulization is the concentration of the agonist during nebulization. With the Wright nebulizer, the concentration of solute in the reservoir increases approximately in proportion to the weight loss[18] though the effect is less marked with more efficient nebulizers.[31] It can be predicted that for a typical nebulizer with an aerosol fraction of 0.6 delivering a 50 μl dose from a reservoir volume of 3 ml via a dosimeter, the concentrating effect will be a little under 1% per dose. This could have a significant effect on airway responsiveness measurements if repeated challenges are performed without changing the nebulizer solution.

Care and maintenance of nebulizers

Without proper cleaning and maintenance the performance characteristics of nebulizers deteriorate rapidly, probably because of deposition or crystallization of solutes within the unit. In one study some unwashed nebulizers of each of five models investigated failed to produce aerosol after 30 uses.[31] However, with proper washing nebulizer output has been shown to remain stable over at least 100 uses.[31] In many laboratories carrying out airway responsiveness measurements nebulizers are disassembled, cleaned, reassembled and used several hundred times without showing evidence of deterioration. For an inexpensive 'disposable' device this is a remarkable achievement.

Inhalation challenge with allergens, occupational and other agents

The inhalation of an aerosol of aeroallergen provokes bronchoconstriction in sensitized individuals. This is usually of little clinical diagnostic value as the response to allergens can be predicted from airway responsiveness and skin prick test results.[55] Inhalation challenge tests with aeroallergens have, however, been of great value in studying the pathophysiology of asthma and in evaluating new therapeutic agents. The allergen is usually administered by aerosol via a nebulizer and the principles of dose control are similar to those discussed above though they are potentially more important as allergen challenge can be more hazardous. Doses are usually administered at 10 min rather than 5 min intervals as the immediate reaction to aeroallergens is of longer duration than that with methacholine or histamine, and doses are reduced when a fall in FEV_1 of 10–15% occurs.[1] Cardiopulmonary resuscitation equipment should be available and the tests should be supervised by a physician in a hospital setting. Because allergen challenges are often associated with late asthmatic reactions which peak 6–12 hours after exposure, subjects should monitor lung function regularly for 24 hours following the challenge.

Occupational exposures may account for up to 10% of adult onset asthma[56] and occupational asthma is an important diagnosis to establish because it can have profound implications for an individual's future health and employment.[57] The diagnosis cannot be established reliably from the clinical history

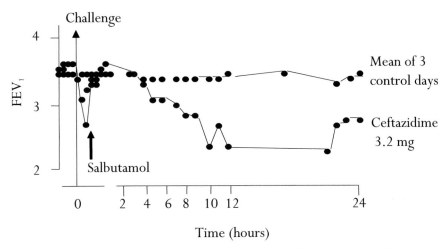

Figure 9.5 *Inhalation challenge test in the diagnosis of occupational asthma. Ceftazidime solution was administered via a jet nebulizer. There was an immediate asthmatic reaction which was followed by a typical late reaction and an increase in airway responsiveness (Figure 9.3). FEV$_1$, forced expiratory volume in one second. (Adapted from Stenton SC et al.* Eur Respir J *1995; 8:1421–3[8] with permission from European Respiratory Society Journals Limited.)*

and although serial peak expiratory flow measurements can help, inhalation challenge tests with the agent thought to be responsible for the asthma are considered to be the diagnostic gold standard (Figure 9.5). Attention to control of the inhaled dose and safety is of vital importance because of the risk of severe reactions, and inhalation challenge tests with occupational agents should only be carried out in specialist centers. Often the potency of the agent is not known, and occupational agents frequently cause isolated late asthmatic reactions so that if an incremental schedule is used doses might need to be increased daily rather than at 5–10 min intervals.[8,58]

Capsaicin, citric acid and hyposmolar solutions are used in the investigation of chronic cough.[59] The capsaicin challenge test is now the most widely used as it is better tolerated than the others and it allows the characterization of a dose–response relationship. The test is carried out using a dosimeter similar to that used for methacholine challenge testing.[60] No specific evaluation of nebulizers for this type of challenge has been carried out.

Considerable thought must be given to safety and delivery of the correct dose before any novel agent is administered in an inhalation challenge test. The addition of allergens and occupational agents to nebulizer solutions can affect both their output and particle size distribution.[61] Solutions of increasing viscosity decrease nebulizer output whereas surface active agents increase output.[62,63] Salbutamol nebulizer solution lowers surface tension and can increase the output of other agents if it is administered concurrently.[64] Ultrasonic nebulizers can disrupt large molecules and denature proteins because of the heat generated by high frequency vibration,[66] and a suspension may not be nebulized at all.[66]

Bronchodilator reversibility

Bronchodilator reversibility testing is useful in the evaluation of COPD to help rule out asthma, and to establish a patient's best attainable lung function. This in turn acts as a guide to prognosis and the potential response to treatment. The tests are often carried out using bronchodilators such as salbutamol administered via a metered dose inhaler (MDI) but nebulizers are recommended when there are doubts about a patient's ability to use an MDI correctly and to ensure that the dose administered is high on the dose–response curve.[66]

The test should be performed when the patient is clinically stable and has not taken inhaled short acting bronchodilators in the previous 6 hours, or longer acting agents in the previous 12–24 hours. FEV_1 is measured, the bronchodilator is administered and FEV_1 is remeasured after 30–45 min depending on the agent administered. Most normal individuals and patients with COPD show small bronchodilator responses. There is considerable variability of the response from one day to the next and the response to bronchdilator on one day is not a good guide to future response to treatment in COPD. Very marked responses to bronchodilators suggest asthma.

Little attention has been paid to the choice and characteristics of nebulizers for bronchodilator reversibility testing. The test depends on the administration of a high dose of bronchodilator which is likely to have its effect on a shallow part of the dose–response curve (Figure 9.6). Minor changes in drug delivery are likely to have little influence on the test outcome but there are quality control issues that are similar to those associated with aerosol delivery in other situations.

Sputum induction

The inhalation of non-isotonic saline solutions can provoke coughing and the production of a small amount of airway secretion that can be expectorated

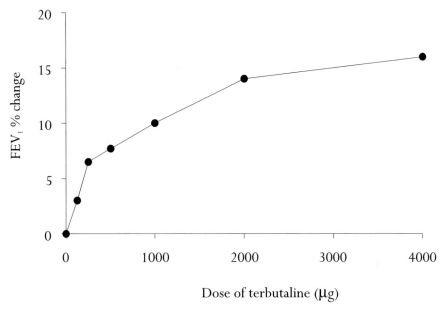

Figure 9.6 *Dose–response relationship to bronchodilator in COPD. When reversibility is tested using a nebulizer, a relatively large dose is administered producing a response on the flatter part of the dose–response curve. Precision of the administered dose is not critical to the test. FEV$_1$, forced expiratory volume in one second. (Redrawn from Lipworth BJ.* Am Rev Respir Dis *1990; **142**:338–42[67] with permission.)*

and analyzed. It also provokes bronchoconstriction and can be used as a method of measuring airway responsiveness. The mechanisms through which this occurs are poorly understood but probably include increased water fluxes across the airway epithelium, stimulation of cough receptors, and stimulation of the mucociliary escalator.[68]

The ability of hypertonic saline to provoke coughing and induce sputum production was exploited from the early 1980s as an alterative to bronchoscopy to detect *Pneumocystis carinii* infection in immunocompromised human immunodeficiency virus (HIV)-infected individuals.[69] Patients with *Pneumocystis* infection do not usually produce sputum spontaneously but induced coughing can produce samples from which the infecting organism can be detected.[70] Pin and colleagues then developed hypertonic saline challenges in the early 1990s to obtain specimens from normal and asthmatic subjects to investigate inflammatory cell and mediator profiles.[71] The technique is now widely used in research and occasionally to provide diagnostic information in individuals.[72]

Little attention has been paid to the standardization of techniques for sputum induction and a variety of protocols are used.[73] Specimens may be induced by nebulizing saline for a predetermined duration, or by incremental challenge either with increasing concentrations of saline or with increasing durations of nebulization. The method described by Pin involves premedication with 200 µg salbutamol 10 min before the start of the challenge and nebulization for six periods of 5 min using an ultrasonic nebulizer (Fisoneb; Fisons, Pickering, Ontario) with an output of 0.6 l/min and mean particle size of 5.9 µm. The saline concentration in the nebulizer is increased every 10 min from 3% to 4% to 5%. FEV_1 is monitored after each period of nebulization and the subject attempts to cough sputum into a container every 5 min after the initial 10 min. Adequate specimens can be obtained in about 80% of individuals.[71]

Although sputum induction can usually be carried out safely some precautions are necessary. Non-isotonic saline can provoke marked bronchoconstriction and one fatality has been reported.[74] Premedication with salbutamol is generally recommended and FEV_1 should be monitored during the procedure to avoid excessive bronchoconstriction. Monitoring of oxygen saturation is recommended if there is a risk of hypoxemia, for example, if patients with COPD are being studied.[73] When sputum is being induced to detect infection there is a risk of infecting staff and other patients particularly with tuberculosis and the procedure must be carried out in an appropriately ventilated room.

Ultrasonic nebulizers are generally preferred for sputum induction because of their higher mass output and denser aerosol which provokes greater coughing.[75] High output (3 ml/min) and low output (0.4 ml/min) nebulizers appear to be equally effective in inducing sputum samples[76] but the degree of bronchoconstriction is related to the amount of hypertonic saline inhaled and low output nebulizers are preferred when this might be a problem.[76] Many subjects find the procedure uncomfortable[75] but it is better tolerated with low output nebulizers and as they appear to provide adequate specimens their use is likely to become standard.[77] Hypertonic solutions are reportedly more effective than isotonic saline but it is possible to induce sputum samples with the latter.[75]

There is evidence that the method used for sputum induction can influence mediator concentrations in the specimens obtained and, potentially, the interpretation of immunological studies. Samples obtained with low output nebulizers contain higher concentrations of mediators such as eosinophilic cationic protein and interleukin (IL)-8 possibly because the

178

mediators are less diluted in the volume of inhaled saline.[78] Cell profiles alter with the duration of nebulization possibly because different parts of the lung are being sampled[78,79] and can be influenced by the saline concentration.[80] Other characteristics of the saline challenge such as particle size distribution of the aerosol might affect the test outcome by influencing the site of deposition. Further characterization and standardization of the technique are required.[73]

Radioaerosols

Radioactive aerosols have a number of important medical diagnostic uses. They are produced by a variety of means including jet and ultrasonic nebulizers.[81,82] Technegas is an aerosol of very small particles which is produced by evaporating a solution and heating it to very high temperatures and has physical properties similar to those of a gas.[83] Technetium-99 (^{99}Tc) is the most commonly used radionuclide for inhalation studies. Its chemistry allows it to be labeled to a wide variety of materials, it has an appropriate half life of 6 hours, it emits gamma rays of appropriate energy to allow counting, and it has negligible beta ray emission.

Ventilation scanning is the most commonly used application and in combination with perfusion scanning it has a high sensitivity for detecting pulmonary thromboembolism.[84] The technique can also be used to quantify regional lung function in patients undergoing assessment for lung surgery and in obstructive lung disease. The overall dose of aerosol delivered to the lung is of little importance and one common technique when both ^{99}Tc ventilation and perfusion images are required is to make the radioactivity of the second image much greater than that of the first so that any residual activity from the first image is swamped by the second. Small particle size distribution on the other hand is critical to avoid central airway deposition as this will result in poor quality images. Settling bags and gravitational settling techniques are commonly used for filtering the larger particles.

The characteristics of radioactive aerosols needed to measure mucociliary clearance are quite different from those required for ventilation scanning. Mucociliary clearance is impaired in a variety of conditions including cystic fibrosis and bronchiectasis. It is assessed by depositing ^{99}Tc sulfur colloid or similar particles in the central airways and observing the rate of clearance of the radioactivity. This is usually achieved with relatively large particles of

4–7 μm diameter produced using a spinning top generator and delivered as a bolus towards the end of inspiration. Lung permeability measurements assess the integrity of the alveolar–capillary interface. This requires soluble particles usually of ^{99}Tc diethylenetriaminepentaacetic acid (DTPA) with a small diameter of 0.5–1 μm delivered during tidal breathing over several minutes to allow peripheral alveolar deposition. A variety of nebulizers and filtering techniques have been used to achieve the correct particle size. Jet nebulizers might be preferable to ultrasonic nebulizers as concerns have been expressed about the dissociation of technetium DTPA by the latter[85] although this has not been found in all studies.[86]

Conclusions

The control of the output of nebulizers and the extent and site of aerosol deposition in the lungs are complex matters but are critical to a number of diagnostic uses of nebulizers. The issues have been most extensively investigated in relation to airway responsiveness measurements and the knowledge gained has had important implications for therapeutic as well as other diagnostic uses of nebulizers. New diagnostic uses for nebulizers continue to be developed, for example, sputum induction to assess airway inflammation and immunology. Characterizing the influence of the method of aerosol delivery still lags behind the clinical application of these tests yet, as with airway responsiveness measurements, subtle differences in aerosol characteristics might have marked influences on the test outcome. Further standardization of all clinical diagnostic uses of nebulizers is required.

References

1. American Thoracic Society. Guidelines for methacholine and exercise challenge testing – 1999. *Am J Respir Crit Care Med* 2000; **161**:309–29.
2. Barraclough R, Devereux G, Hendrick DJ, Stenton SC. Apparent but not real increase in asthma prevalence during the 1990s. *Eur Respir J* 2002; **20**:826–33.
3. Beach JR, Dennis JH, Avery AJ et al. An epidemiologic investigation of asthma in welders. *Am J Respir Crit Care Med* 1996; **154**:1394–400.
4. Devereux G, Hendrick DJ, Stenton SC. Asthmatic symptoms, airway hyperresponsiveness and the perception of bronchoconstriction. *Eur Respir J* 1998; **12**:1089–93.

5. Tashkin DP, Altose MD, Bleeker ER et al. The Lung Health Study: airway responsiveness to inhaled methacholine in smokers with mild to moderate airflow obstruction. *Am Rev Respir Dis* 1992; **145**:301–10.

6. Hendrick DJ, Burge PS. Occupational asthma. In: Hendrick DJ, Burge S, Beckett WS, Churg A eds. *Occupational disorders of the lung*. London: WB Saunders, 2002.

7. Perrin B, Lagier F, l'Archeveque J et al. Occupational asthma: validity of monitoring of peak expiratory flow rates and non-allergic bronchial responsiveness as compared to specific inhalation challenge. *Eur Respir J* 1992; **5**:40–8.

8. Stenton SC, Dennis JH, Hendrick DJ. Occupational asthma caused by ceftazidime. *Eur Respir J* 1995; **8**:1421–3.

9. Magnus P, Jaakkola J. Secular trend in the occurrence of asthma among children and young adults: critical appraisal of repeated cross sectional surveys. *BMJ* 1997; **314**:1795–9.

10. Chinn S, Burney P, Jarvis D, Luczynska CM. Variation in bronchial responsiveness in the European Community Respiratory Health Survey (ECRHS). *Eur Respir J* 1997; **10**:2495–501.

11. Chinn S, Arossa WA, Jarvid DJ, Luczynska CM, Bruney PGJ. Variation in nebulizer aerosol output from the Mefar dosimeter: implications for multicentre studies. *Eur Respir J* 1997; **10**:452–6.

12. Ward RJ, Reid DW, Walters EH, Hendrick DJ. Calibration of aerosol output from the Mefar dosimeter. Implications for epidemiological studies. *Eur Respir J* 1992; **5**:1279–82.

13. Hartley-Sharpe CJ, Booth H, Johns DP, Walters EH. Differences in aerosol output and airways responsiveness between the DeVilbiss 44 and 45 hand held nebulizers. *Thorax* 1995; **50**:635–8.

14. Sterk PJ, Fabbri LM, Quanjer PH et al. Airway responsiveness. Standardized challenge testing with pharmacological, physical and sensitizing stimuli in adults. *Eur Respir J* 1993; Suppl 16:53–83.

15. Beach JR, Young CL, Stenton SC et al. Measurement of airway responsiveness to methacholine: the relative importance of the precision of drug delivery and the method of assessing the response. *Thorax* 1993; **48**:133–5.

16. Stenton SC, Dennis JH. Diagnostic uses of nebulizers. *Eur Respir Rev* 2001; **10**:567–70.

17. Ryan G, Dolovich MB, Obminski G et al. Standardization of inhalation provocation tests: influence of nebulizer output, particle size, method of inhalation. *J Allergy Clin Immunol* 1981; **67**:156–61.

18. Cockroft DW, Hursst TS, Gore BP. Importance of evaporative water losses during standardized nebulized inhalation provocation tests. *Chest* 1989; **96**:505–8.

19. Dennis JH, Stenton SC, Beach JR et al. Jet and ultrasonic nebulizer output: use of a new method for direct measurement of aerosol output. *Thorax* 1990; **45**:728–32.

20. Tandon R, McPeck M, Smaldone GC. Aerosol production vs gravimetric analysis. *Chest* 1997; **111**:1361–5.

21. Dennis JH, Avery AJ, Walters EH, Hendrick DJ. Calibration of aerosol output from the Mefar dosimeter: implications for epidemiological studies. *Eur Respir J* 1992; **5**:1279–82.

22. Gatnash AA, Chandler ST, Connolly CK. A new method for measuring aerosol nebulizer output using radioactive tracers. *Eur Respir J* 1998; **12**:467–71.

23. Ward RJ, Reid DW, Leonard RF, Johns DP, Walters EH. Nebulizer calibration using lithium chloride: an accurate, reproducible, user-friendly method. *Eur Respir J* 1998; **11**:937–41.

24. Ward RJ, Ward C, Johns DP et al. European Community Respiratory Health Survey calibration project of dosimeter driving pressures. *Eur Respir J* 2002; **19**:252–6.

25. Ward RJ, Liakakos P, Leonard RF et al. A critical evaluation of the Mefar dosimeter. *Eur Respir J* 1999; **14**:430–4.

26. Devereux G, Hendrick DJ, Stenton SC. Asthmatic symptoms, airway hyperresponsiveness and the perception of bronchoconstriction. *Eur Respir J* 1998; **12**:1089–93.

27. Nerbrink O, Dennis JH, Pagel J, Pieron C. Technical aspects of nebulizers used in dosimetry. *Eur Respir J* 2000; **10**:232–7.

28. Peat JK, van der Berg RH, Green WF et al. Changing prevalence of asthma in Australian children. *BMJ* 1994; **308**:1591–6.

29. Hartley-Sharpe CJ, Booth H, Johns DP, Walters EH. Differences in aerosol output and airways responsiveness between the DeVilbiss 44 and 45 hand held nebulizers. *Thorax* 1995; **50**:635–8.

30. Sterk PJ, Plomb A, van de Vate JF, Quanjier PH. Physical properties of aerosols produced by several jet and ultrasonic nebulizers. *Bull Eur Physiopathol Respir* 1984; **20**:65–72.

31. Standaert TA, Morlin GL, Williams-Warren J et al. Effects of repetitive use and cleaning techniques of disposable jet nebulizers on aerosol generation. *Chest* 1998; **114**:577–86.

32. Thomas SHL, O'Docherty MJ, Page CJ, Nunan TG. Variability in the measurement of nebulized aerosol deposition in man. *Clin Sci* 1991; **81**:767–75.

33. Hollie MC, Malone RA, Skufca RM et al. Extreme variability in aerosol output of the De Vilbiss 646 jet nebulizer. *Chest* 1991; **100**:1339–44.

34. Mercer TT, Goddard RF, Flores RL. Effect of auxilliary airflow on the output characteristics of compressed air nebulizers. *Ann Allergy* 1969; **27**:211–17.

35. Clay ME, Clarke SW. Effect of nebulised aerosol size on lung deposition in patients with mild asthma. *Thorax* 1987; **42**:190–4.

36. Clarke AR. The use of laser defraction for the evaluation of the aerosol clouds generated by medical nebulizers. *Int J Pharm* 1995; **115**:69–78.

37. Nerbrink O, Dahlback M. Basic nebulizer function. *J Aerosol Med* 1994; **7**(Suppl 1): S7–S11.

38. Rudolph G, Kobrich R, Stahlhofen W. Modelling and algebraic formulation of regional aerosol deposition in man. *J Aerosol Sci* 1990; **21**(Suppl 1):S306–S406.

39. Clay MM, Pavia D, Newman SP, Lennard-Jones T, Clarke SW. Assessment of jet nebulizers for lung aerosol therapy. *Lancet* 1983; **2**:592–4.

40. Ruffin RE, Dolovich MB, Wolff RK, Newhouse MT. The effects of preferential deposition of histamine in the human airway. *Am Rev Respir Dis* 1978; **117**:485–92.

41. Brain JD, Valberg PA, Sneddon S. Mechanisms of aerosol deposition and clearance. In: Moren F ed. *Aerosols in Medicine*. London: Elsevier, 1985.

42. Ferron GA. Modelling of aerosol solution droplets between production by jet nebulizers and human respiration. *Eur Respir Rev* 2000; **10**:192–8.

43. Ferron GA, Haider B, Kreyling WG. Inhalation of salt aerosol particles – I. Estimation of the temperature and relative humidity in the upper human airways. *J Aerosol Sci* 1988; **19**:343–63.

44. Ferron GA, Soderholm SC. Estimation of the times for evaporation of pure water droplets and for stabilization of salt solution particles. *J Aerosol Sci* 1990; **21**:415–29.

45. Phipps PR, Gonda I. Droplets produced by medical nebulizers. Some factors affecting their size and solute concentration. *Chest* 1990; **97**:1327–32.

46. Nerbrink OL, Lindstrom M, Meurling L, Svartengren M. Inhalation and deposition of nebulized sodium cromoglycate in two different particle size distributions in children with asthma. *Pediatr Pulmonol* 2002; **34**:351–60.

47. Stapleton KW, Finlay WH. Errors in characterizing nebulized particle size distributions with cascade impactors. *J Aerosol Med* 1998; **11**(Suppl 1):S80–S83.

48. Dennis JH, Pieron CA, Nerbrink O. Standards in assessing in vitro nebulizer performance. *Eur Respir Rev* 2000; **10**:178–82.

49. Ilowite JS, Gorvoy JD, Smaldone GC. Quantitative deposition of aerosolised gentamycin in cystic fibrosis. *Am Rev Respir Dis* 1987; **136**:1445–9.

50. Madsen F, Frolund L, Nielsen NH, Svendsen UG, Weeke B. Bronchial challenge: ventilation during 'tidal volume breathing' inhalation is not constant. *Bull Eur Physiopathol Respir* 1986; **22**:517–22.

51. Laube BL, Adams GK, Norman PS, Rosenthal RR. The effect of inspiratory flow rate regulation on nebulizer output and on human airway response to methacholine aerosol. *J Allergy Clin Immunol* 1988; **76**:708–13.

52. Wanner A, Brodnan JM, Perez J, Henke KG, Kim CS. Variability of airway responsiveness to histamine aerosol in normal subjects. Role of deposition. *Am Rev Respir Dis* 1985; **131**:3–7.

53. Clay MM, Pavia D, Newman SP, Clarke SW. Factors influencing the size distribution of aerosols from jet nebulizers. *Thorax* 1983; **38**:755–9.

54. Kongerud J, Soyseth V, Johansen B. Room temperature influences output from the Wright jet nebulizer. *Eur Respir J* 1989; **2**:681–4.

55. Stenton SC. Determinants of whether occupational agents cause early, late, or dual asthmatic responses. *Occup Med* 2000; **15**:431–44.

56. Blanc P, Toren K. How much asthma can be attributed to occupational factors. *Am J Med* 1999; **107**:580–7.

57. Weir D, Obertson AS, Jones S, Burge PS. The economic consequences of developing occupational asthma. *Thorax* 1987; **42**:209.

58. Stenton S, Dennis JH, Walters EH, Hendrick DJ. The asthmagenic properties of a newly developed detergent ingredient – sodium iso-nonoyl oxybenzene sulphonate. *Br J Industr Med* 1990; **47**:405–10.

59. Doherty MJ, Mister R, Pearson MG, Calverley PMA. Capsaicin responsiveness and cough in asthma and chronic obstructive pulmonary disease. *Thorax* 2000; **55**:643–9.

60. National Institutes of Health. Global initiative for chronic obstructive lung disease. Publication number 2701. 2001.

61. Thomas SHL, O'Docherty MJ, Page CJ, Nunan TG. Variability in the measurement of nebulized aerosol deposition in man. *Clin Sci* 1991; **81**:767–75.

62. Dahlback M. Behaviour of nebulizing solutions as suspensions. *J Aerosol Med* 1997; **7**(Suppl 1):S13–S18.

63. Coates AL, MacNeish CF, Meisner D et al The choice of jet nebulizer, nebulizing flow, and addition of albuterol affects the output of tobramycin aerosols. *Chest* 1997; **111**:1206–12.

64. Wagner MH, Wiethoff S, Friedrich W et al. Ultrasonic surfactant nebulization with different exciting frequencies. *Biophys Chem* 2000; **84**:35–43.

65. Takanami C, Goto Y. Physical properties of antibiotic aerosols produced by jet and ultrasonic nebulizers. *J Aerosol Med* 1990; **3**:45–52.

66. Chung KF. Measurement and assessment of cough and the cough reflex. *Eur Respir Rev* 2002; **12**:226–30.

67. Lipworth BJ, Clark RA, Dhillon DP, McDevitt DG. Comparison of the effects of prolonged treatment with low and high doses of inhaled terbulaline on beta-adrenoceptor responsiveness in patients with chronic obstructive pulmonary disease. *Am Rev Respir Dis* 1990; **142**:338–42.

68. Pavord ID, Pizzichini MM, Pizzichini E, Hargreave FE. The use of induced sputum to investigate airway inflammation. *Thorax* 1997; **52**:498–501.

69. Pitchenik AE, Gaanjei P, Tporres A et al. Sputum examination for the diagnosis of *Pneumocystis carinii* pneumonia in the acquired immunodeficiency syndrome. *Am Rev Respir Dis* 1986; **133**:226–9.

70. Shimomoto H, Hasegawa Y, Takagi N et al. Detection of *Pneumocystis carinii*, *Mycobacterium tuberculosis*, and cytomegalovirus in human immunodeficiency virus (HIV)-infected patients with hemophilia by polymerase chain reaction of induced sputum samples. *Intern Med* 1995; **34**:976–81.

71. Pin I, Gibson PG, Kolendowicz R et al. Use of induced sputum cell counts to investigate airway inflammation in asthma. *Thorax* 1992; **1145**:1265–9.

72. Hargreave FE. Induced sputum for the investigation of airway inflammation: evidence for its clinical application. *Can Respir J* 1999; **6**:169–74.

73. Paggiaro PL. Sputum induction. *Eur Respir J* 2002; **20**(Suppl 37):3S–8S.

74. Saetta M, Di Stefanon A, Turato G et al. Fatal asthma attack during inhlation challentge with ultrasonically nebulized distilled water. *J Allergy Clin Immunol* 1995; **95**:1285–7.

75. Popov TA, Pizzichini MMM, Pizzichini E. Some technical factors influencing the induction of sputum for cell analysis. *Eur Respir J* 1995; **8**:559–65.

76. Kelly MG, Brown V, Martin SL, Ennis M, Elborn JS. Comparison of sputum induction using high-output and low-output ultrasonic nebulizers in normal subjects and patients with COPD. *Chest* 2002; **122**:955–9.

77. Hunter CJ, Ward R, Woltman G, Wardlaw AJ, Pavord ID. The safety and success rate of sputum induction using a low output ultrasonic nebulizer. *Respir Med* 1999; **93**:345–8.

78. Belda J, Hussack P, Dolovich M, Efthimiadis A, Hargreave FE. Sputum induction: effect of nebulizer output and inhalation time on cell counts and fluid-phase measures. *Clin Exp Allergy* 2001; **31**:1740–4.

79. Gershman NH, Liu H, Wong H, Liu JT, Fahy JV. Fractional analysis of sequential induced sputum samples during sputum induction: evidence that different lung com-

partments are sampled at different time points. *J Allergy Clin Immunol* 1999; **104**:322–8.

80. Bacci E, Carnevali S, Cianchetti S et al. Comparison between hypertonic saline and normal saline-induced sputum in asthmatic subjects. *Am Rev Respir Dis* 1994; **149**:A571.

81. Taplin GV, Poe ND. A dual lung scanning technique for the evaluation of pulmonary function. *Radiology* 1965; **85**:365–8.

82. O'Docherty MJ, Miller RF. Aerosols for therapy and diagnosis. *Eur J Nucl Med* 1993; **200**:1201–13.

83. Burch WM, Sullivan PJ, McLaren CJ. Technegas – a new ventilation agent for lung scanning. *Nucl Med Comm* 1986; **7**:865–71.

84. The PIOPED Investigators. Value of the ventilation/perfusion scan in acute pulmonary embolism. Results of the prospective investigation of pulmonary embolism diagnosis (PIOPED). *JAMA* 1990; **263**:2753–9.

85. Waldman DL, Weber DA, Oberdorster G et al. Chemical breakdown of technetium-99m DTPA during nebulization. *J Nucl Med* 1987; **28**:378–82.

86. Groth S, Funch-Rosenberg H, Mortensen J, Rossing N. Technetium-99m DTPA does not break down during ultrasound nebulization. *Clin Physiol* 1989; **9**:151–9.

10. PEDIATRIC USES OF NEBULIZERS

Peter W Barry

Introduction

Nebulizers are useful devices for delivering inhaled medications to children. In contrast to many other inhalation drug delivery devices, much less patient cooperation is required – a resource that is often in short supply with younger patients! Furthermore, almost any drug can be delivered by nebulization, and nebulized therapy provides a potential portal of entry for systemic drug treatment as well as for the direct treatment of respiratory diseases.

Specific factors need to be borne in mind when considering nebulizer therapy for children. Anatomical, physiological and developmental differences mean that data derived from adult studies cannot necessarily be used to guide choice of device or therapy. Practical difficulties arise in pediatric therapy that require specific and innovative responses from the device manufacturer and the care-giver. These issues will be discussed in this chapter.

Why use nebulizers?

Traditional nebulizers are bulky, expensive and inconvenient to use, requiring a power source and prolonged treatment time. In the routine treatment of pediatric asthma, metered dose inhalers (MDIs) with spacer devices or dry powder inhalers have been shown to have a similar efficacy to nebulizers, and have largely replaced them. However, in the treatment of acute severe asthma the nebulizer is still commonly used, and programs to replace them may be resisted by staff and parents.[1,2] Traditional nebulizer use should be limited to delivering high-dose therapy, to delivering therapy not available in other forms or special situations where other drug delivery devices are not tolerated by the patient or are not practical.

Newer nebulizers – smaller, perhaps with their own power source, and with added features, such as compliance monitors or end of treatment indicators – are being developed, and their place in the family of drug delivery devices is yet to be fully established. They may be particularly useful in delivering drug to uncooperative patients like children, and in delivering high cost drugs or those with a narrow therapeutic window where dosage needs to be more tightly controlled.

Where nebulizers are used, careful attention should be paid to optimizing delivery by selecting an appropriate nebulizer, using an adequate driving gas flow, and ensuring that the face mask or mouthpiece is used correctly. The success of therapy will depend on selecting a device and regime that the patient will comply with, and giving clear written guidelines for nebulizer use.

Inhalation therapy in children[3,4]

A number of problems arise in evaluating and administrating nebulized therapy in children. These include anatomical and physiological variations due to age, difficulty in knowing the dose received by the patient and compliance with nebulized therapy.

Anatomical and physiological differences between children and adults

Children differ from adults in size, in the relative proportions of the structures of the lung and upper airway, and in their lung function. These factors all change during childhood and affect the deposition and response to inhalation therapy in children of different ages.

Size

The upper airway is relatively large in children compared to adults, although the nose is an effective filter in children, and is often blocked with secretions. Nasal inhalation reduces lung deposition of aerosols,[5] and inhalation through the mouth is preferred to nasal inhalation. However, in childhood the oral cavity and oropharynx are themselves crowded with a relatively large tongue and tonsils. The effect of these structures on inhaled therapy is not known.

The lower airways of infants are narrow, and a small amount of airway narrowing due to bronchospasm, inflammation or secretions may result in a marked increase in airway resistance, encouraging central airways deposition.[6] Nebulized aerosols are more unevenly distributed with more central deposition in subjects with bronchoconstriction compared to those with normal lung function.[7,8] For these reasons, the optimum particle size for inhaled therapy may be smaller in children than adults, and smaller still for children with lung disease. Producing aerosols with smaller droplets will mean selecting an appropriate nebulizer design and usually lengthening nebulization times – issues that may affect cost and compliance. Also, it may be impossible to nebulize some medications in small enough particles to produce a therapeutic effect.[9]

Lack of effect of certain drugs in children compared to adults

Not all drugs used in adult practice will have the same effects when administered to children. For instance, young children may wheeze when they get an upper respiratory tract infection, and there may be little response to beta-2-agonists, even though infants do have functional beta-2 receptors. The administration of bronchodilators may lead to a worsening of symptoms, as the infant's small airways lose their tone and collapse, particularly during expiration. A reduction in oxygen saturation following nebulized beta-2-agonists has also been described in young infants, possibly because the drug opens up airways leading to underperfused alveoli, and worsening ventilation–perfusion mismatching.

Breathing pattern

For most traditional nebulizers, aerosol output is fixed by the driving gas flow and the design of the nebulizer, and is constant throughout drug delivery. A child's inspiratory flow, by contrast, will vary according to the respiratory pattern. Thus any aerosol released during expiration will not be inhaled and will be wasted (Figure 10.1). Children who spend longer in expiration, for instance with a prolonged expiratory phase due to airways obstruction or crying[10] will inhale less drug from conventional jet nebulizers. The breathing pattern of a particular child may be variable, with periods of irregular breathing when little aerosol is inhaled.[11] If at all possible, quiet breathing with slow inhalation from residual volume should be encouraged.

Children may also not cooperate whilst receiving their medication, and may breathe through the nose. Another problem with nasal breathing was highlighted in older children using the mouthpiece of a spacer device, where therapeutic failures were attributed to inappropriate inhalation through the nose rather than the mouthpiece.[12] These factors may explain the large variability in lung deposition and drug effects in children. Inhalation training is necessary for all children prescribed a nebulizer.

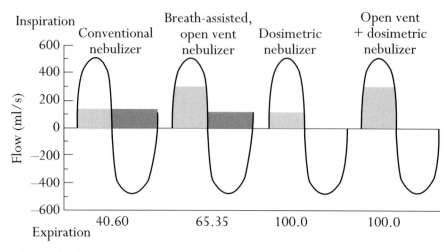

Figure 10.1 *Graph showing aerosol output, which is fixed by the driving gas flow and the design of most traditional nebulizers, and is constant throughout drug delivery. However, a child's inspiratory flow will vary according to the respiratory pattern. Therefore, any aerosol released during expiration will not be inhaled, and will be wasted. (Modified from Nikander K. Drug delivery systems. J Aerosol Med 1994; 7:519–24.)*

Breathing pattern may also affect the site of deposition within the respiratory tract. Fast inspiration encourages inertial impaction of drug in the upper airways, and more central deposition.[13] Slow inspiration increases lung delivery of drug from conventional jet nebulizers.[14] Breath holding at the end of inspiration increases deposition by giving time for drug particles to settle in the lung with gravity, but will also lessen the total dose inhaled from continuously running nebulizers as proportionally less time is spent in inhalation (see above).

Entrainment
This occurs when the child's inspiratory flow rate exceeds the nebulizer output. In conventional jet nebulizers, the aerosol is carried in a volume of air dependent upon the driving gas flow and the nebulizer design. If the child's inspiratory flow exceeds this, additional air will be entrained from the surrounding atmosphere. Only the youngest children have peak inspiratory flows lower than commonly used nebulizer outputs (Figure 10.2), and for the others aerosol will be diluted by entrained air.[15] For this type of nebulizer, the mass of drug inhaled with each breath remains constant throughout most of childhood, despite the fact that the body mass increases five-fold or more. So the mass of drug inhaled per

190

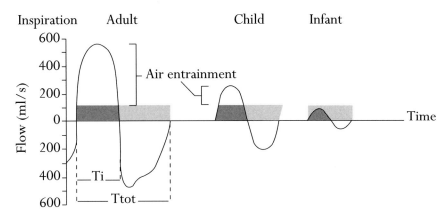

Figure 10.2 *If the child's inspiratory flow exceeds the nebulizer output, additional air will be entrained from the surrounding atmosphere. Only the youngest children have peak inspiratory flows lower than commonly used nebulizer outputs, so for older children aerosol will be diluted by entrained air. Ti, inspiratory time; Ttot, total time for one breath.*

kilogram body weight is constant until air entrainment occurs, and then reduces with size (Figure 10.3). A consequence is that small children may be overdosed and larger children undertreated if this is not taken into account. Some centers recommend age, weight or surface area correcting the concentration of drug placed in the nebulizer, and this is further discussed below. Another approach is to nebulize the medication into a spacer or holding chamber, so that all of the child's inspiration consists of aerosol cloud.[16]

With 'breath-enhanced' nebulizers, aerosol output is increased during inspiration. Where this enhancement is proportional to or greater than the child's inspiratory flow, drug delivery per kilogram body weight will be constant as the child gets bigger. However, once inspiratory flow increases above the (enhanced) nebulizer output, reduction of dose relative to weight again occurs, in a way similar to constant output nebulizers.

Newer designs of nebulizers have been produced, which electronically control drug output, only delivering drug during inspiration, at flows less than the peak inspiratory flow (so no drug is wasted), and calculate from the breathing parameters when a preset mass of drug has been inhaled.[17] Such devices are, however, costly, and it may be difficult to justify their use to deliver drugs that are inexpensive and have a wide therapeutic ratio.

191

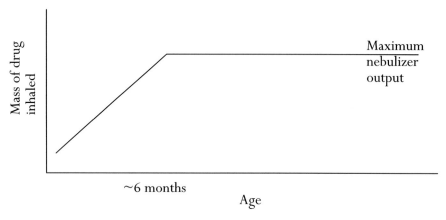

Figure 10.3 *Graph showing that the mass of drug inhaled increases with size until air entrainment occurs, and then is constant.*

Should the nominal drug dose be varied with age or size?

It is clear that the amount of drug placed in the nebulizer chamber is not the only determinant of the amount of drug reaching the desired site in the patient. Patient age and size may affect drug dosage, and it is routine practice in many units to vary the nominal prescribed dose with patient size. The published data on this are conflicting.

Assuming that approximately 10% of a nebulized dose is deposited in the lungs of an adult, the dose per kilogram body weight can be calculated. For example, a 70 kg adult will receive 0.14%/kg (i.e. 10% ÷ 70). Data from pediatric studies[18] suggest that up to 1.5% of drug nebulized from a conventional jet nebulizer will be deposited in the lungs of infants and young children (6–36 months of age). A 1-year-old, weighing, for instance 10 kg, would receive 0.15%/kg. This suggests that although there may be poor drug deposition in infant lungs, this is compensated for by their small size, so that the final dose reaching the lungs per kilogram body weight may be very similar to that of an adult. This further suggests that the same nominal drug dose should be used in all age groups.

Conversely, considering the effect of entrainment (discussed above), others have suggested a different approach[19] (Figures 10.3 and 10.4), reducing the nominal drug dose for infants who do not dilute inhaled aerosol with entrained air. For conventional jet nebulizers, this is the most appropriate dosing strategy.

In practice, most inhaled medications in current use in pediatrics are relatively non-toxic with a wide therapeutic ratio, so large doses may be placed

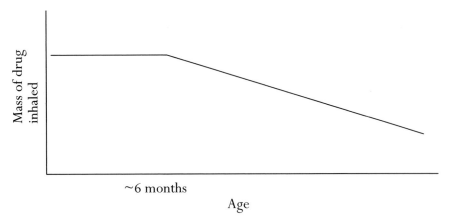

Figure 10.4 *Graph showing that the mass of drug inhaled per kilogram body weight is constant until air entrainment occurs, and then reduces with size.*

in a nebulizer to get adequate doses in the lung. For newer, more expensive medications, or those with greater toxicity, more accurate knowledge of the dose actually delivered to the patient will be needed.

Compliance[20]

Patient compliance with inhaled medication is poor. In clinical studies, irrespective of whether drug administration was undertaken by children themselves or supervised by a parent, compliance with inhaled medication was less than 50%.[21,22] Patients whose compliance is poor have an increased risk of exacerbations, and this may increase the risks of fatal asthma.[23-25]

The most effective inhaler for any given patient is the one that the patient will use on a regular basis and in an effective manner. Nebulizer design factors that improve compliance are not known. Factors that *may* improve compliance are listed in Box 10.1[20] and those of particular relevance to children are discussed below.

Size: Small, unobtrusive devices are often marketed on the basis that they are more acceptable to the patient, and will therefore be used more. They may also be less frightening to patients. There is, however, little evidence that compliance is improved by changing to a different nebulizer.

Appearance: There is no doubt that the appearance and style of an object can affect its acceptability by a consumer, and also affect perceptions of the object's

---

Box 10.1 Factors that may improve compliance for inhalers.

Size (portability, obtrusiveness)
Color (material, decoration)
Noise
Power (battery/car adaptor/mains)
Administration time
Multiple dosage
End of life/treatment/dose remaining indicators
Effectiveness?
Interaction with patient/feedback?
Fashion

---

effectiveness. In pediatric practice, one company produces attachments for their nebulizers that give them the appearance of a cartoon character.[26] Many therapists advise children and parents to 'personalize' their devices with stickers of famous television or film characters. Although there is no research evidence to suggest that this affects device acceptability or compliance, it seems to be a reasonable tactic and is widely accepted by parents in relation to other commodities.

Noise: Jet nebulizers can be noisy and this may frighten children, and reduce acceptability and compliance. As noted above, crying during nebulization reduces lung deposition.

Administration time: Despite research documenting the reduction in nebulizer output after a relatively short period of time,[27,28] nebulizers continue to be used 'until dryness' or 'until spluttering occurs'. High output nebulizers have been developed that deliver medication quickly, and are said to improve patient acceptability. However, the high output may also lead to increased drug wastage to the environment and paradoxically reduce drug delivery,[28] particularly to infants with small tidal volumes.

End of life/end of treatment/dose remaining indicators: The facility available in some devices that indicates when drug administration is completed may also improve device acceptability. This may take the form of a simple on/off indicator after a certain time, a detector when the nebulizer chamber is empty or a more sophisticated detector that measures the volume of aerosol leaving the device.[29]

Face masks, mouthpieces and nose clips

Nebulizers should be used with a mouthpiece or a tightly fitting face mask. A mouthpiece is preferred, as its use has been shown to improve lung deposition and changes in lung function compared with use of a face mask.[30]

It is important to ensure that the mouthpiece is used properly, as children may inhale around it, block it with their tongue, or inhale through their nose. The carer should be instructed to observe the aerosol cloud arising from the exhalation area of the mouthpiece. If there is no difference in the appearance of this during inhalation and exhalation, it is likely that the child is not breathing through the mouthpiece. Nose clips may be used to promote mouth breathing, but these are not often tolerated. The type of nebulizer is also important. For children using jet nebulizers with mouthpiece, breath-synchronized nebulization may improve delivery compared to constant output nebulizers.[31]

Face masks may be used in those children too young to use mouthpieces. However, face masks are poorly tolerated by many children, and are associated with crying in a significant number of patients, particularly the youngest. Crying is known to reduce lung deposition of nebulized drug. In one study, crying also influenced the acceptance of the face mask, reduced parental compliance and made the use of inhalation devices more difficult.[32]

Not all face masks are equally effective, with some providing a poor seal with the face, leading to reduced or more variable dose delivery.[33] Inhalation through a face mask 2–3 cm from the face, which is often seen, will reduce drug delivery to the patient by approximately 50% in school children, with a corresponding increase in release of aerosol to the environment.[34] The face mask seal is critical for efficient aerosol delivery to infants and young children, and this should be stressed to patients and their parents.[35]

Choice of nebulizer

Factors to consider when choosing a nebulizer for children are summarized in Table 10.1[3] and further discussed below.

Table 10.1 Factors to consider when choosing a nebulizer.

Patient factors

Age	'Open vent' nebulizers may be unsuitable for young children
	Is a mouthpiece or face mask to be used?
Compliance	What is the optimum nebulization time with the proposed drug and nebulizer? Can treatment frequency be minimized?
Lifestyle	Are size and portability important?
Breathing pattern	The optimum breathing pattern is not known, but children should at least be encouraged to mouth breathe, and light nose clips should be considered. A low respiratory rate with high tidal volumes and mouth breathing may be preferred.

Drug factors

Suspension or solutions	Some nebulizers are inappropriate for drug suspensions (e.g. budesonide) – i.e. ultrasonic nebulizers and jet nebulizers that produce particularly small particles
Viscosity	Viscous solutions are not nebulized by some nebulizers
Site of deposition	Smaller particles for alveolar deposition, but are these needed for steroids or beta-2-agonists?
Bioavailability	Increasing the dose to the lungs may also increase systemic drug effects

Technical factors

Drug output	Choose the nebulizer with the highest respirable output in the shortest time.
Optimum compressor	Choice of compressor may vary the output of the nebulizer considerably, and should be chosen with a particular drug and nebulizer in mind.
Volume fill	The larger volume fill will deliver more drug, but will increase the nebulization time.
Nebulization time	The patient should use the nebulizer for a specific time, not 'to dryness' or 'until spluttering occurs'

Other factors

Cost	
Durability	
Cleaning	Single patient use – wash in soap and hot water after use, rinse and dry. How often?
Servicing	Regular checks of compressors needed – who will do them and how much will it cost?
Patient education	Written and oral instructions to include: how and when to use the nebulizer, how much drug to be used and how long to continue nebulization; what to do if the nebulizer does not provide the usual therapeutic benefit or malfunctions

Patient factors

Age: As discussed above, nebulizer output should ideally be tailored to inspiratory flow, with increased output during inspiration, and minimal output during expiration or respiratory pauses. High output 'open vent' nebulizers may be unsuitable for young children, as drug is lost during both inspiration and expiration.

A mouthpiece should be used where possible, but in younger children this may not be used correctly and a nebulizer with a comfortable, close fitting face mask should be chosen. Not all face masks are the same, and drug delivery from a particular device may vary by a factor of 10 or more, depending on the face mask used.

Breathing pattern: The optimum breathing pattern is not known, but children should at least be encouraged to mouth breathe, and light nose clips should be considered, if tolerated (they rarely are!). A low respiratory rate with short expiratory times and mouth breathing will optimize drug delivery, but it may be difficult to teach this, and quiet tidal breathing, aided by distraction therapy such as a story, video or computer game, is a good compromise.

Compliance: Where possible, choose a nebulizer with a short administration time, and consider whether treatment frequency can be minimized. Compliance with nebulized therapy may be improved by allowing the patient or family to be involved in device selection.

Lifestyle: Are size and portability important to the patient or their family? It may be necessary to compromise on other areas of device selection in order to pick a device that the family will actually use.

Is the nebulizer to be used for prophylactic therapy at home, or is it needed for emergency treatment, or treatment outside, for instance prior to sports in exercise-induced asthma? In this case, an alternative to mains power is important, and issues such as battery life, practicalities of recharging and battery cost must be considered.

Drug factors

Suspension or solutions: Some nebulizers are inappropriate for drug suspensions (e.g. some steroid formulations). For instance ultrasonic nebulizers do not aerosolize suspensions effectively. Jet nebulizers that produce small particles may only release particles of solvent, leaving the larger drug particles in the nebulizer.

Viscosity: Viscous solutions such as some antibiotic solutions are not aerosolized effectively by lower powered nebulizers.

Complex drugs and formulations: The force of jet nebulization may degrade complex drugs, as may the heating of nebulized liquid that occurs with some ultrasonic nebulizers. Certain drugs may have been assessed with particular nebulizers in clinical trials. If alternative nebulizers are used, it is important to ensure that they have also been adequately assessed and are capable of nebulizing that particular drug.

Site of deposition: Nebulizer choice may be used to crudely target drug delivery. For instance, nebulizers producing smaller particles may be preferred for alveolar deposition. Often, however, the optimal site of drug deposition is not known.

Bioavailability: Drug depositing in the lungs may be absorbed into the circulation and be distributed around the body. Changing to a more effective nebulizer or drug delivery system may, by increasing the dose to the lungs, also increase systemic drug effects. This is particularly important with children when using drugs such as inhaled steroids that may have serious systemic effects.

Other factors
Cost: Depending on the healthcare system, this may be a significant consideration for the patient and their family.

Patient and parent education: The nebulizer and compressor should be simple to assemble and use. Written and oral instructions should be given to the patient and his or her carers. These should include: how and when to use the nebulizer; how much drug to be used and how long to continue nebulization; what to do if the nebulizer does not provide the usual therapeutic benefit or if it malfunctions.

Clinical indications for nebulized therapy[3]

Clinical indications for nebulized therapy, grouped by disease process, are discussed below. The indications are not exhaustive, but do cover the majority of cases where nebulized therapy may be considered. Cystic fibrosis is covered elsewhere in this book (Chapters 7 and 8).

Severe acute asthma

In the treatment of asthma, nebulizers are used for acute attacks and to treat children unable or unwilling to cooperate with spacers or other handheld inhalers. Frequent nebulization of bronchodilators to children with severe acute asthma has become common practice in many centers in the first hours after admission. Continuous nebulized therapy may be used in the intensive care setting for those with very severe asthma. It improves clinical scores and gas exchange in children with severe asthma and may reduce hospitalization time,[36,37] although not all studies have found continuous nebulization to be preferable.[38] Nebulizers with large volume fills may be used, specifically designed for continuous nebulization,[39] or the nebulizer chamber may be constantly refilled from a syringe pump (Figure 10.5).

Hypoxia and ventilation–perfusion mismatching may occur in severe acute asthma. For this reason, oxygen should be used as the driving gas for nebulizers used to deliver therapy. Recent reports have shown some benefit of using helium–oxygen mixtures (heliox) as the driving gas.[40,41] The lower density of the gas improves the deposition profile of the inhaled medication, and reduces the patient's work of breathing. Equipment calibrated for use

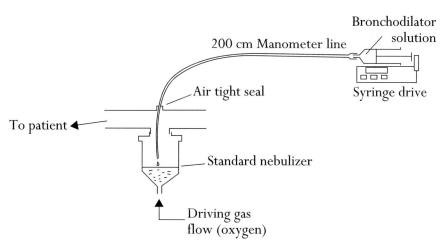

Figure 10.5 *System for giving continuously nebulized bronchodilators in severe acute asthma. The syringe pump continuously replaces bronchodilator solution that is lost by either nebulization or evaporation. The rate of the syringe pump delivery required will depend on the type and make of nebulizer used.*

with heliox should be used, and the driving gas flow will need to be altered to maintain nebulizer output. Another disadvantage is that high concentrations of oxygen cannot be given without reducing the concentration (and hence the effect) of helium. Studies demonstrating significant benefit of heliox to deliver aerosols in children are awaited.

MDIs used with spacer devices provide an effective and cheaper alternative to nebulizers. Bronchodilators delivered by MDI and spacer are as effective as those delivered via nebulizer and have fewer side effects. They may be used both in acute asthma for drug delivery to infants and to deliver inhaled steroids to infants and older children. Delay between MDI actuation and inhalation and multiple actuations into the spacer prior to inhalation should be avoided. The use of a spacer and MDI in preference to a nebulizer is cheaper, but changing the practice of parents and medical staff who have previously viewed nebulizer therapy as the 'gold standard' may be difficult.

There have been anecdotal suggestions that young children respond less well to bronchodilators given by spacer and MDI than nebulizer, possibly because young children cannot produce sufficient flow rates to open the spacer valve. It is important for carers to check this during drug administration. In any comparison of nebulizers and spacer devices, it is important to be aware of the different factors that affect drug output from spacers, to avoid inappropriate conclusions being drawn.[43]

Beta-2-agonists

Beta-2-agonists are the mainstay of therapy in severe acute asthma. They act rapidly, may be given in different doses according to clinical need, and have a wide therapeutic ratio. Mention has already been made of their use in continuous nebulization, but frequent, repeated nebulization is also effective.

Anticholinergics

Anticholinergics are also effective when given in addition to beta-2-agonists in the emergency department, particularly in older children where they reduce the time to discharge and medication requirements in hospital. Their role in younger children is less clear,[44] with little evidence of additional benefit compared with beta-2-agonists alone in children under 2 years of age. Outside the emergency department, studies suggest that the use of anticholinergic drugs does not reduce the overall admission rate of children with severe acute asthma.[45,46] Nevertheless, current practice and guidelines

200

would suggest that they be added to beta-2-agonist therapy in acute pediatric asthma.

Corticosteroids

A short course of a systemic corticosteroid, such as prednisolone, is normally given in a severe asthma attack. Although inhaled steroids have been used as a treatment of severe acute asthma in some studies via dry powder inhalers or MDI and spacers[47,48] they have not replaced oral or intravenous therapy.

Chronic asthma

Beta-2-agonists

As in acute asthma, beta-2-agonists may be more easily given via MDI and spacer or dry powder inhaler than via a nebulizer. In clinical studies these delivery methods have been found to be similar,[49,50] and in a deposition study equivalent percentages of total lung deposition were observed in children aged 2–8 years after aerosolization of radiolabeled salbutamol administered either by a nebulizer or an MDI and holding chamber.[51] Nebulizers may be preferable for those unable to correctly use other delivery methods, or for those who require high-dose inhaled therapy. It is important to ensure that whatever device is used it is used correctly.

Anticholinergics

Anticholinergics are not routinely used in the treatment of chronic childhood asthma, although in wheezy infants under 2 years of age (excluding acute bronchiolitis) symptoms improved following nebulized anticholinergic aerosols compared with placebo.[52]

Corticosteroids

Corticosteroids are the first-line preventive therapy in asthma, but may be more easily given via MDI and spacer or dry powder inhaler than via a nebulizer.

Bronchiolitis[53,54]

When interpreting studies of nebulized therapy for bronchiolitis care should be taken not to confuse those which have included patients with recurrent wheeze (often following a coryzal illness) with those which include only patients with respiratory syncytial virus (RSV) positive bronchiolitis. The therapy for and the clinical course of these conditions may be different, and this may confuse the findings of studies.

Beta-2-agonists

Although there is a lack of evidence of efficacy of inhaled beta-2-agonists in bronchiolitis,[54–56] in practice a trial of inhaled beta-2-agonists may be given. Therapy should be continued only if there is a clear and repeatable improvement in symptoms.

Epinephrine

Inhaled epinephrine causes transient improvement in clinical score and oxygen saturation. Early randomized controlled trials suggest a reduction in hospitalization rates for children given epinephrine compared with salbutamol.[57,58] The regimes used were 3 ml of 1/1000 epinephrine nebulized at arrival and 30 min later, followed by observation for at least 2 hours,[57] and 0.1 mg/kg per dose given at 20 min intervals three times followed by observation for 3 hours.[58] There are no good placebo-controlled trials showing a reduction in mortality or the need for assisted ventilation. Caution is needed in the repeated and frequent use of inhaled epinephrine, as systemic effects including myocardial infarction in a child have been described.[59]

Corticosteroids

Corticosteroids are not effective in the acute phase of bronchiolitis, and do not prevent post-bronchiolitis wheezing.[60]

Ribavirin

Use of ribavirin in infants with RSV positive lower respiratory tract infection is not supported by evidence of significant benefit[61] even in infants with severe bronchiolitis requiring mechanical ventilation.[62] It is also controversial because of difficulties in its administration, the generally self-limiting course of RSV infection, the cost of the drug and its potential toxicity. Ribavirin is mixed with sterile water and aerosolized using a small particle aerosol generator (SPAG) which consists of a modified Collison nebulizer and drying chamber to reduce the aerosol particle size (median aerosol diameter, 1–2 μm). Aerosol is administered by means of a headbox or hood, and much of the drug is deposited on the patient rather than in the lungs. For ventilated patients, the aerosol is given into the inspiratory limb of the ventilator circuit. The SPAG is an inefficient nebulizer and it is not clear how much drug actually reaches the patient. Ribavirin is administered for 12–20 hours a day for a mean duration of 4–5 days, although shorter administration times have been used.

Previous studies showing benefit of ribavirin in RSV positive bronchiolitis have been criticized on methodological grounds. Ribavirin appears to be safe, although there have been anecdotal reports of increased bronchospasm with its use and concerns about blockage of filters in mechanical ventilator circuits. It is, however, expensive and neither efficacy nor effectiveness have been clearly demonstrated in large randomized trials. Routine use of ribavirin at this time cannot be recommended.

Croup (laryngotracheobronchitis)

Epinephrine

Epinephrine may transiently improve croup scores, but the effect is short lived, and rebound symptoms may occur. No effect on the need for intubation has been demonstrated.[63]

Corticosteroids

Inhaled corticosteroids reduce the rate of hospitalization in croup, but oral dexamethasone is associated with at least equal clinical improvement.[64] Some authors feel that the low cost of oral dexamethasone makes it the treatment of choice. Further studies are awaited to determine if there are clinically important systemic side effects from dexamethasone given for the treatment of croup.

Neonatology

Beta-2-agonists

Short-term improvements in lung mechanics in infants with chronic lung disease of prematurity (bronchopulmonary dysplasia, BPD) have been demonstrated,[65] but inhaled salbutamol does not prevent BPD,[66] and is not effective in the treatment of hyaline membrane disease.

Anticholinergics

Anticholinergics may also have short-term effects on bronchial hyperresponsiveness in BPD,[67,68] but no proven longer-term effect.

Surfactant

Intratracheal instillation of surfactant is standard treatment for surfactant deficient respiratory distress (hyaline membrane disease). Nebulization may offer more uniform distribution of surfactant and avoid the transient hypoxia, hypercapnia and cerebrovascular changes associated with surfactant instillation,[69,70] although it is technically difficult due to the lipid nature of the product and lung deposition of nebulized surfactant is poor (approximately 2% of the nebulized dose). It is also dependent on the surfactant preparation and nebulizer used,[71] and these should be chosen with care.

Corticosteroids
Systemic corticosteroids may be used in established BPD to aid weaning from mechanical ventilation.[72] There is no evidence that they improve long-term outcome, and there is concern over the possible effects of systemic doses of corticosteroids on the developing neonatal brain. A number of small trials show that inhaled corticosteroids aid weaning from mechanical ventilation and supplemental oxygen, and reduce the need for systemic corticosteroids.[73,74]

Furosemide
Inhaled furosemide has been shown to improve pulmonary mechanics in infants with BPD in some but not all trials.[75,76] The difference in results between these trials has been attributed to problems with drug delivery, and differences in the age and severity of illness in the study population. Inhaled furosemide cannot be recommended at present as a routine therapy in the treatment of BPD.

Pediatric intensive care

DNase
Anecdotal reports suggest that direct instillation of DNase may be useful to help clear retained secretions in children undergoing mechanical ventilation. Randomized trials are awaited.

N-acetylcysteine
There is only anecdotal evidence that *N*-acetylcysteine is effective in reducing sputum retention, and it may lead to bronchoconstriction. A recent systematic review found no evidence to support its use as a mucolytic in patients with cystic fibrosis.[77]

Surfactant
Instilled surfactant has been used in a number of reports for the treatment of term infants with acute lung injury (i.e. meconium aspiration syndrome) and older children and adults with acute respiratory distress syndrome. Results have been conflicting, with some showing benefit and others not. Aerosolized surfactant may be preferentially delivered to less damaged areas

of the lung, and this may explain its lack of efficacy. There is currently no consensus supporting the use of nebulized surfactant in childhood respiratory distress.

Corticosteroids for post-extubation stridor

Intravenous dexamethasone (administered 6–12 hours before extubation) reduces the incidence of post-extubation stridor and the re-intubation rate in children and infants at high risk of extubation failure, and is cheaper than nebulized therapy. The prophylactic use of systemic or inhaled corticosteroids in routine elective extubation where there are no risk factors for extubation failure is not recommended.

Epinephrine

Nebulized epinephrine reduces the incidence and severity of post-extubation stridor, but does not reduce the re-intubation rate. Both the laevo isomer and the racemic formulation are effective.

Conclusions

In the author's opinion, nebulizers are overused both in hospitals and in the community for the treatment of childhood respiratory diseases. As noted above, they can often be replaced by an MDI and spacer. Where nebulizers are recommended, their use should follow recognized guidelines.

Very little work has been done on the important factors that need to be considered when choosing a nebulizer for children. The nebulizer/compressor combination proposed must deliver an adequate amount of the prescribed drug in appropriately sized particles to the patient. Breath-controlled open vent nebulizers improve drug delivery, but require further evaluation before they can be recommended for infants and young children.

If children use nebulizers at home, oral and written instructions should be given to the patient or parent on the method of use, the action to be taken in the event of worsening asthma, the cleaning and maintenance of the nebulizer and compressor, and when to attend for follow-up. The child should be supervised in a clinic with expertise in the delivery of inhaled medications such as an asthma clinic. Such supervision should include measurement of peak flow, monitoring of prescriptions and regular servicing of the compressor.

Where possible, a mouthpiece should be used with a nebulizer as this increases pulmonary deposition of drug. If a face mask is used, it should be closely applied to the face. Different face mask designs may not be equally effective.

The patient should be given a maximum time for nebulization (based where possible on specific studies). This time will depend on the nebulizer and drug being used, but for some medications administered for asthma, little drug may be delivered after 5 min.

The most effective inhaler for any given patient is the one that will be used on a regular basis and in an effective manner. Compliance with asthma medications is poor, and the factors that affect compliance under researched. Nebulizer designs that improve the acceptability of therapy to children and their parents are awaited, but must be cost effective before they can be recommended.

References

1. Powell CV, Maskell GR, Marks MK et al. Successful implementation of spacer treatment guideline for acute asthma. *Arch Dis Child* 2001; **84**:142–6.
2. Dunbar H, Barry PW. The use of metered dose inhalers and spacer devices in the treatment of acute severe childhood asthma – changing clinical practice. *Eur Respir J* 1998; **12**:339S.
3. Barry PW, O'Callaghan C, Pedersen S, Fauroux B. Nebulizers in childhood. *Eur Respir Rev* 2000; **10**:527–35.
4. Barry PW, O'Callaghan C. Nebuliser therapy in childhood. *Thorax* 1997; **52**:S78–S88.
5. Everard ML, Hardy JG, Milner AD. Comparison of nebulised aerosol deposition in the lungs of healthy adults following oral and nasal inhalation. *Thorax* 1993; **48**:1045–6.
6. Love RG, Muir DCF. Aerosol deposition and airway obstruction. *Am Rev Respiv Dis* 1976; **114**:891–7.
7. O'Doherty MJ, Thomas SHL, Gibb D et al. Lung deposition of nebulised pentamidine in children. *Thorax* 1993; **48**:220–6.
8. Alderson PO, Secker-Walker RH, Strominger DB et al. Pulmonary deposition of aerosols in children with cystic fibrosis. *J Pediatr* 1974; **84**:479–84.
9. O'Callaghan C. Particle size of beclomethasone dipropionate produced by two nebulisers and two spacing devices. *Thorax* 1990; **45**:109–11.
10. Iles R, Lister P, Edmunds AT. Crying significantly reduces absorption of aerosolised drug in infants. *Arch Dis Child* 1999; **81**:163–5.
11. Bisgaard H. Patient related factors in nebulized drug delivery to children. *Eur Respir Rev* 1997; **7**:376–7.
12. Pedersen S, Ostergaard PA. Nasal inhalation as a cause of inefficient pulmonal aerosol inhalation technique in children. *Allergy* 1983; **38**:191–4.

13. Dolovich M, Ryan G, Newhouse MT. Aerosol penetration into the lung: influence on airway responses. *Chest* 1981; **80**:834–6.

14. Cardellicchio S, Ferrante E, Castellani W et al. Influence of inspiratory flow rate on the bronchial response to ultrasonic mist of distilled water in asthmatic patients. *Respiration* 1989; **56**:220–6.

15. Collis GG, Cole CH, Le Souef PN. Dilution of nebulised aerosols by air entrainment in children. *Lancet* 1990; **336**:341–3.

16. Thomas SH, Langford JA, George RD, Geddes DM. Improving the efficiency of drug administration with jet nebulisers. *Lancet* 1988; **1**:126.

17. Nikander K. Adaptive aerosol delivery: the principles. *Eur Respir Rev* 1997; **7**:385–7.

18. Salmon B, Wilson NM, Silverman M. How much aerosol reaches the lungs of wheezy infants and toddlers? *Arch Dis Child* 1990; **65**:401–3.

19. Coates AL, Allen PD, MacNeish CF et al. Effect of size and disease on estimated deposition of drugs administered using jet nebulization in children with cystic fibrosis. *Chest* 2001; **119**:1123–30.

20. Barry PW. The future of nebulisation. *Respir Care* 2002; **47**:1459–70.

21. Coutts JA, Gibson NA, Paton JY. Measuring compliance with inhaled medication in asthma. *Arch Dis Child* 1992; **67**:332–3.

22. Gibson NA, Ferguson AE, Aitchison TC, Paton JY. Compliance with inhaled asthma medication in preschool children. *Thorax* 1995; **50**:1274–9.

23. Milgrom H, Bender B, Ackerson L et al. Noncompliance and treatment failure in children with asthma. *J Allergy Clin Immunol* 1996; **98**:1051–7.

24. Spitzer WO, Suissa S, Ernst P et al. The use of b-agonists and the risk of death or near death from asthma. *N Engl J Med* 1992; **326**:501–6.

25. Birkhead G, Attaway NJ, Strunk RC et al. Investigation of a cluster of deaths of adolescents from asthma: evidence implicating inadequate treatment and poor patient adherence with medications. *J Allergy Clin Immunol* 1989; **84**:484–91.

26. Vance R. Hands on: gear, gadgets and great ideas. Nic the magic dragon: nebulizer calms children. *J Emerg Med Services* 2002; **27**:97–8.

27. O'Callaghan C, Clark AR, Milner AD. Why nebulise for more than five minutes? *Arch Dis Child* 1989; **64**:1270–3.

28. Barry PW, O'Callaghan C. An in vitro analysis of the output of salbutamol from different nebulisers. *Eur Respir J* 1999; **13**:1164–9.

29. Nikander K. Adaptive aerosol delivery: the principles. *Eur Respir Rev* 1997; **7**:385–7.

30. Kishida M, Suzuki I, Kabayama H et al. Mouthpiece versus facemask for delivery of nebulized salbutamol in exacerbated childhood asthma. *J Asthma* 2002; **39**:337–9.

31. Nikander K, Agertoft L, Pedersen S. Breath-synchronized nebulization diminishes the impact of patient-device interfaces (face mask or mouthpiece) on the inhaled mass of nebulized budesonide. *J Asthma* 2000; **37**:451–9.

32. Marguet C, Couderc L, Le Roux P et al. Inhalation treatment: errors in application and difficulties in acceptance of the devices are frequent in wheezy infants and young children. *Pediatr Allergy Immunol* 2001; **12**:224–30.

33. Hayden JT, Smith N, Woolf DA et al. Choice of facemask attached to a spacer may markedly affect drug delivery to children. *Arch Dis Child* (in press).

34. Everard ML, Clark AR, Milner AD. Drug delivery from jet nebulisers. *Arch Dis Child* 1992; **67**:586–91.

35. Amirav I, Newhouse MT. Aerosol therapy with valved holding chambers in young children: importance of the facemask seal. *Pediatr* 2001; **108**:389–94.

36. Moler F, Hurwitz M, Custer J. Improvement of clinical asthma scores and $PaCO_2$ in children with severe asthma treated with continuously nebulised terbutaline. *J Allergy Clin Immunol* 1988; **81**:1101–9.

37. Portnoy J, Aggarwal J. Continuous terbutaline nebulisation for treatment of severe asthma in children. *Ann Allergy* 1988; **60**:368–71.

38. Khine H, Fuchs SM, Saville AL. Continuous vs intermittent nebulized albuterol for emergency management of asthma. *Acad Emerg Med* 1996; **3**:1019–24.

39. McPeck M, Tandon R, Hughes K, Smaldone GC. Aerosol delivery during continuous nebulization. *Chest* 1997; **111**:1200–5.

40. Kress JP, Noth I, Gelbach BK et al. The utility of albuterol nebulized with heliox during acute asthma exacerbations. *Am J Respir Crit Care Med* 2002; **165**:1317–21.

41. Henderson SO, Acharya P, Kilaghbian T et al. Use of heliox driven nebulizer therapy in the treatment of acute asthma. *Ann Emerg Med* 1999; **33**:141–6.

42. Cates CJ. Holding chambers versus nebulisers for beta agonist treatment of acute asthma (Cochrane Review). In: the *Cochrane Library*, Issue 1. Oxford: Update Software, 1999.

43. O'Callaghan C, Barry PW. Spacer devices in the treatment of asthma. *BMJ* 1997; **314**:1061–2.

44. Everard ML, Matthew K. Anticholinergic drugs for wheeze in children under the age of two years (Cochrane Review). In: the *Cochrane Library*, Issue 1. Oxford: Update Software, 1999.

45. Qureshi F, Pestian J, Davis P, Zaritsky A. Effect of nebulized ipratropium on the hospitalization rates of children with asthma. *New Engl J Med* 1998; **339**:1030–5.

46. Schuh S, Johnson DW, Callahan S et al. Efficacy of frequent nebulized ipratropium bromide added to frequent high-dose albuterol therapy in severe childhood asthma. *J Pediatr* 1995; **126**:639–45.

47. Volovitz B, Bentur L, Finkelstein Y et al. Effectiveness and safety of inhaled corticosteroids in controlling acute asthma attacks in children who were treated in the emergency department: a controlled comparative study with oral prednisolone. *J Allergy Clin Immunol* 1998; **102**:605–9.

48. Rowe BH, Bota GW, Fabris L et al. Inhaled budesonide in addition to oral corticosteroids to prevent asthma relapse following discharge from the emergency department: a randomized controlled trial. *JAMA* 1999; **281**:2119–26.

49. Schuh S, Johnson DW, Stephens D et al. Comparison of albuterol delivered by a metered dose inhaler with spacer versus a nebulizer in children with mild acute asthma. *J Pediatr* 1999; **135**:22–7.

50. Pierce RJ, McDonald CF, Landau LI et al. Nebuhaler versus wet aerosol for domiciliary bronchodilator therapy. A multi-centre clinical comparison. *Med J Aust* 1992; **156**:771–4.

51. Wildhaber JH, Dore ND, Wilson JM et al. Inhalation therapy in asthma: nebulizer or pressurized metered-dose inhaler with holding chamber? In vivo comparison of lung deposition in children. *J Pediatr* 1999; **135**:28–33.

52. Everard ML, Matthew K. Anticholinergic drugs for wheeze in children under the age of two years (Cochrane Review). In: the *Cochrane Library*, Issue 1. Oxford: Update Software, 1999.

53. Barry PW. Aerosols in bronchiolitis. *J Aerosol Med* 2002; **15**:109–16.

54. Kellner JD, Ohlsson A, Gadomski AM, Wang EEL. Bronchodilator therapy in bronchiolitis (Cochrane Review). In: the *Cochrane Library*, Issue 1. Oxford: Update Software, 1999.

55. Flores G, Horwitz RI. Efficacy of beta 2 agonists in bronchiolitis: a reappraisal and meta analysis. *Pediatrics* 1997; **100**:233–9.

56. Dobson JV, Stephens-Groff SM, McMahon SR et al. The use of albuterol in hospitalized infants with bronchiolitis. *Pediatrics* 1998; **101**:361–8.

57. Menon K, Sutcliffe T, Klassen T. A randomised trial comparing the efficacy of epinephrine with salbutamol in the treatment of acute bronchiolitis. *J Pediatr* 1995; **126**:1004–7.

58. Ray MS, Singh V. Comparison of nebulized adrenaline versus salbutamol in wheeze associated respiratory tract infections in infants. *Indian J Pediatr* 2002; **39**:12–22.

59. Butte MJ, Nguyen BX, Hutchison TJ, Wiggins JW, Ziegler JW. Pediatric myocardial infarction after racemic epinephrine administration. *Pediatrics* 1999; **104**:E9.

60. Richter H, Seddon P. Early nebulized budesonide in the treatment of bronchiolitis and the prevention of postbronchiolitic wheezing. *J Pediatrics* 1998; **132**:849–53.

61. Randolph AG, Wang EEL. Ribavirin for RSV lower respiratory tract infection (Cochrane Review). In: the *Cochrane Library*, Issue 1. Oxford: Update Software, 1999.

62. Guerguerian A, Gauthier M, Farrell CA, Lacroix J. Ribavirin in ventilated respiratory syncytial virus bronchiolitis. A randomized, placebo-controlled trial. *Am J Respir Crit Care Med* 1999; **160**:829–34.

63. Anonymous. Inhaled budesonide and adrenaline for croup. *Drug Ther Bull* 1996; **34**:23–4.

64. Klassen TP, Craig WR, Moher D et al. Nebulized budesonide and oral dexamethasone for treatment of croup: a randomized controlled trial. *JAMA* 1998; **279**:1629–32.

65. Yuksel B, Greenhough A. Effect of nebulized salbutamol in preterm infants during the first year of life. *Eur Respir J* 1991; **4**:1088–92.

66. Denjean A, Paris-Llado, J, Zupan V et al. Inhaled salbutamol and beclomethasone for preventing broncho-pulmonary dysplasia: a randomised double-blind study. *Eur J Pediatr* 1998; **157**:926–31.

67. Kao LC, Durand DJ, Nickerson BG. Effects of inhaled metaproterenol and atropine on the pulmonary mechanics of infants with bronchopulmonary dysplasia. *Pediatr Pulmonol* 1989; **6**:74–80.

68. Brundage KL, Mohsini KG, Froese AB, Fisher JT. Bronchodilator response to ipratropium bromide in infants with bronchopulmonary dysplasia. *Am Rev Respir Dis* 1990; **142**:1137–42.

69. Cowan F, Whitelaw A, Wertheim D, Silverman M. Cerebral blood flow velocity changes after rapid administration of surfactant. *Arch Dis Child* 1991; **66**:1105–9.

70. Dijk PH, Heikamp A, Bambang Oetomo S. Surfactant nebulisation prevents the adverse effects of surfactant therapy on blood pressure and cerebral blood flow in rabbits with severe respiratory failure. *Intensive Care Med* 1997; **23**:1077–81.

71. Fok TF, al-Essa M, Dolovich M et al. Nebulisation of surfactants in an animal model of neonatal respiratory distress. *Arch Dis Child* 1998; **78**:F3–F9.
72. The Collaborative Dexamethasone Trial Group. Dexamethasone therapy in neonatal chronic lung disease: an international placebo controlled trial. *Pediatrics* 1991; **88**:421–7.
73. Cloutier MM. Nebulised steroid therapy in bronchopulmonary dysplasia. *Pediatr Pulmonol* 1993; **15**:111–16.
74. Arnon S, Grigg J, Silverman M. Effectiveness of budesonide aerosol in ventilator dependent preterm babies: a preliminary report. *Pediatr Pulmonol* 1996; **21**:231–5.
75. Ohki Y, Nako Y, Koizumi T, Morikawa A. The effect of aerosolized furosemide in infants with chronic lung disease. *Acta Paediatr* 1997; **86**:656–60.
76. Kugelman A, Durand M, Garg M. Pulmonary effect of inhaled furosemide in ventilated infants with severe bronchopulmonary dysplasia. *Pediatrics* 1997; **99**:71–5.
77. Duijvestijn YC, Brand PL. Systematic review of N-acetylcysteine in cystic fibrosis. *Acta Paediatr* 1999; **88**:38–41.

11. USE OF NEBULIZERS IN PRIMARY CARE: ISSUES AND CHALLENGES

Jennifer Cleland, David Price and Mike Thomas

Introduction

The principal use of nebulizers in primary care is for the treatment of asthma and chronic obstructive pulmonary disease (COPD), mainly for bronchodilation and, to a lesser extent, for delivery of anti-inflammatory corticosteroids. Other uses of nebulizers are to deliver antibiotics in cystic fibrosis, bronchiectasis and human immunodeficiency virus/acquired immune deficiency syndrome (HIV/AIDS) and for symptom relief in palliative care. The latter uses are most frequent in secondary care settings and will not be discussed in this chapter, which focuses on the current issues and challenges of using nebulizers in primary care.

Asthma is a chronic inflammatory disorder of the airways characterized by variable or reversible airflow obstruction of 15% or greater. It is a common health problem which affects approximately 130 million people worldwide[1] and which requires long-term management, often involving taking preventive medications every day. Guidelines and primary care-based research have led to a shift to predominantly primary care delivered asthma care in the United Kingdom (UK) and in many other countries, although with enormous variations.[2–5] In the UK, 80.6% of people with asthma are managed in primary care alone, a further 17.5% in combined primary and secondary care and only 1.9% solely in secondary care.[6]

COPD is a chronic, slowly progressive disorder characterized by airways obstruction which does not change markedly over several months.[7] Most of the lung impairment is fixed, although some reversibility can be produced by bronchodilator therapy. COPD is usually associated with a history of smoking and is generally limited to patients aged over 45 years. It is currently the fourth leading cause of death in the world[8] with prevalence and mortality predicted to increase in the coming decades. Again, guidelines and research stress the role of primary care in identifying and managing COPD, including reducing risk factors such as smoking.[9–11]

Nebulizer use in asthma and COPD

Most treatment for asthma and COPD is by the inhaled route, delivering medication to the site of the disease process and minimizing potential for side effects. In asthma, anti-inflammatory agents, particularly inhaled corticosteriods, are currently the most effective long-term preventive medications, with inhaled bronchodilators prescribed for quick relief (Global Initiative for Asthma, GINA)[2] with adjuvant inhaled or oral agents if control is not achieved.[12] Recommended treatment for COPD involves regular and as needed bronchodilators for symptom relief and prevention. The role of inhaled corticosteroids in COPD is less clear[7] but studies have shown these to have a beneficial effect on reducing exacerbations in subsets of patients.[13]

Delivery to the site of the disease process can be achieved by three broad categories of different inhalation devices. These are: pressurized metered dose inhalers (MDIs) used with or without a spacer, dry powder inhalers (DPIs) and nebulizers. Each method of inhalation has its advantages and disadvantages. For example, nebulizers are relatively easy to use but expensive, bulky and require maintenance. MDIs are cheap and 'everyday' but patient inhalation technique is often poor even with training. DPIs resolve the need to coordinate actuation and inspiration, but need a minimum inspiratory flow rate generation.[14] They are more expensive than MDIs in most countries.

The general term 'nebulizer' usually implies the combination of nebulizer chamber, compressor and mouthpiece or face mask. There are at least 40 000 nebulizer systems in use for adult domiciliary treatment in the UK with an associated drug cost of over £40 million annually.[15] Elsewhere in Europe usage may be even higher.[16]

Possible uses of nebulizers in the treatment of asthma and COPD in primary care are for the delivery of drugs to the airways in acute exacerbations and in maintenance therapy. In acute asthma, bronchodilator drugs (short acting beta-agonist and anticholinergic drugs) have been delivered by the nebulized route extensively in the past, although as discussed below there is a paucity of evidence of superior clinical efficacy of nebulizer over the same drugs delivered by MDI and spacer systems.[17] High-dose corticosteroid drugs to treat acute exacerbations have also been delivered by the nebulized route in some studies, with evidence of comparable efficacy[18] (although also with comparable systemic effects to oral corticosteroids) and currently not standard practice.

212

Nebulized bronchodilators and corticosteroids are occasionally used in the maintenance treatment of asthma in the community, and are generally employed under expert supervision in exceptional circumstances, such as severe and brittle asthma or in patients with difficulties in mastering inhaler techniques.[19] Also, some patients and parents are keen to have home nebulizers for the delivery of bronchodilator drugs in the maintenance or acute situation[20] based sometimes on personal experience or on misunderstanding of the effectiveness of different delivery systems, and have obtained the equipment themselves. Prior to the availability of guidelines, clinicians did at times collaborate with such patients by prescribing nebules for their equipment.

Similarly, nebulized bronchodilators have been widely used in the treatment of acute exacerbations of COPD in the community.[21] There is no evidence of efficiency of nebulizers concerning the use of nebulized corticosteroids in acute exacerbations of COPD in the community. Maintenance nebulized bronchodilators may play a role in the community management of severe COPD. However, current COPD guidelines suggest that the use of nebulized maintenance therapy in COPD should be undertaken only after full specialist assessment, and consideration of a home nebulizer is an indication for referral to a respiratory specialist.[22]

Nebulizers versus handheld inhalers

In clinical practice, the fundamental principle of prescribing is to prescribe the most clinically and cost effective drug. Are nebulizers any more clinically effective than, or at least equivalent to, alternative forms of inhaler in the treatment of asthma and COPD? Evidence from systematic reviews suggests not. A systematic review of randomized controlled trails (RCTs) found no difference in the efficacy of nebulizers and an MDI with spacer for delivering beta-agonists in people with acute asthma.[17] Similar results have been found for treatment of patients with acute exacerbations in COPD.[21] Neither has there been shown any clinical difference between inhalers and nebulizers for delivery of bronchodilators in stable asthma in children, adults or stable COPD.[18] However, as discussed later in this chapter, this final evidence may be limited in its applicability to patients in primary care as most patients at the severe end of the spectrum and those with poor inhaler technique are excluded from many studies. These are the very

Table 11.1 Community-based prescribing and cost data for inhaled therapies used for all respiratory conditions in England in 1998.

Drug		Prescriptions in millions	Net ingredient cost in million pounds (£)	NIC/Pxs in pounds (£)
Salbutamol	DPI	1375	15 249	11
	pMDI	12 806	46 997	4
	Nebulizer	726	14 856	20
Terbutaline	DPI	1062	11 153	11
	pMDI	477	3520	7
	Nebulizer	1539	14 673	10
Ipratropium	DPI	13	209	16
	pMDI	1192	8006	7
	Nebulizer	1539	14 673	33
Budesonide	DPI	1226	31 527	26
	pMDI	520	10 997	21
	Nebulizer	136	17 919	131
Fluticasone	DPI	613	20 983	34
	pMDI	931	41 224	44
Beclometasone	DPI	871	21 926	25
	pMDI	7336	119 256	16
All	DPI	5160	101 047	20
	pMDI	23 262	229 999	10
	Nebulizer	2822	61 525	22
	Total	31 244	392 572	13 (average)

All inhaler therapies recorded as prescribed under Chapter 3 of the *British National Formulary*, 'Respiratory system'.
Excludes combined or compound inhaler therapies, which are not recommended.
DPI, dry powder inhaler; pMDI, pressurized metered dose inhaler; Pxs, prescriptions; NIC, net ingredient cost.
(Reproduced from Brocklebank et al. *Health Technol Assess* 2001; 5: 1–149[14] with permission of National Coordinating Centre for Health Technology Assessment.)

groups of patients that many clinicians with an interest in this area feel may benefit from the use of a nebulizer.

Are nebulizers a generally cost-effective method of treating asthma and COPD compared to alternative forms of inhaler device? Again, it appears not. Table 11.1 summarizes community-based prescribing and cost data for inhaled therapies used for all respiratory conditions in England in 1998. The net ingredient cost was over £392 million, varying from £4 to £131 depending on the combination of device, drug and dose. The average cost of a prescription varied from £10 for MDI inhaler treatment, £20 for DPI inhaler treatment, and £22 for nebulizer inhaler treatment. Brocklebank et al also provided the standardized 28-day costs of the devices by classification and drug, including resource use, unit cost and cost of each class of drug, and found that both MDIs and DPIs cost less than nebulizers.[14]

This and other evidence has led to guidelines supporting the use of inhalers, rather than nebulizers, as treatment of first choice in asthma and COPD on the basis that nebulized treatment costs more and is of only equivalent efficacy to inhaler treatment.[23] However, prescribing costs for asthma are outweighed by costs resulting from poor asthma control, such as hospitalization costs and indirect costs.[24] Although nebulizer-associated costs are undoubtedly high, they may still be cost effective if they allow better asthma control to be achieved. There is a need for health economic evaluations in a primary care setting with appropriate subgroup analyses as it may be that nebulizers are cost effective in some patient subgroups.

Additionally, guidelines are based on the conclusions of 2 RCTs and systematic reviews of these trials. There is evidence that patients who take part in RCTs are not typical and selection of these patients may not reflect usual practice. For example, trials tend to focus on select patients (often with a prescribed level of disease) and often exclude patients with comorbidity.[25] Patients who have physical and learning disabilities that affect inhaler use are generally excluded from such studies, as are patients with poor compliance. This population does not reflect primary care patients who have a range of disease severity and frequent comorbidity.[26]

Another common inclusion criterion for clinical trials is that the participants should already have a good inhalation technique[19] although inhaler technique in many patients is poor[27] – again supporting the hypothesis that patients in clinical trials may not be typical. As a consequence, the conclusions drawn from these studies may not be generalizable.

Some of the conclusions in frequently cited systematic reviews may be based on small numbers or poor studies. For example, Brocklebank et al concluded that, in children with asthma nebulizers are not clinically superior to other inhaler devices on the basis of three trials with a total of 51 individuals. The duration of two of the studies was short: one day[28] and 3 × 4 hours,[29] and in the latter a non-clinically valid comparison was carried out (Rotahaler DPI (Allen and Hanburys Ltd, Middlesex, UK) vs a nebulizer). The authors identified similar weaknesses in studies on adult patients comparing inhalers with nebulizers. More methodologically robust studies are needed before we can safely conclude that inhalers should always be first choice treatment in asthma and COPD. Further studies on typical primary care populations, undertaken in 'real-life' primary care settings and utilizing a range of outcome measures, including health economic evaluations, are needed to identify the role of nebulizers in the treatment of such groups.

Finally, patients often comment that nebulizer therapy improves their breathing although objective evidence is absent.[30] Symptom scores and quality of life measures may indicate benefits other than bronchodilator effect for patients. Data of this nature are likely to be relevant when assessing patients for treatment.

Clinical indications for nebulizer treatment

At this point in time, the absolute indications for treatment with nebulizers are few. Box 11.1 outlines the indications for nebulizer treatment.[16] The absolute indicators outlined in Box 11.1 are situations most often encountered in secondary care (other than being incapable of managing a handheld inhaler). This is seen in all groups of patients but is most common in young children and the elderly and is an issue for primary care (see later).

With regard to relative indicators for nebulizer use, the need for a large dose (usually in emergency situations) can be achieved with multiple actuations of a handheld inhaler.[31] However, the patient may prefer the relative ease of a nebulizer to taking a large number of actuations of a handheld inhaler for an equivalent drug dose.[16] Anecdotal evidence suggests that staff also prefer the use of nebulizers in emergency situations due to their convenience and the reassurance that the drug is being inhaled. There is some

---

Box 11.1 Indications for treatment with nebulizers.

Absolute indications
- Too sick or incapable of managing handheld inhalers
- Drug not available in handheld inhalers
- Need to target treatment to particular generation of bronchi or the alveoli

Relative indications
- Need for a large drug dose
- Patient preference
- Practical convenience

(Reproduced from Muers MF. *Thorax* 1997; **52** (Suppl 2): S25–S30[16] with permission from the BMJ Publishing Group.)

---

evidence that patients prefer nebulizers even in non-emergency situations. For example, Pierce et al compared the use of a MDI with a nebulizer for domiciliary bronchodilator therapy.[20] Adults preferred the nebulizer despite an equivalent clinical response.

Why do patients prefer nebulizers to handheld inhalers? It could well be that using a nebulizer is easier than using an inhaler. Table 11.2 shows that a high proportion of patients exhibit inadequate inhaler technique – even very experienced inhaler users – supporting the hypothesis that patients may find inhalers difficult to use.[19] The widespread use of nebulizers in acute situations, particularly in secondary care and emergency situations, may have resulted in patient expectation of this treatment modality in severe asthma and COPD exacerbations, rather than the more 'everyday' devices that they may associate with the treatment of stable disease. Similarly, the undoubted efficacy of nebulized bronchodilation and the perception that this method of drug delivery is widely used in secondary care inpatient and accident and emergency situations may encourage their use by clinicians who are unaware of the current evidence and guidelines recommendations.

Ease of use is likely to impact on adherence to therapy which will, in turn, affect the efficacy of therapy. Patient perception of efficacy may also be an important factor. Patients prescribed high-dose bronchodilators often comment that nebulizer therapy improves their breathing although objective evidence of bronchodilation is absent.[30] Muers suggests that while this may be due to these drugs having a non-respiratory effect, it is also possible this is a placebo effect.[32] Thus, nebulizers may be more effective than inhalers in real life because patients find them easy to use, so they use the nebulizer, feel better and are thus encouraged to adhere to their nebulizer treatment.

Bearing in mind that inhalers are less costly than nebulizers and, with reference to the existing evidence base, at least as effective as nebulizers, would teaching patients the correct inhaler technique allow us to minimize the use of nebulizers? Much research has investigated the educational needs of patients with handheld inhalers. This has indicated that verbal and written instructions[33] accompanied by practical demonstrations,[34] frequent reassessment and re-education (as correct technique usually deteriorates over time[33,35]) are necessary. Thus, the educational needs of patients with inhalers are great and, clearly, necessitate dedicated resources which may be a problem in the current cost containment climate. Unfortunately, in addition, poor patient knowledge is often compounded by poor understanding of technique by nurses and doctors.[36]

Table 11.2 Prevalence of inadequate inhaler technique in selected studies.

Authors	No. of patients	Inhaler device	Inadequate technique	Comment on methodology
Erickson et al	159	MDI	82% (>2 of 9 steps incorrect)	Patients had ≥6 months prior MDI experience. Self-assessment and observation
Larsen et al	12	MDI	58% actuated the MDI too early or too late	Patients with asthma used an MDI for ≥3 months prior to study. Healthy volunteers were naïve to MDIs. Written instructions for device use provided, performance judged by 2 observers
Schmid et al	25	DPI (Turbuhaler, Astra Zeneca, Luton, UK)	64% made errors on an 8-point scale	Regular Turbuhaler users. Performance graded on an 8-point scale
Shrestha et al	125	MDI	79% made errors in series of 7 steps	Patients already on inhaler therapy. Time taken to perform all 7 steps correctly measured
Thompson et al	72	MDI	76% made errors in series of 8 steps	Patients already receiving MDI therapy. Errors persisting over the 2-day period counted as misuse
van Beerendonk et al	316	MDI (19% of patients) or DPI (81%)	89% made at least 1 mistake in inhalation technique	Patients' existing therapy included an MDI or DPI. Excluded those who had previously received instruction. Assessment by standardized inhaler checklist

MDI, metered dose inhaler; PDI, dry powder inhaler.
(Reproduced from Duerden M et al. New Ethics J 2001, **4**: 31–42[19] with permission from New Ethics Journal.)

While training in technique is likely to impact positively on the effective use of inhalers by many patients, there are other problems. Some patients using inhalers, especially the elderly and children, may have physical and/or cognitive difficulties. In these circumstances, nebulizers may be a more suitable method of drug administration.[16]

Nebulizer use in preschool children

Nebulized bronchodilators have been traditionally used for the treatment of severe asthma and acute exacerbations of asthma in preschool children, and many studies have supported their effectiveness.[37,38] However, therapy with an MDI plus spacer and mask is as effective as nebulizer therapy in preterm infants,[39] infants[40] and children[41] with acute wheezing or asthma. Studies have demonstrated adequate lung deposition of medication delivered by MDI when compared to nebulizer although it is worth noting that the lung deposition may be as much as 60% lower if the child is crying.[42] Thus, there is both clinical and physiologic evidence to support the use of MDI therapy in place of nebulization[43] in this category of patients. In addition, when used in acute, severe asthma, air-driven nebulized bronchodilators may result in increased hypoxemia if used without supplementary oxygen due to worsened ventilation–perfusion mismatch. Some authorities recommend that nebulized bronchodilators should only be used in acute asthma with oxygen-driven nebulizers – seldom available in the community setting.[44]

Given this evidence, what is the case for continuing to use nebulizers for treatment of childhood asthma in primary care? The National Institute for Clinical Excellence (NICE) guidelines state that an MDI with spacer is the first-line treatment and nebulized therapy may be considered where this combination is not clinically effective dependant on the child's condition.[45] The main indication for nebulized treatment is that effective use of the MDI under real life conditions is not easy for young children.[46] Another factor, especially in the under-5-year-olds, may be poor inspiratory flow rate which supports the use of a device that does not require the child's active cooperation, although in most circumstances adequate benefit may be achieved with a large volume spacer and mask. Parents[47] and nurses[48] often state that they find a nebulizer easier to use, or that they find an MDI impossible to administer to children. Thus, compliance (by parents) may be better given the powerful placebo effect of a nebulizer.[47] These factors may add to nebulizers being more effective in real life than inhalers due to patient/parent preference and ease of use. Table 11.3 summarizes the advantages and disadvantages of nebulizers in pediatric practice.[48]

Table 11.3 Advantages and disadvantages of nebulizers in pediatric practice.

Advantages	Disadvantages
Minimal cooperation needed	Time-consuming
Easy to administer when unwell, better tolerated than pMDI	Inconvenient (size, weight, electrical supply)
	Expensive
Easy to administer when asleep	Expense of purchasing compressor
No close facial contact essential	Expense of servicing compressor
No unpleasant taste	Expensive drugs
Drug delivered over a longer period?	Correct compressor and nebulizer equipment
Powerful placebo effect	necessary
Patient/parent confidence	Questionable efficiency; efficiency increases with age
	Patient/parent dependency
	Perceived as a mechanism for claiming DLA

pMDI, pressurized metered dose inhaler; DLA, disability living allowance.
(Reproduced from Brownlee KG. *Eur Respir J* 1997; **44**: 177–9,[47] with permission from the publisher.)

Clearly, where nebulized treatment is used for treatment of childhood asthma, it is important that attention is given to choosing the correct equipment, parental training and an infrastructure to support the servicing and maintenance of the system (see later).[47] Again, good clinical trials, undertaken in primary care with 'typical' patients, using a range of outcome measures and evaluating health economics, are needed.

Nebulizer use in the elderly

Nebulizers in the elderly are mainly used to administer inhaled bronchodilators to patients with asthma and in patients with COPD. There is a lack of published data on the efficacy and use of nebulizers in this age group, and clinical decisions tend to be based on results from studies in younger patients.[49] However, studies have shown that patients over the age of 65 are significantly less likely to learn inhaler technique than younger patients,[50] probably due to hand strength.[51] Cognitive impairment is also an important aspect in the management of older patients who require inhaled therapy[52] suggesting that a nebulizer would be a useful option in patients with deficits in memory or other cognitive functions.[49] Nebulized beta-agonists should be used with caution in elderly patients with known ischemic heart disease as the incidence of dysrhythmias following nebulised beta-agonists is well recognized, particularly in those who have had a previous myocardial infarction.[53] Ideally, an elechocardiogram recording should be taken before drug administration in this group of patients.[49]

There is increasing evidence that the bronchodilator response to anti-cholinergic agents is less age-dependent than the response to beta-agonists.[54] This evidence, and the relative lack of side effects from inhaled anticholinergics, suggests that anticholinergic drugs and beta-agonists should always be considered in a nebulizer assessment of an elderly patient.

Pounsford suggests that elderly patients who are being considered for treatment should always be assessed over a period of 2 weeks with an MDI and 2 weeks with a nebulizer.[49] Nebulizers should be reserved for those patients who remain symptomatic despite treatment with MDIs or DPIs.

Variables impacting on effective use of nebulizers

Few reviews or audits of nebulizer use have been published and, unfortunately, these few do not inspire confidence. For example, Craig et al found that only 7% of nebulizer prescriptions reviewed on five medical wards in an English teaching hospital were correct.[55] In primary care settings, national comparisons have shown unreasonable differences in clinical practice. In a UK regional survey, for instance, compressor use for domiciliary treatment varied between districts from four to 213 per 10 000 population.[15] The 1992 European international asthma survey showed similar variation in reports by physicians on their use of nebulizers for airway disease.[56] Thus, in practice, the use of nebulizers is variable and poor. While this picture is disturbing, it is perhaps not unexpected given the many variables impacting on effective use of nebulizers.

Assessment of patients

The first step in appropriate prescribing is formally assessing the patient for a nebulizer. The European Respiratory Society (ERS) guidelines[57] for the use of nebulizers include guidelines for assessing patients, as do British Thoracic Society guidelines for management of asthma and COPD.[22,58] In brief, diagnosis should be confirmed via spirometry, the patient's inhaler technique should be assessed and a large volume spacer tried, oral steroids tried and patient compliance assessed, treatment with a handheld inhaler versus a nebulizer should be formally trialled, ideally over at least 2 weeks each. After this assessment process, the clinician must decide with the patient if the nebulizer treatment has produced subjective and objective benefits. The patient and doctor need to discuss whether the degree of benefit is sufficient to justify the high cost of home nebulizer therapy.

It is hard to argue with these guidelines. Unfortunately, however, anecdotal evidence suggests that formal assessment of patients for a nebulizer varies depending on who is carrying out the assessment. Within secondary care, respiratory physicians differ in their method of assessment with home trials ranging from 1 week to 1 month, and criteria for a positive assessment are also variable.[15]

The assessment of pulmonary function by general practitioners in primary care may be haphazard if they do not have a special interest in respiratory disease. Not all generalists will have, or indeed, wish to provide, the level of expertise required to carry out such an assessment. A full assessment in primary care may require the availability of appropriate specialist services in the community, perhaps through trained generalist or nurse specialists, or a GP with a special interest (GPwSIs).

An added complication is that many patients commence home nebulizer treatment after having used a nebulizer during an emergency hospital admission. This does not imply that patients leave hospital having been formally assessed by a respiratory physician as suitable for nebulized treatment. Rather, it seems that, having experienced a nebulizer in hospital, many patients may decide that this is their preferred method of treatment without consulting with a healthcare professional. These patients may have bought their own nebulizer before presenting at their general practitioner for nebules to use with this equipment.

Anecdotal evidence suggests that a general practitioner, faced with a patient with poorly controlled asthma or COPD who has decided to use a nebulizer rather than a handheld inhaler, is likely to collude with the patient. This is probably in the belief that compliance with treatment, and therefore management of the respiratory disease in question, will improve given the patient preference for treatment has been acknowledged and accepted.[59] However, patients should be discouraged from buying their own system as the many possible combinations of nebulizer, compressor, etc,[60] makes selection of an appropriate system suitable for the treatment of choice extremely complex.

Selecting a nebulizer (see also Chapter 13)

If it has been decided that a nebulizer is the most appropriate method of treatment for a patient, then which nebulizer is the most appropriate for the

---

Box 11.2 Parameters to be standardized in the use of nebulizer systems.

Nebulizer type

Choice of driving gas

Driving gas pressure

Driving gas flow rate

Drug and formulation

Nebulizer fill volume (as recommended by manufacturer)

Time of nebulization

Accessories (mouthpiece/face mask, etc)

Residual solute volume (amount of drug left in chamber)

(Reproduced from Boe J et al. *Eur Respir J* 2001; **18**: 228–42[57] with permission from the publisher.)

---

required treatment? Which compressor will best match that nebulizer chamber to achieve the optimal clinical effect? The recent ERS guidelines on the use of nebulizers recognize that all the components of a nebulizer system will affect performance.[57] If one component of the system is changed, the performance and efficiency of the drug delivery also changes and it is then necessary to redefine the nebulizer system. Box 11.2 outlines the parameters to be considered and, ideally, standardized in the use of nebulizer systems. Table 11.4 illustrates that selecting a nebulizer system is no easy task.[60] Note that the compressors and nebulizers listed in Table 11.4 are only examples of what is available, not a comprehensive guide to equipment.

Who in primary care has the expertise necessary to select the most appropriate combination of nebulizing equipment for a particular patient? We suggest that it is unrealistic to expect this level of knowledge in primary care other than from nurse or GP specialists. Selection is probably based on ad hoc factors such as previous experience, knowledge of a system the patient used while in hospital with an exacerbation, etc. While healthcare professionals should base their prescribing of nebulizers on the interpretation of present evidence, again it is unrealistic to expect individual primary care practitioners to have the level of knowledge and time required to select an appropriate nebulizing system. Protocols based on evidence are needed, and should be reviewed regularly to ensure best practice by primary care specialists.

The European Respiratory Task Force guidelines recommend that a standard operating practice be adopted for each nebulizer in local use as this will provide a baseline in determining the clinical effectiveness of that system for the given application.[57] This would allow any changes to the

Table 11.4 Examples of combinations of compressors and nebulizer chambers supplied for bronchodilator therapy based on flow rate.

Flow rate	Compressor	Nebulizer chambers sold with compressor unit	Multivolt
High flow rate (>6.0 l/min)	AFP Classic	MicroMist	No
	AFP Aquillon	MicroMist	No
	AFP Ultima	MicroMist	Rechargeable battery
	AFP Tourer	MicroMist	Yes
	Flaem Nuova Combineb	Flaem Nuova Type 3	Yes
	Flaem Nuova Micelfluss Pro	Flaem Nuova Type 2	Yes
	Medic-Aid CR50	Medic-Aid Sidestream	No
	Medic-Aid CR60*	Medic-Air Ventstream	No
	Medic-Air Freeway		Yes
	Gast*†		?
	Inspiron	MiniNeb, Incenti-Neb	No
	Medix M Flo	Medix A11	No
	Medix AC2000*	Medix A11	No
	Medix World Traveller	Medix A11	Yes
	Medix Econoneb	Medix A11	No
	Medix Minor*†	Cirrus	No
	Medix Turboneb	Cirrus	No
	Porta-Neb	Medic-Aid Sidestream Medic-Aid Ventstream	No
	Porta-Neb Multi	Medic-Aid Sidestream	Yes
	SunMist Plus	Perma Neb	No
Medium flow rate (4.0–6.0 l/min)	Aeroneb HP†	Cirrus	No
	Atomolette†	Own	No
	Flaem Nuova M70	Flaem Nuova Type 2	No
	NebuPump†	Acorn	No
	Novair II	Cirrus	No
	Pari Inhaler Boy†	Own	No
	Pari Turbo Boy	Pari LC Plus, LC Plus Junior	No
	Pari Junior Boy	Pari LC Plus, LC Plus Junior	No
	Pulmo-Aide†	Own	No
	SunMist	Perma Neb	No
	DeVilbiss Traveller	Perma Neb	Yes
Low flow rate (<4.0 l/min)	Aeroneb Standard†	Own, Cirrus	No
	Pari Walk Boy	Pari LC Plus	Yes
	Aeroneb HP†	Own	No

Table 11.4 *(Continued)*			
Flow rate	Compressor	Nebulizer chambers sold with compressor unit	Multivolt
Others	Aerolyser CF1B[†]	Wright	Yes
	Aerolyser CF1R[†]	Respi-Neb	Yes
	Aerolyser 216[†]	Respi-Neb	Yes
	Flaem Nuova Travelneb	Flaem Nuova Type 3	Yes
	Henley HCU-1[†]	Hudson MK II	Yes

*Wilson and Steventon[64] have tested these compressors with 19 nebulizer chambers: Acorn, Aerflo, Cirrus, De Vilviss, Econoneb, Hudson II, Jet set, MicroNeb III, MiniNeb, Sandoz, Suremist, Turret Turbo, Unicorn, Unimist, Unineb, Upmist and Wee Neb. With these compressors they all achieved flow rates at the nebulizer of >6.0 l/min.
† These devices may not be currently available but are included since they may still be in use.
(Reproduced from Kendrick AH et al. *Thorax* 1997; **52**(Suppl 2): S92–S101[60] with permission from the BMJ Publishing Group.)

standard operating practice to be supported by appropriate follow-up of outcomes such as clinical benefits or side effects. While these guidelines are welcome, the question of who collects the data required to formulate standard operating practices, and how these data are disseminated effectively to primary care practitioners, remains unanswered. Collaboration is needed between health service administrators, the medical profession and allied professions, and the pharmaceutical and equipment manufacturing industries. National and international respiratory societies are in a good position to take the lead in establishing such ventures.[16] The provision of evidence-based protocols and information for selecting a nebulizing system will aid appropriate prescribing in the future. It may be that a centralized service, accessible to both primary and secondary care, is needed to achieve this task efficiently.

Monitoring of equipment use and maintenance of equipment

Smith et al have discussed how staff must be educated to instruct patients in the knowledge required to use and clean the equipment, the principles of operation, maintenance and servicing issues to do with nebuliser systems, and what advice to give when the system malfunctions.[61] Other service issues include loan of compressors, repairs, routine maintenance, replacements, emergency out-of-hours needs. Clearly, effectively supporting home use of nebulizer systems is costly[62] and this must be taken into account when deciding to prescribe a nebulizer. Who holds the necessary funding?

Servicing and maintenance of nebulizers may be particularly haphazard in self-obtained systems. While patient wishes regarding choice of treatment should be recognized and acknowledged, it is undesirable that patients choose a method of treatment without consultation with a healthcare professional. Closely associated with this caveat is the need for formal assessment of nebulizer use, discussed earlier in the chapter. This is unlikely to happen, or if it does occur, the patient is unlikely to accept that a nebulizer may not be the most appropriate treatment of choice if they have already purchased equipment.

It is worth noting that patients choosing to change from an inhaler to a nebulizer may be looking for secondary gain. For example, a nebulizer is an obvious sign of 'illness' and use of a nebulizer allows a patient to access additional financial support via disabled living allowance in the UK.

Staff education

Education of those involved in prescribing, supplying and supervising nebulizer therapy is essential. Primary healthcare professionals dealing with nebulizer therapy should have the required knowledge and skills to provide an optimal service.[62] Unfortunately, research indicates considerable variation in the level of service offered to patients. Districts with coordinated services appear to offer a more comprehensive (secondary care-led) service.[15] We are unaware of any centralized primary care-led nebulizer service in the UK. However, such a service would provide comprehensive and coordinated facilities for patients, and a reliable source of information for staff. It would require adequate funding to meet the costs of equipment purchase, a maintenance/repair/replacement service and staffing. Research and audit are needed to assess if a centralized, appropriately funded nebulizer service for primary care would successfully address these practical issues.

Care pathways

Even with the provision of a centralized service, how would care be delivered to patients within a practice? Which member(s) of the primary care team are best placed to interface with patients regarding assessment for and use of a nebulizer system? Figure 11.1 presents various models of delivery of respiratory care which could be primary care-led.[63] While these models refer specifically to COPD, they are equally applicable to asthma.

There is a need for appropriate research and audit to ascertain which model of delivery of care is most clinically and cost effective. This research needs to take into account the patients' views of treatment, and primary

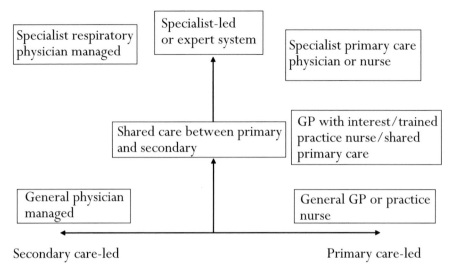

Figure 11.1 *Models of delivery of respiratory care. GP, general practitioner. (Reproduced from Price DB et al.* Primary Care Respir J *2001;* ***10****:47–39[63] with permission from GPIAG Publishing.)*

care staff's attitudes to changes in practice. No matter which care pathway is developed, changes in practice must be supported by continuing education, not one-off directives, to both staff and patients.[55]

Patients who are considered for domiciliary nebulizers will generally be at the severe end of the disease spectrum, and it is important that provision of a nebulizer is made as part of an overall review of the condition and optimization of treatment. Clinicians providing such care therefore need to have appropriate and ongoing medical education in respiratory diseases. It is also important that the supervising clinician provides such patients with a written, personalized management plan that includes instructions on when to call for medical assistance, as inappropriate reliance on nebulized bronchodilators may otherwise result in delay by the patient in calling for help in a life-threatening situation.

The decision to use nebulized treatment and referral

For the many reasons outlined above, not least of which is the considerable cost associated with nebulized therapy, the decision to use nebulizers in the community and, in particular, to provide a patient with a domiciliary nebulizer is an important and complicated one. Nebulized bronchodilators are still widely used in primary care in the acute setting, although, for the reasons outlined above, their use is declining. It is important that general practitioners and nurses who treat acute asthma and COPD are aware of the effectiveness of multiple actuations of bronchodilators delivered by an MDI and spacer system, and are appropriately trained in their use and in educating patients. Decreased use of nebulized therapy in the acute situation may lessen inappropriate pressure from patients and parents for the inappropriate provision of home nebulizers in situations where other delivery systems are safer and more appropriate.

There will be patients in the community who, for a variety of reasons will benefit from nebulized therapy. These patients need full assessment, the provision of a detailed management plan and regular review from an adequately trained clinician. It is apparent that not all generalists will have (or indeed wish to provide) the level of expertise required to meet this demand. We feel, therefore, that there is a need for the availability of appropriate specialist services in the community for such patients: this may be through appropriately trained and accredited general practitioners or nurses, or through 'shared care' protocols and management structures with a local secondary care respiratory clinic. There is at present, increasing interest in the training and accreditation of primary care specialists, i.e. of doctors and nurses with a special interest and special training in particular clinical areas. An appropriately trained primary care respiratory specialist would be ideally placed, in conjunction with the patient's usual general practitioner and nurse, to assess and monitor patients with domiciliary nebulizers.

Potential impact of future devices

In the future we are likely to see the emergence of nebulizers that can reduce the dosage of drug required due to monitoring of and adapting to an individual patient's breathing pattern. Such devices may also be able to monitor adherence with planned treatment regimes and even provide reminders that treatment is due. Such developments may broaden the use of nebulizers in primary care to regular preventative use in a larger group of patients, especially the very young and those with poor adherence.

Summary

- Asthma and COPD are currently and increasingly managed predominantly in primary care.
- More evidence is needed before we unequivocally accept that for all patients inhalers should be first-line treatment for bronchodilation in asthma and COPD
- There are few absolute or objective indicators for nebulizer use in primary care *at this point in time*. Treatment is based on patient preference, ease of use and placebo effect.
- Education in inhaler technique is likely to be beneficial to many patients but some patients may have particular difficulty with inhalers – supporting more use of nebulizers in carefully assessed and selected groups.
- Assessment of symptoms and lung function should be carried out, and treatment with a handheld inhaler and nebulizer tried and compared, before deciding to issue a nebulizer.
- Care should be taken with elderly patients with a history of ischemic heart disease when deciding to issue a nebulizer.
- Evidence-based protocols for selecting nebulizer systems for particular treatments are urgently required.
- Patients should be actively discouraged from buying their own equipment.
- Centralized services for nebulizer provision, maintenance, information and education to primary care teams may be effective.
- Whatever primary care pathway is adopted, best practice should involve evidence and continuing education.
- Advances in nebulizer technology may broaden its use, especially in the very young and in those with poor adherence with regular asthma and COPD therapy.

References

1. Sears MR. Descriptive epidemiology of asthma. *Lancet* 1997; **350**(Suppl 2):S11–S14.
2. NHLBI/WHO workshop report. NIH: Global Initiative for Asthma: Global strategy for asthma management and prevention. NIH Publication No. 95–3659. Bethesda, MD: National Institutes of Health, 1995.
3. Neville RG, Hoskins G, Smith B et al. Observations of the structure, process and clinical outcomes of asthma care in general practice. *Br J Gen Pract* 1996; **46**:583–7.

4. Antic R. Asthma in Australia: the current understanding. Overview of a national series of interactive meetings for general practitioners. Sydney: Excerpta Medica, 1993.

5. Barnes G, Partridge MR. Community asthma clinics: 1993 survey of primary care by the National Asthma Task Force. *Quality Health Care* 1994; **3**:133–6.

6. The Health of Adult Britain 1841–1994. London: Stationery Office, 1997.

7. British Thoracic Society. Guidelines for the management of chronic obstructive pulmonary disease. *Thorax* 1997; **52**(Suppl 5):S1–S28.

8. World Health Organization. World Health Report. Geneva: World Health Organization, 2000.

9. NHLBI/WHO workshop report. NIH: Global Initiative for Chronic Obstructive Lung Disease: Global strategy for the diagnosis, management and prevention of chronic obstructive pulmonary disease. Bethesda, MD: National Institutes of Health, 1996.

10. Britten J, Know A. Helping people to stop smoking: the new smoking cessation guidelines. *Thorax* 1999; **54**:1–2.

11. Pauwels R. Global strategy for the diagnosis, management, and prevention of COPD. Geneva: World Health Organization, 2001.

12. National Heart LaBINIoH. International consensus report on diagnosis and management of asthma (GINA). Publication No 92–3091. Bethesda, MD: National Heart, Lung and Blood Institute, National Institutes of Health, 1992.

13. Burge PS, Calverley PMA, Jonas PW et al. Randomised, double blind, placebo controlled study of fluticasone propionate in patients with moderate to severe chronic pulmonary disease: the ISOLDE study. *BMJ* 2000; **320**:1297–303.

14. Brocklebank D, Ram F, Wright J et al. Comparison of the effectiveness of inhaler devices in asthma and chronic obstructive airways disease: a systematic review of the literature. *Health Technol Assess* 2001; **5**:1–149.

15. Hosker HSR, Teale C, Greenstone MA, Muers MF. Assessment and provision of home nebulisers for chronic obstructive pulmonary disease (COPD) in the Yorkshire region of the UK. *Respir Med* 1995; **89**:47–52.

16. Muers MF. Overview of nebuliser treatment. *Thorax* 1997; **52**(Suppl 2):S25–S30.

17. Cates C. Holding chambers versus nebulisers for B agonist treatment of acute asthma. *Cochrane Database Syst Rev* 2000; 3:CD001491.

18. Brocklebank D, Wright J, Cates C. Systematic review of clinical effectiveness of pressurised metered dose inhalers versus other hand held inhaler devices for delivering corticosteroids in asthma. *BMJ* 2001; **323**:1–7.

19. Duerden M, Price DB. Training issues in inhaler use. *New Ethicals J* 2001; **4**:31–42.

20. Pierce RJ, McDonald CF, Landau LI et al. Nebuhaler versus wet aerosol for domiciliary bronchodilato therapy (adults). *Med J Aust* 1992; **156**:771–4.

21. Turner JR, Corkery KJ, Eckman DE et al. Equivalence of continuous flow nebuliser and metered dose inhaler with reservoir bag for treatment of acute airflow obstruction. *Chest* 1988; **93**:476–81.

22. British Thoracic Society. Guidelines for the management of chronic obstructive pulmonary disease. *Thorax* 1997; **52**(Suppl 5):S1–S28.

23. Eccles M, Rousseau N, Higgins B, Thomas L. Evidence-based guideline on the primary care management of asthma. *Fam Pract* 2001; **18**:223–9.

24. Barnes PJ, Jonsson B, Klim JB. The costs of asthma. *Eur Respir J* 1996; **9**:636–42.

25. Lacasse Y, Wong E, Guyatt GH et al. Meta-analysis of respiratory rehabilitation in chronic obstructive pulmonary disease. *Lancet* 1996; **348**:1115–19.

26. Stewart AL, Greenfield S, Hays RD et al. Functional status and well being of patients with chronic conditions: results from the medical outcomes study. *JAMA* 1989; **262**:907–13.

27. Crompton GK. The adult patient's difficulties with inhalers. *Lung* 1990; **168**(Suppl):658–62.

28. Blackhall MI. A dose response study of inhaled terbutaline administered via Nebuhalar or nebuliser to asthmatic children. *Eur J Respir Dis* 1987; **71**:96–101.

29. Grimwood K, Johnson-Barrett JJ, Taylor B. Salbutamol: tablets, inhalational powder or nebuliser? *BMJ* 1981; **282**:105–6.

30. Wijkstra PJ, Van Altena R, Kraan J et al. Quality of life in patients with chronic obstructive pulmonary disease improves after rehabilitation at home. *Eur Respir J* 1994; **7**:269–73.

31. Freelander S, Van Asperen N. Nebuhaler vs nebulizer in children with acute asthma. *BMJ* 1984; **288**:1873–4.

32. Muers MF. The rational use of nebulizers in clinical practice. *Eur Respir J* 1997; **7**:189–97.

33. Nimmo CJ, Chen DNM, Martinusen SM et al. Assessment of patient acceptance and inhalation technique of a pressurised aerosol inhaler and two breath-actuated devices. *Ann Pharmacother* 1993; **27**:922–7.

34. van der Palen J, Klein JJ, Kerkoff AHM et al. Evaluation of the long-term effectiveness of three instruction modes for inhaling medicines. *Patient Educ Counsel* 1997; **32**:S87–S95.

35. Kesten S, Elias M, Cartier A et al. Patient handling of a multidose dry powder inhalation devices for albuterol. *Chest* 1994; **105**:1077–81.

36. Newman SP. Efficient use of nebulisers. *Update* 1988; **36**:381–8.

37. Ilangovan P, Pederson S, Godfry S et al. Treatment of severe steroid-dependent preschool asthma with nebulised budesonnide suspension. *Arch Dis Child* 1993; **68**:356–9.

38. De Blic J, Delacourt C, Bourgeois J. A double-blind, parallel-group study of nebulised budesonide in severe infantile asthma. *Am Rev Respir Dis* 1993; **147**(Suppl 4, part 2):A266.

39. Fok TF, Lam K, Ng PC et al. Delivery of salbutamol to nonventilated preterm infants by metered-dose inhaler, jet nebulizer and ultrasonic nebulizer. *Eur Respir J* 1998; **12**:159–64.

40. Closa RM, Ceballos JM, Gomez-Papi A et al. Efficacy of bronchodilators administered by nebulizer versus spacer devices in infants with wheezing. *Pediatr Pulmonol* 1998; **26**:344–8.

41. Lin YZ, Hsieh KH. Metered dose inhaler and nebuliser in acute asthma. *Arch Dis Child* 1995; **72**:214–18.

42. Tal A, Golan H, Grauer N et al. Deposition pattern of radiolabeled salutamol inhaled from a metered-dose inhaler by means of a spacer with mask in young children with airway obstruction. *J Pediatr* 1996; **128**:479–84.

43. Callahan CW. Wet nebulization in actue asthma: the last refrain? *Chest* 2000; **117**:1226–8.

44. Inwald D, Roland M, Kuitert L, McKenzie SA, Petros A. Oxygen treatment for acute severe asthma. *BMJ* 2001; **323**:98–100.

45. National Institute for Clinical Excellence. Guidance on the use of inhaler systems (devices) in children under the age of 5 years with chronic asthma. Technological Appraisal Guidance No. 10. London: NICE, 2000.

46. Boccuti LT, Geller RJ, Celano M, Phillips KM. Development of a scale to measure children's metered-dose inhaler and spacer technique. *Ann Allergy Asthma Immunol* 1996; **77**:217–21.

47. Brownlee KG. A rationale for the use of nebulized steroids in children. *Eur Respir J* 1997; **44**:177–9.

48. Parkin PC, Saunders NR, Diamond SA et al. Randomised trail spacer vs. nebuliser for acute asthma. *Arch Dis Child* 1995; **72**:239–40.

49. Pounsford JC. Nebulisers for the elderly. *Thorax* 1997; **52**(Suppl 2):S53–S55.

50. Armitage JM, Williams SJ. Inhaler technique in the elderly. *Age Ageing* 1988; **17**:272–8.

51. Buckley D. Assessment of inhaler technique in general practice. *Irish J Med Sci* 1989; **158**:297–9.

52. Allen SC, Prior A. What determines whether an elderly patient can use a metered dose inhaler correctly? *Chest* 1986; **80**:45–9.

53. Lim R, Walshaw MJ, Saltissi S, Hind CRK. Cardiac arrhythmias during acute exacerbations of chronic airflow limitation: effect of fall in plasma potassium concentration induced by nebulised beta agnoist therapy. *Postgrad Med J* 1989; **65**:449–52.

54. Ullah MI, Newman GB, Suanders KB. Influence of age on response to ipratropium and salbutamol in asthma. *Thorax* 1981; **36**:523–9.

55. Craig IR, Riley MR, Cooke NJ. Prescribing of nebulized bronchodilators – can we change bad habits? *Respir Med* 1989; **83**:333–4.

56. Vermiere P. European trends in inhalation therapy. *Eur Respir J* 1994; **4**(Suppl 18):89–91.

57. Boe J, Dennis JH, O'Driscoll BR and members of the European Respiratory Society Task Force. European Respiratory Society guidelines on the use of nebulizers. *Eur Respir J* 2001; **18**:228–42.

58. British Thoracic Society, National Asthma Campaign, Royal College of Physicians of London et al. The British guidelines on asthma management. *Thorax* 1997; **52**(Suppl 1):S1–S21.

59. Stewart M, Brown JB, Weston WW et al. Patient-centred medicine: transforming the clinical method. Thousand Oaks: Sage Publications, 1995.

60. Kendrick AH, Smith EC, Wilson RSE. Selecting and using nebuliser equipment. *Thorax* 1997; **52**(Suppl 2):S92–S101.

61. Smith EC, Kendrick AH, Brewin A. Staff education. *Thorax* 1997; **52**(Suppl 2):S102–S103.

62. Dodd ME, Hanley SP, Johnson SC, Webb AK. Costs of a district nebuliser compressor service. *Thorax* 1992; **47**:863P.

63. Price DB, van der Molen T. The Aberdeen primary care COPD research needs statement, March 2001. *Primary Care Respir J* 2001; **10**:47–9.

Section C.

Practical Considerations

12. PRACTICAL USE

Louise Lannefors and Jacob Boe

Introduction

Nebulization therapy: a multifactorial route for drug administration

Inhalation therapy administered by a nebulizer system encompasses many different practical aspects each of which may affect the outcome of the treatment.[1-3] Information and instructions regarding what is effective treatment, as well as practical training in how to handle the drug(s), how to use and clean the nebulizer, effective inhalation technique (Figure 12.1) and timing the inhalations are often omitted when nebulizer systems are prescribed/delivered to patients.[4,5] Most healthcare professionals have little or no knowledge or training when it comes to the practical applications of this kind of treatment that comprises so many potentially undermining steps.

Individually tailored choice of inhalation device

A physician who is often not a specialist in respiratory medicine usually signs the prescription for inhalation therapy. However, the choice of a dry powder inhaler, a handheld metered dose inhaler (MDI) with a spacer, a handheld breath-activated inhaler or a nebulizer system (if the drug is available for all forms of administration) can be made by the prescribing physician, a nurse or a physiotherapist/respiratory therapist. One good way of choosing a device is to follow an optimization protocol, where the needs and the capability of the patient are assessed and some possible alternatives are tried.[2] The questions that need to be answered before a nebulizer system is prescribed are whether the patient can handle a nebulizer system in the first place and which type of system would be most suitable.[6,7]

Purchase and delivery options for nebulizer systems

The purchase and delivery options for nebulizer systems differ a great deal from one country or region to another. These options range from a patient who has been prescribed a nebulizer system collecting it from a

(a)

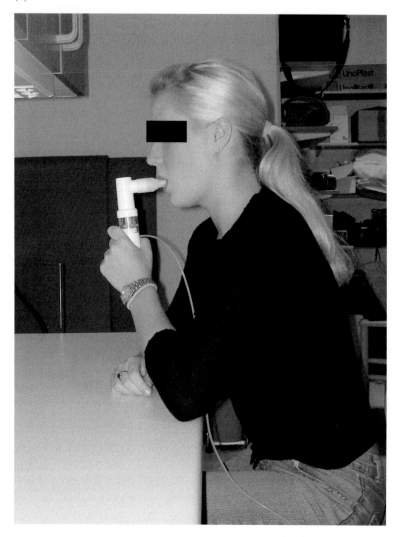

Figure 12.1a,b Patients inhaling with the help of a nebulizer system.

specialized unit to a pharmacy handing out the device, or the patient collecting it directly from the manufacturer or supplier. Rarely, but nonetheless it can happen that patients obtain access to a nebulizer system by purchasing one in a shop or at a secondhand market. The extent to which adequate practical information and supervision is included when the therapy is prescribed and/or the device is supplied varies tremendously (if it is included at all).

(b)

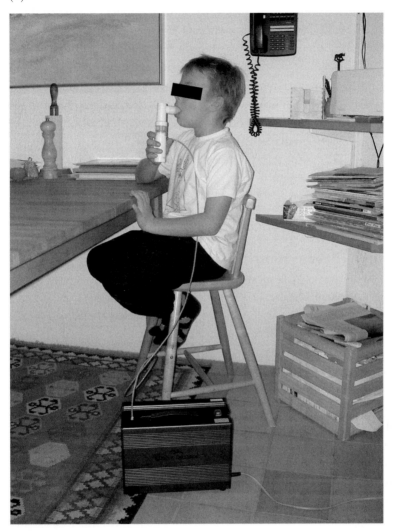

Figure 12.1a,b (Continued)

Organized nebulizer system service unit

Healthcare professionals who are educated in and involved in inhalation therapy are often not available or do not receive funding to provide an inhalation therapy clinic or at least a nebulizer system service unit.[1,2,8] However, whenever possible, patients who are prescribed inhalation therapy should be referred to a specialist unit to define the optimal administration device. If nebulization therapy appears to be the optimal method,

237

the choice of the optimal nebulizer system, the delivery of the system and the instruction/training of the patient in its use must be worked through to secure effective and safe treatment conditions.[2,7–12]

Thus, a good comprehensive education in the practical use of nebulizer systems is needed, but not only for patients. Healthcare professionals involved in nebulization therapy often know too little about the different practical factors that produce effective therapy and reduce the risks of undesirable effects.[2,4,8,10,13] This is the situation both in hospital and in home care. This chapter will mainly focus on the latter.

Nebulization therapy in practice

The nebulizer system

A jet nebulizer system consists of a nebulizer, a driving source and a tube connecting them (Figure 12.2). There are many different types of nebulizer systems on the market and more are in the pipeline. The most common are still the jet nebulizer systems, but ultrasonic nebulizer systems are increasing in number and new types of systems are being developed. Most of the information mentioned here is based on studies and experience of jet nebulizer systems, unless otherwise specified. However, the information applying to jet nebulizers is usually also applicable to ultrasonic nebulizer systems.

The quality of the aerosol produced and the volume nebulized per unit time is a result of the performance of the driving source and the performance of the nebulizer when combined to create one nebulizer system. The capacity of the system is changed if either the driving source or the nebulizer is replaced with another type or model.[14] The capacities of many different types of nebulizer systems or combinations of driving sources and nebulizers are well known. Combinations other than these should be avoided until the capacity has been properly measured and defined. One system might be heavy and difficult to move, but it may also rapidly produce an aerosol of good quality. Another system might be very mobile, but the nebulizer may consist of several small parts that are difficult to put together and clean and could also perhaps be easily lost. A compromise is needed in which not only the type of drug prescribed is taken into account. Practical and functional factors are equally important in the struggle to make the nebulization therapy as easy as possible for the patient to carry out, a factor which will most probably affect compliance with the treatment.

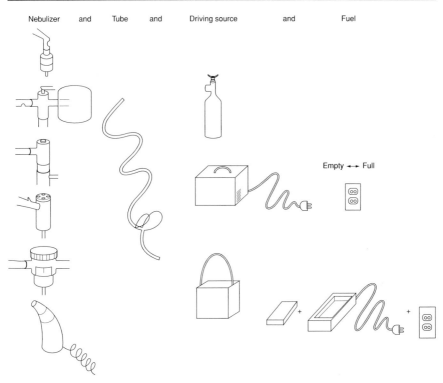

Nebulizer   and   Tube   and   Driving source   and   Fuel

Empty ←→ Full

Figure 12.2 *Schematic drawing of the different parts of a 'nebulizer system'.*

Pharmaceutical companies that produce new drugs for nebulization therapy nowadays often recommend a suitable nebulizer system to use with the drug. One undesirable effect of this is that patients who are prescribed more than one drug for nebulization might need to acquire more than one type of nebulizer system for their treatment!

The driving source
Jet nebulizers for home care can be powered by an electrical compressor connected to a plug, or using a chargeable battery as the power supply, or by a bottle of compressed gas containing either air or oxygen. In hospital, jet nebulizers can be powered by compressed gas supplied through back-pressure-compensated flow regulators or by pressure regulators connected to the air or oxygen lines. One compressor might be heavy yet powerful, while another could be easy to carry but underpowered. Compressors are noisy, while bottles containing compressed gas are quiet. However, bottles become empty and a system in which empty bottles are replaced by full ones needs to be organized, and the patient must master moving the flow regulator from an empty bottle to a full one.

239

The nebulizer

Different kinds of nebulizer have different aerosol delivery characteristics (Figure 12.3). The amount of the loaded dose that can be deposited within the lungs is highly dependent on these characteristics. This is one factor that is often neglected when prescribing the dose and/or filling volume to be loaded into the nebulizer. The dose might need to be corrected if the type of nebulizer system is changed. Some nebulizers offer more than one delivery pattern, which gives the patient an opportunity to choose. Patients must know which delivery pattern to use and how to use it. Loss of drug into the room might be of less importance in relation to the effect in certain situations than in others. If the lost aerosol affects staff, parents/carers and surroundings, the nebulizer should be equipped with an expiratory filter. Connecting a tube to the expiratory outlet of the nebulizer and letting the expired air out of the window is sometimes recommended. This could be an alternative, but only if re-breathing of the expired air is avoided. The delivery pattern and nebulizer characteristics that are suitable for the patient and the drug prescribed depend on several practical and functional factors, such as the produced aerosol quality, nebulization time, drug output and the desired proportion of the dose that can be deposited within the lungs. Other factors of importance, which affect the choice of nebulizer systems are listed in Box 12.1

Requirements for information and practice

Patients need information about the nebulizer system in order to be able to handle it correctly (Box 12.2). They also need to see the equipment being handled and to practice the handling procedure together with the instructor.[1,2,14,15] An optimal teaching situation could involve the patient bringing the prescribed drug and performing the first inhalation procedure, including all the different practical elements, under supervision. The information about how to use and maintain a nebulizer system should be provided in writing as well.

The drug(s)

Patients need practical information about the drug(s) that are prescribed. They need to understand which symptom the drug is targeted at, the expected effect, which dosage to use, whether to use it regularly and/or when needed, and also which side effects can appear.[11] They also need more practical information about how to handle the drug(s) (Box 12.3). If patients have not inhaled the prescribed drug before, the first inhalation

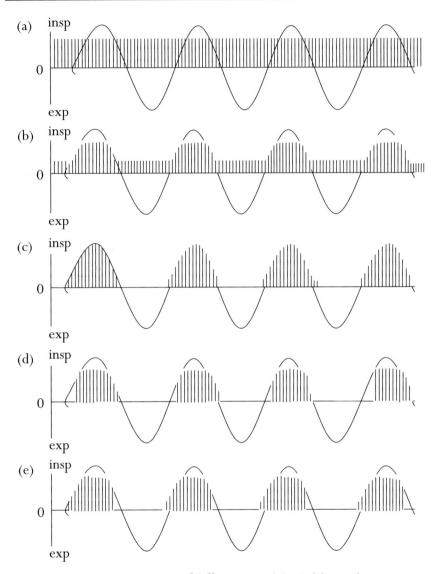

Figure 12.3 *Schematic drawing of different aerosol (▦) delivery characteristics for different types of nebulizer. (a) Continuous aerosol production and continuous delivery. (b) Continuous aerosol production with a Venturi effect and continuous delivery. (c) Continuous aerosol production and continuous delivery into a spacer from where the aerosol is inhaled. (d) Breath-enhanced aerosol production and delivery (passive). (e) Manually activated / interrupted aerosol production and delivery (either active or passive).*

241

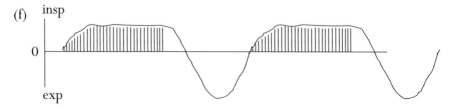

Figure 12.3 (Continued) *(f) An optimal aerosol delivery characteristic inhaled with an optimal inspiratory flow. The y-axis represent flows and the x-axis time.*

Box 12.1 Practical and functional factors that affect a patient's choice of nebulizer system.

The patient's:
  capability to cooperate and coordinate
  capability to handle small parts and several parts
  desire/need to take small pauses while inhaling a dose
  desire/need to put the nebulizer away during these small pauses (to be able to handle coughing, sputum, tissues and so on)
  need to combine the spontaneous breathing pattern with deep inspirations and deep expirations
  need/desire to inhale some of the dose while lying on their side

---

ought to be carried out at a medical unit. All the information about how to handle the drug(s) should be provided to them in writing as well.

Oxygen supply
One way of supplying hypoxic patients with oxygen is to use compressed oxygen as the nebulizer driving source. This can be done through the oxygen lines in hospital or through bottles of compressed oxygen at home. Due to the working mechanism of jet nebulizers, the oxygen is diluted with room air and its concentration leaving the nebulizer is never 100%. However, oxygen is a drug and its effects/side effects should always be monitored closely, especially in emergency situations. The occurrence of negative side effects, such as increased $PaCO_2$, reduced consciousness or irregular breathing pattern during oxygen supply, would make it necessary to reconsider both the dose and the indication for further oxygen therapy. A situation like this should not, however, be confused with patients falling asleep. In dyspneic patients who might lack sleep for long periods, perhaps several days, one sign of effective treatment is that they actually dare to fall asleep. Sleep is often what they need most, secondary to the effective treat-

---

Box 12.2 Information necessary for a patient to be able to handle the nebulizer system and the drug adequately for therapy in different situations.

How the nebulizer system works and the names of the different parts of the system (for future communication)

The main function of the driving source and

    if powered by compressed gas, how long a bottle lasts, when to replace empty bottles with full ones, how to transfer the pressure regulator from one to another, security regulations at home and when traveling

    if powered by rechargeable batteries, what kind of battery, how long it lasts when fully charged, how to charge it and service life

    if and how to change a compressor input filter regularly

    how to clean and exchange the tubing connecting the driving source with the nebulizer

    how to wipe the compressor

    if abroad, different voltage requirements and plugs in different countries

The function of the nebulizer and

    how to connect it to the driving source

    how to dismantle and put it together

    how to clean the different parts

    service life, recommended exchange (single-use, single-patient-use, durable)

    choice of mouthpiece or face mask, if both are delivered with the system

    nebulizing into a spacer, how often to exchange the spacer

    whether or not an expiratory filter is needed and how often to change it or its pad

Adequate nebulization time for the prescribed drug, to be able to judge dysfunction

Other signs/sounds of malfunction

Suppliers, access to spare parts and repairs, replacement equipment

Maintenance, how often and where, replacement equipment

What to do with the nebulizer system when it is not needed any more

---

ment of their lung disease. If there is any doubt, blood gases can be checked during nebulized therapy to exclude sleepiness due to hypercapnia.

Inhalation technique

Ventilation

Drugs administered as an aerosol are carried into the lungs during inspiration. Therefore inhaled drugs can only be deposited in ventilated airways, where air enters during inspiration and leaves during expiration.[16–18] Inhaled aerosol is homogeneously distributed throughout the airways in healthy lungs.[19] However, the deposition pattern in patients with different

---

Box 12.3 Practical information for the patient about the drug(s) prescribed for nebulization therapy and how to handle drugs.

How to store the drug

The benefits of warming up (if possible) a refrigerator-cold drug to room temperature before nebulizing it

How long a multidose bottle lasts when opened; where to discard a bottle which still contains drug

Are a syringe and needle needed to load the nebulizer with the prescribed dose, how long can each syringe and needle be used, where to get them and how/where to discard them

Whether to dilute the drug and what to dilute it with

If used in combination with other inhaled drugs, in what order should they be inhaled

If used in combination with mucus evacuating therapy, what drugs to inhale before and/or during airway clearance and what to inhale when as much mucus as possible has been evacuated

If used in combination with other nebulized drugs, whether to mix them

If used in combination with other nebulized drugs, whether a clean nebulizer is needed for each drug, or perhaps a totally different nebulizer system

Define an adequate endpoint for each inhalation treatment: options include running the nebulizer totally empty, stopping when the first 'spitting sounds' occur, running it for a certain number of minutes, stopping when symptoms have disappeared and so on

Action to take if dyspnea continues; whether to increase the inhaled dose or contact the hospital

---

degrees of pulmonary disease varies a great deal, depending on both the ventilation pattern and the breathing pattern (Figure 12.4). The breathing pattern and the technique with which the aerosol is inhaled have been shown to be essential for the optimal share of the dose to be deposited within the lungs.[20] Perhaps the importance of training a patient to use an optimal technique increases with the degree of lung damage and an abnormal breathing pattern.

Inhalation
The term inhalation technique has many aspects, such as mouth breathing (independent of using a mouthpiece of face mask), how to place the mouthpiece in the mouth, relaxed breathing, inspiratory flow, inspired volume, varying FRC (functional residual capacity) level, body positioning, aerosol loss during expiration and perhaps others (Figures 12.5 and 12.6).[3,20,21] The potential for adjusting the spontaneous breathing pattern depends on many factors, such as age, degree of lung disease, body position and the patient's

(a)

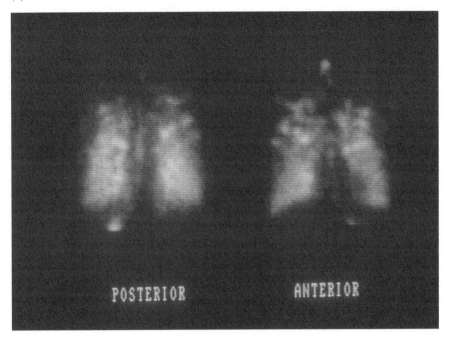

Figure 12.4 *Radioactive aerosol MMD (mean median diameter) 3 μm inhaled in a sitting position with ordinary tidal volume breaths. Deposition patterns in (a) a 24-year-old man with mild chronic obstructive pulmonary disease and (b) a 28-year-old man with severe chronic obstructive pulmonary disease.*

ability to cooperate. The extent to which an improved breathing pattern results in an improved pulmonary deposition pattern and an increased amount of drug being deposited depends to a great extent on the characteristics of the nebulizer. More knowledge is needed about ways of optimizing the deposited dose and the deposition pattern of nebulized drug(s), especially when included as part of the daily treatment at home for long periods. It is also not known whether the inhalation technique itself is equally important for all kinds of drug.

Dose deposited within the lungs and deposition pattern
It is not always obvious how much of the dose needs to be deposited in the lungs to achieve the desired/expected effects. When inhaling bronchodilators, the effect is usually easy to measure and it is possible to define an optimal individual dose. However, the safety margins for the prescribed bronchodilator dose for nebulizers are usually large and the level of ambition for the inhalation

(b)

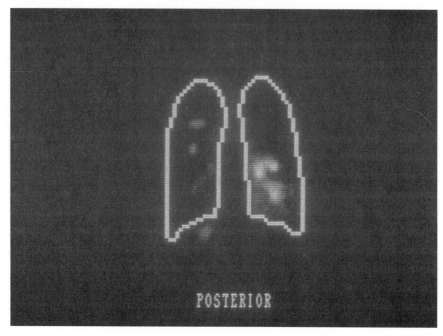

POSTERIOR

Figure 12.4 (Continued)

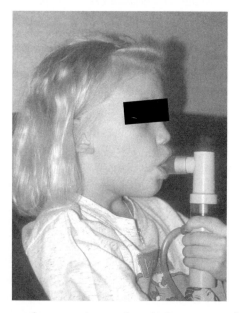

Figure 12.5 *The mouthpiece in the mouth with the tongue underneath and the teeth and lips around it.*

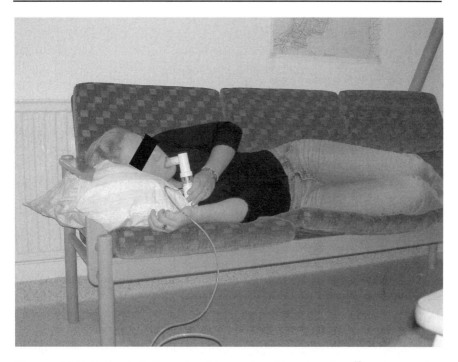

Figure 12.6 *Patient inhaling when lying on her side, using the effects that gravity has on regional ventilation.*

technique can probably therefore be at a minimum level. Defining the optimal dose is much more difficult when it comes to mucolytics, corticosteroids, antibiotics and other drugs, where it is still not possible to measure the immediate effects. Too low a dose of inhaled antibiotics deposited within the lungs might have a negative effect, due to the risk of developing microbiological resistance. In addition, some of the newer drugs (like antibiotics and mucolytics) are very expensive. Depositing as large a share as possible of the prescribed dose in the lungs is of greater interest in these situations. Viscous airway mucus and micro-organisms can appear all over the lungs and/or in poorly ventilated parts of the lungs. For these patients, as even a deposition pattern as possible might be necessary to obtain a good effect from the treatment. The less ventilated the airways, the smaller the amount of drug deposited.[22] In closed airways, the inhaled drug has no access at all. In these situations, the level of ambition for an optimal inhalation technique might need to be high, with the aim of improving regional deposition (Box 12.4).

To summarize, the definition of a sufficiently good inhalation technique has to take account of the drug prescribed, age, severity of lung disease, the

---

Box 12.4 Factors to be considered when training a patient inhalation technique using a nebulizer system.

Always start using a mouthpiece regardless of the functional age, always (when possible) inspire through the mouth, even if a face mask needs to be used (using a mouthpiece gives information about mouth breathing or not and it could be easier for the patient/parent to correct)

Sit in a comfortable position, leaning forward with the elbows on a table. Other body positions can be of interest if the treatment is aimed at specific parts of the lungs that are less well ventilated when sitting or if the most possible uniform deposition pattern in the whole of the lungs is desired

Relaxed breathing forms the base from which patients learn

   not to hyperventilate

   to slow inspirations to improve the deposition within the lungs and reduce the deposition in the throat and central airways

   to match inspirations to TLC in between the ordinary breaths to open up clogged or collapsed airways

   if lungs are hyperinflated, to breathe at a lower FRC level during parts of the inhalation to deposit aerosol in otherwise poorly ventilated airways

   if using a manually interrupted nebulizer, to coordinate optimally with the inspirations to lose as little aerosol as possible during expiration

---

TLC, total lung capacity; FRC, functional residual capacity.

---

home situation and the patient's ability to cooperate. The extent to which the spontaneous inhalation technique needs to be improved is individual. Improving an inhalation technique requires instructions and practice. Sometimes a great deal of training is required, but improvements are almost always possible to achieve and are also worthwhile.

Cleaning and maintenance

A nebulizer system forms a unit that changes fluid to an aerosol of a certain quality as rapidly as possible, according to the data presented by the manufacturer. As the compressor filters become dirty and channels become clogged, and as some exposed parts of the nebulizer wear out the unit will not be able to live up to its original standard. The cleaning and maintenance of all nebulizer systems are therefore essential to optimize the effects of the nebulizing therapy and avoid unnecessary dysfunction or undesirable or negative effects.[23]

It has been shown and it is also well known that nebulizer systems are frequently not cleaned and maintained as recommended (Figure 12.7).

(a)

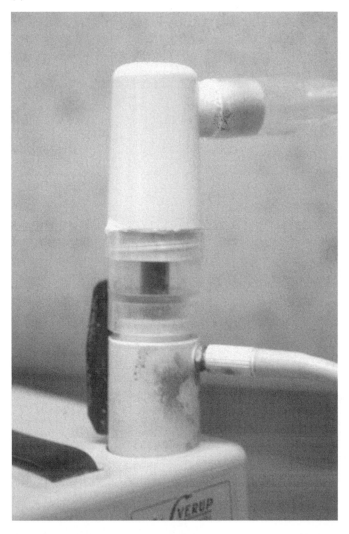

Figure 12.7(a–e) *Examples of dirty nebulizer systems where effectiveness and hygienic safety of the inhilation therapy are affected.*

Undesirable or negative effects of these include malfunction, contamination and cross-infection.[5] In some countries, the healthcare organization is responsible for the formulation of and compliance with cleaning recommendations. Elsewhere, the responsibility for providing cleaning recommendations lies with each manufacturer.[23]

249

(b)

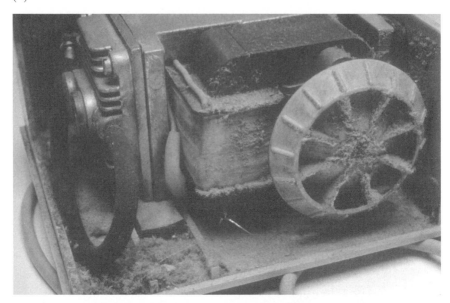

(c)

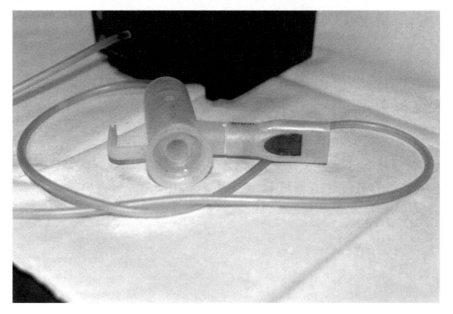

Figure 12.7(a–e) (Continued)

(d)

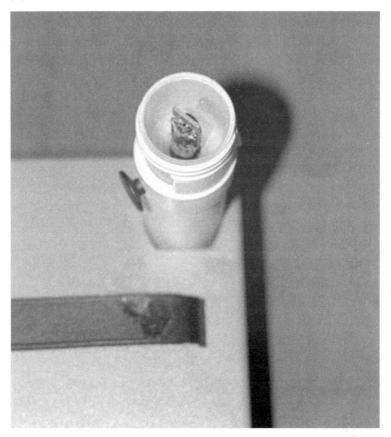

Figure 12.7(a–e) (Continued)

Cleaning

A single-use nebulizer is by definition designed to be used only once and then thrown away. A single-patient nebulizer can be used for several inhalation sessions by one patient for a limited time. A limited time is usually defined as 1 week. A durable nebulizer can be used for many inhalation sessions over a much longer period. Producers usually recommend that the use of durable nebulizers should be limited; a common recommendation is 1 year.

It is naturally important to respect the recommendations for use – whether a nebulizer unit is prescribed for single use, single-patient use or is of a durable type. Single-use nebulizers are not designed for cleaning; they may not even withstand cleaning. However, single-patient-use

(e)

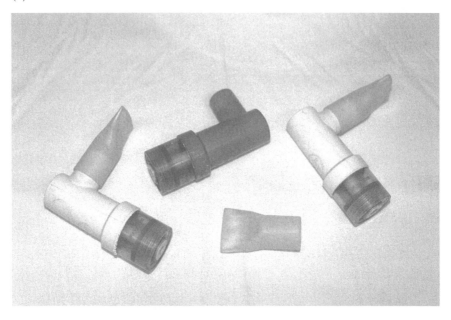

Figure 12.7(a–e) (Continued)

nebulizers can usually withstand usage and cleaning for a limited period of time. Even in hospitals, it has been shown that single-patient nebulizers are not always cleaned between inhalation sessions, as the staff have experienced the risk of confusing the nebulizers with those of other patients in the cleaning process. They further report lack of time or fear that small parts will get lost during the cleaning procedure.[5] In home care, single-use or single-patient nebulizers are sometimes used with no time limit, although the quality of these nebulizers will never be as good as that of the durable ones.[24]

The cleaning procedure needs to be well described to the patient. It includes the whole nebulizer system, the driving source, the nebulizer, the tubing and the wire for electricity supply, if there is one.[23] Cleaning includes removing sticky drug residues and getting rid of microbial growth and ordinary dust and dirt (Figure 12.8).[2] Suboptimal function has been reported in situations in which the nebulizer has not been cleaned at all and in which the nebulizer has been cleaned too vigorously.[25,26] Even though different situations (hospital and home care) require the same high standards, they require different routines, which are possible to adhere to in the long term.

Box 12.5 Suggested hygienic procedures for nebulization therapy.

Loading

the loading procedure should be kept uncontaminated by simply washing the hands prior to handling the drug(s). If needles and syringes are needed, change them both when changing the drug bottle if it is kept as a closed unit. At hospital, the loading procedure should follow the hygiene rules for other non-intravenous drugs

Nebulizers (single-patient or durable nebulizers)

empty the nebulizer after each use and if possible nebulize some water or NaCl (sodium chloride) to get the sticky drug out of the thin channels or just run the nebulizer dry, dismantle and rinse it in warm water

at home, disinfect once a day in boiling water for 2 min. In hospital, after each use, disinfect in a 10-min disinfection program at ≥85 °C. To ensure the inactivation of mycobacteria, 97 °C for at least 3 min must be achieved

at home, wipe the lower part (the handle of the jet nebulizer and the membrane of the ultrasonic nebulizer) with a mild detergent once a day. In hospital, wipe with a disinfectant after each use

tap off all water and leave the different parts of the nebulizer to dry on a clean, dry cloth. If possible, have the nebulizer dried in a drying chamber in hospital

Tubing

if there is moisture in the tube, change the tubing frequently

Driving source

wipe dust and dirt from the driving source, the tube and the wire at home with a damp cloth once a week. In hospital, clean with a disinfectant between different patients

change the air inlet filter on the compressor according to recommendations

---

The ideal standards for hygienic procedures, cleaning methods and cleaning frequency have not yet been well established, but some procedures are suggested in Box 12.5 (see also Figure 12.8).[23] Many prescribing units or hospitals have specified their own hygiene recommendations, while others recommend their patients to stick to the cleaning regime recommended by the manufacturer.

If nebulization therapy is carried out more than once a day, the optimal solution for the patient would be to have more than one nebulizer for the driving source. The nebulizer that is used should be emptied and rinsed after each treatment session. However, all the nebulizers used during the past 24 hours can be disinfected at the same time, once a day. This would save some time for the patient. The same goes for those patients who are prescribed more than one drug for nebulization, where the drugs should not be mixed. Patients might have been taught to use a clean nebulizer for

(a)

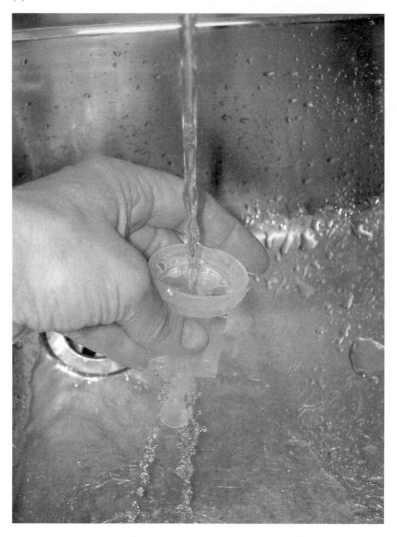

Figure 12.8 *This dismantled nebulizer is (a) rinsed in warm water (b) disinfected in boiled water and (c) the different parts are then left to dry on a clean cloth.*

the second drug and they will therefore use more than one nebulizer at each treatment session.

Maintenance

It is usually recommended that service and check-ups should be carried out annually, following a specific protocol.[1,2,23] The whole nebulizer system

(b)

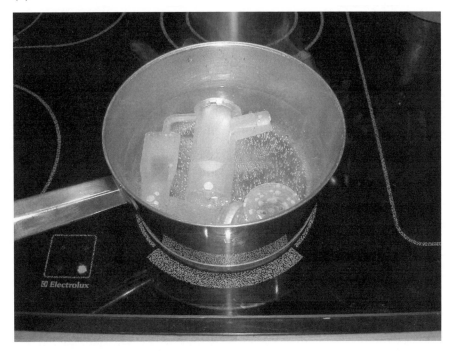

Figure 12.8 (Continued)

should be checked in one piece, as this is how it is used. It is important to measure the working pressure during nebulization for the whole system. Checking the output is essential. A malfunction might be found in either the driving source or the nebulizer itself. The nebulizer, tube and filters should be exchanged as often as necessary or as recommended by the manufacturer.

Follow-up, assessment and compliance with therapy
Repeated evaluation of the effects of treatment is necessary to assess the need for continued inhalation therapy, and to justify the nebulizer system as the optimal way of administering the drug(s). A change to another inhalation system should be considered at regular intervals.

Compliance with the nebulized treatment varies considerably among patients.[27,28] The extent to which this is associated with the indication for and the knowledge of the treatment can be discussed. Most patients need help to remain motivated to carry out the treatment and/or maintain high-quality treatment in the long term. Individually adapted education could form the basis for helping patients to stay motivated and it could be

(c)

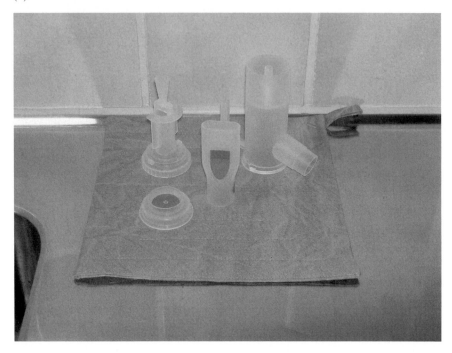

Figure 12.8 (Continued)

followed up by regular contact with the nebulizer system service unit, which can also help to achieve a safe treatment procedure.[8,12]

The effects of the treatment should be monitored both objectively and subjectively. This could also include a functional parameter chosen by the patient. Apart from assessing the effects of the treatment, the regular follow-ups should include evaluating the practical aspects, how patients handle the nebulizer system and the drug(s), their inhalation technique, and the condition of the nebulizer system.[2,3] The first follow-up should be offered at an early stage: perhaps 1 week after the treatment begins. The effects of the treatment and the way it is carried out are then reassessed regularly, following a standard protocol, but individually adapted when needed.

One effective way of checking the practical aspects of the treatment is to ask patients to bring their nebulizer system and their drug(s) with them during routine visits to their nebulizer system service unit. Patients are then asked to perform an inhalation treatment session as they do at home. After finishing the inhalation procedure, they are asked to dismantle the nebulizer and describe the cleaning procedures used at home.

A situation like this gives patients a good opportunity to bring up both positive and negative experiences and ask for help if they are dissatisfied. It also gives the instructor an effective opportunity to answer questions and to clarify misunderstandings, if there are any, and to optimize the treatment.

An optimal way of following up and assessing the effects of the treatment would be to use 'follow-up protocols', including parameters such as lung function, symptom protocol, side effects, sense of wellbeing and quality of life.[2]

References

1. Muers MF, Corris PA eds. British Thoracic Society: Guidelines. *Thorax* 1997; **52**(Suppl 2):S4–S24.

2. Boe J, Dennis JH, O'Driscoll BR et al. European Respiratory Society guidelines on the use of nebulizers. *Eur Respir J* 2001; **18**:228–42.

3. Le Brun PP, de Boer AH, Heijerman HG, Frijlink HW. A review of the technical aspects of drug nebulization. *Pharm World Sci* 2000; **22**:75–81.

4. Caldwell NA, Milroy R. Optimizing nebulization practice within a large teaching hospital: easier said than done. *Respir Med* 1995; **89**:57–9.

5. Heslop K, Harkawat R. Nebulizer therapy from a practical perspective. *Eur Respir Rev* 2000; **10**:213–15.

6. Dautzenberg B, Nikander K. Choice of a device for each disease and medicine. *Eur Respir Rev* 2000; **10**:545–8.

7. Porter-Jones G, Francis S, Benfield G. Running a nurse-led nebulizer clinic in a district general hospital. *Br J Nurs* 1999; **8**:1079–84.

8. Heslop K, Lannefors L, Dautzenberg B. Local nebulizer services. *Eur Respir Rev* 2000; **10**:549–51.

9. Dodd ME, Hanley SP, Johnson SC, Webb AK. District nebuliser compressor service: reliability and costs. *Thorax* 1995; **50**:82–4.

10. Smith EC, Kendrick AH, Brewin A. Staff education. *Thorax* 1997; **52**(Suppl 2):S102–S103.

11. Wilson RSE, Muers MF. Running a domiciliary nebuliser service. *Thorax* 1997; **52**(Suppl 2): S104–S106.

12. O'Driscoll BR, Bernstein A. A long-term study of symptoms, spirometry and survival amongst home nebulizer users. *Respir Med* 1996; **90**:561–6.

13. Caldwell NA, Milroy R, McCabe J, Banham SW, Moran F. An audit of nebulisation techniques in a major teaching hospital: scope for improvement. *Pharm J* 1991; **247**:706–8.

14. Kendrick AH, Smith EC, Wilson RSE. Selecting and using nebuliser equipment. *Thorax* 1997; **52**(Suppl 2):S92–S101.

15. Tiddens HAWM, Van der Broek E, Struycken VHJ, Dzoljic-Danilovic G, De Jongste JC. Maintenance, bacterial contamination and performance of jet nebulizers used by out-patients. *Am J Respir Crit Care Med* 1995; **151**:A362.

16. O'Callaghan C, Barry PW. The science of nebulised drug delivery. *Thorax* 1997; **52**(Suppl 2): S31–S44.

17. Nikander K, Denyer J. Breathing patterns. *Eur Respir Rev* 2000; **10**:576–9.

18. Denyer J. Adaptive aerosol delivery in practice. *Eur Respir Rev* 1997; **7**:388–9.

19. Goldstein I, Wallet F, Robert J et al. Lung tissue concentrations of nebulized amikacin during mechanical ventilation in piglets with healthy lungs. *Am J Respir Crit Care Med* 2002; **165**:171–5.

20. Kumazawa H, Asako M, Yamashita T, Ha-Kawa SK. An increase in laryngeal aerosol deposition by ultrasonic nebulizer therapy with intermittent vocalization. *Laryngoscope* 1997; **107**:671–4.

21. Kishida M, Suzuki I, Kabayama H et al. Mouthpiece versus facemask for delivering of nebulized salbutamol in exacerbated childhood asthma. *J Asthma* 2002; **39**:337–9.

22. Elman M, Goldstein I, Marquette CH et al. Influence of lung aeration on pulmonary concentrations of nebulized and intravenous amikacin in ventilated piglets with severe bronchopneumonia. *Anesthesiology* 2002; **97**:199–206.

23. Lannefors L, Heslop K, Teirlinck C. Nebulizer systems: contamination, microbial risks, cleaning and effect on function. *Eur Respir Rev* 2000; **10**:571–5.

24. Rosenfeld M, Emerson J, Astley S et al. Home nebulizer use among patients with cystic fibrosis. *J Pediatr* 1998; **132**:125–31.

25. Standaert TA, Morlin GL, Williams-Warren J et al. Effects of repetitive use and cleaning techniques of disposable jet nebulizers on aerosol generation. *Chest* 1998; **114**:577–86.

26. Nerbrink O, Dahlbäck M. Basic nebulizer function. *J Aerosol Med* 1994; **7**:S7–S11.

27. Schöni MH, Horak E, Nikolaizik WH. Compliance with therapy in children with respiratory diseases. *Eur J Pediatr* 1995; **154**(Suppl 3):S77–S81.

28. Turner J, Wright E, Mendella L, Anthonisen N. Predictors of patient adherence to long-term home nebulizer therapy for COPD. *Chest* 1995; **108**:394–400.

13. CHOICE OF NEBULIZER DEVICE AND RUNNING A NEBULIZER SERVICE

Karen Heslop and Jim Fink

Introduction

Inhalation is the preferred route of administration of drugs in the treatment of many respiratory disorders. By inhalation, drugs can be delivered to the required site of action, minimizing both unwanted systemic delivery and the total dose administered. Systemic side effects are minimized and the onset of action is rapid.[1] Currently, there are numerous methods of delivering inhaled medication and choosing a device can be problematic. Devices include:

- Pressurized metered dose inhalers (MDIs).
- Pressurized metered dose inhalers with a holding chamber (valved or non-valved).
- Breath actuated pressurized metered dose inhalers (BApMDIs).
- Dry powder inhalers (DPIs).
- Nebulizers.

Within each group there are marked differences with respect to design, construction, aerosol generation, output characteristics, deposition pattern, technique and ease of use.[2,3] Availability also varies from drug to drug and country to country. During 2002 aerosol medications were prescribed for the treatment of 30 million people in the United States of America (USA), representing 16% of the total population diagnosed with asthma, cystic fibrosis or other chronic obstructive pulmonary diseases (COPD). As much as one billion dollars of this inhaled medication was wasted due to poor aerosol device selection, inadequate patient instruction and a mismatch of device to patient.[4]

Aerosol device selection is key to effective therapy. Unfortunately, a broad population of legislators, regulators, pharmacists, medical equipment providers, physicians and clinicians are not well versed in differential selection criteria, and there exist financial incentives to pair the least expensive components, irrespective of performance and ease of use. While the Food and Drug Authority (FDA) guidelines are specific to performance requirements for pressurized MDIs and DPIs, there are no standards of nebulizer performance in the USA to guide the provision of effective nebulizer systems. European standards have been developed through the European Respiratory Society to define consistent testing and performance standards to guide the nebulizer selection process. Unfortunately, such standards have not to date been universally adopted or applied. Until such time, it is incumbent upon the clinician and respiratory care community to understand the key measures of aerosol device performance and to promote device selection which best meets the needs of each individual patient.

Considerations for device selection

Device selection should be based on five key considerations: prescription, patient, payor, provider and performance (Box 13.1).

Prescription

The drug prescribed often dictates the available aerosol delivery device options. Some inhaled drugs are available as a solution or suspension for administration with liquid nebulization systems, as well as pressurized MDI and/or DPI forms. Many formulations are available with only one drug/device formulation. Table 13.1 gives examples of a number of inhaled drugs and their available dosage forms in North America.

Each drug has a primary target or preferred site of action. Sites for aerosol deposition include the nasopharnx (e.g. decongestants, anti-inflammatory agents), hypopharynx (e.g. vasoconstrictors and anesthetics), the conducting airways (e.g. bronchodilators, anti-inflammatory agents, antibiotics and mucoactive agents) and lung parenchyma (e.g. steroids, antibiotics, surfactants, peptides and proteins). Particle size, rate and pattern of aerosol generation, inspiratory flow rate, and breathing pattern are just some of the factors that influence where aerosols deposit in the airways.

The amount of drug to be delivered to the lung should also dictate device selection. Relatively potent drugs requiring only a small quantity to be delivered to the targeted site of action to achieve a therapeutic threshold may lend themselves to the pressurized MDI or DPI. When larger delivered volumes of drug are required (such as mucoactive agents and antibiotics) liquid nebulizers become the clear device of choice.

Box 13.1 Considerations for device selection.

Prescription
  what is the drug
    available drug formulations and device options
  site of action
    lower airways
    central airways
    upper airways
  desired dose to lung
    dose specificity – what is the effect of too much or too little
  toxicity profile
  schedule/frequency of administration
Patient
  disease
  condition
  mobility
  age
  skills
  cognition
  motivation
Payor
  reimbursement policies
    device specific
    drug specific
    environment specific
Provider
  clinician knowledge
  time to provide proper education
  nebulizer support services
    properly organized and staffed
Performance

The specificity of dose is another selection criterion. Total nominal dose placed in the nebulizer being deposited in the lung can range from 3.1% to 23.4%.[5] For drugs with a low therapeutic threshold and a broad range of dose tolerance for most patients (e.g. albuterol, also known as salbutamol), a range of devices may be adequate to achieve therapeutic endpoints. The albuterol pressurized MDI with a recommended label dose of two puffs (200 μg) delivers approximately 20 μg (10% of emitted dose) of drug to the lung (Figure 13.1).[6] This is sufficient to produce the desired level of bronchodilation in mild to moderate asthmatics, with reported incidence

Table 13.1 Commonly used inhaled drugs in North America.

	Form	Dose	No. of doses	Recommended dosage
Bronchodilators				
Beta-adrenergic				
Albuterol	pMDI	90 µg	200	2 doses 4–6 times/day
Albuterol SO$_4$	pMDI(HFA)	90 µg	200	2 doses 4–6 times/day
	DPI	200 µg	1	1–2 capsules 4 times/day
	Solution	0.5%	Unit	2.5 mg 4 times/day
Levalbuterol	Solution	0.02/0.04%	1	0.63–1.25 mg every 6 hours
Metaproterenol SO$_4$	pMDI	650 µg	200	2 doses 4–6 times/day
	Solution	5%	1	10–15 mg
Salmeterol xinafoate	pMDI	21 µg	120	2 doses 2 times/day
	DPI	50 µg	60	2 doses 2 times/day
Pirbuterol acetate	pMDI/Autohaler	200 µg	300/400	2 doses 4–6 times/day
Bitolterol mesylate	pMDI	370 µg	300	2 doses 3 times/day
	Solution	0.2%	1	0.5–3.5 mg
Formoterol fumarate	DPI	12 µg	1	1 dose 2 times/day
Anticholinergic				
Ipratropium bromide	pMDI	18 µg	200	2 doses 4 times/day
	Solution	0.02%	1	0.5 mg
Combination				
Albuterol SO$_4$ +	pMDI	100/18 µg	200	2 doses 4 times/day
ipratropium bromide	Solution	0.083%/0.02%	Unit	2.5/0.5 mg

Table 13.1 (Continued)

	Form	Dose	No. of doses	Recommended dosage
Anti-inflammatory				
Non-steroidal				
Cromolyn sodium	pMDI	0.8 mg	102/200	2 doses 4 times/day
	Solution	1%	1	20 mg 4 times/day
Nedocromil sodium	pMDI	1.75 mg	104	2 doses 4 times/day
Corticosteroids				
Beclomethasone dipropionate	pMDI	42, 84 μg	80/200	2 doses 4 times/day/4 doses 2 times/day
Budesonide	DPI	200 μg	200	1–2 doses 2 times/day
	Solution	250/500 μg	Unit	1–2 doses/day
Flunisolide	pMDI	250 μg	100	2 doses 3 times/day
Fluticasone propionate	pMDI	44, 100, 220 μg	120	2 doses 3 times/day
	DPI	50, 100, 250 μg	4	2 doses 2 times/day
Triamcinolone	pMDI	100 μg	240	2 doses 3–4 times/day
Combination (fluticasone/salmeterol)	DPI	100/50, 250/50		
Fenoterol hydrobromide	MDI (HFA)	500/50 μg	60	1 dose 2 times/day
Antibiotics				
Tobramycin	Solution	300 μg	Unit	1 dose 2 times/day
Mucolytics				
Acetylcysteine	Solution	10/20%	Unit	
Dornase alpha	Solution	2.5 μg	Unit	1 dose daily

pMDI, pressurized metered dose inhaler; pMDI (HFA) DPI, dry powder inhaler.

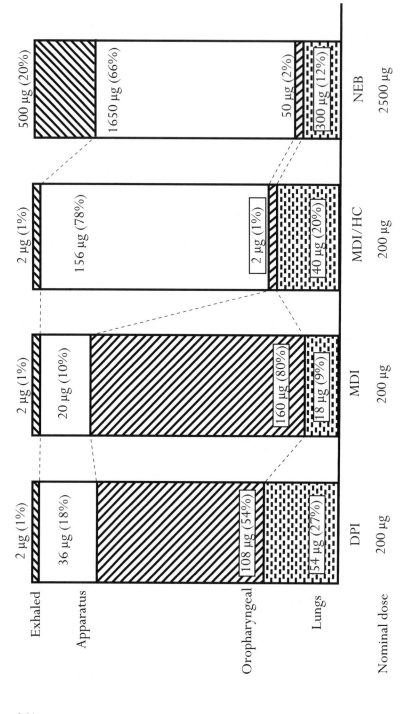

Figure 13.1 *Comparison of quantity and percent of nominal dose of albuterol deposited in the lung, oropharynx, apparatus, and exhaled with dry powder inhaler (DPI), metered dose inhaler (MDI), MDI with valved holding chamber (MDI/HC) and standard jet nebulizer (NEB). (From Fink JB. Respir Care 2000; 45:623–35[6] with permission from Daedalus Enterprises.)*

of adverse effect (tremor, tachycardia, headache, bronchospasm) in up to 17% of subjects. In contrast, the standard nebulizer dose of 2.5 mg of albuterol in 2.5–3.0 ml of diluent, can result in a delivered dose to the lung ranging from 80 μg to 625 μg, with no greater incidence of toxicity reported.

Drugs such as steroids and antibiotics may require considerably larger doses deposited in the lung to reach a therapeutic threshold, and may have a narrower therapeutic range, with greater potential for toxicity. For these drugs it becomes crucial for the clinician to understand the implications of the efficiency of the specific nebulizer prescribed to the patient. With the introduction of drugs that may be more dose sensitive (and expensive) effectiveness and potential for toxicity are far more dose specific.

For drugs available as pressurized MDIs and DPIs, the device and drug formulation have been designed to deliver a predetermined particle size and specific emitted dose. An antibiotic such as TOBI (Chiron, Emeryville, CA, USA) was approved based on use of a specific delivery system consisting of the Pari LC Plus (Pari, Monterrey, CA, USA) driven by a DeVilbis Pulmoaide (Devilbiss Health Care Inc, Somerset, PA, USA) compressor. Indiscriminate substitution of nebulizer and/or compressor can result in the patient receiving a lung dose that is less than half or more than twice that which has been shown to be effective in the clinical trials. Similarly, Pulmocort (Astra Zeneca) was approved based on clinical trials using a specific nebulizer compressor system (inhaled mass of approximately 13% of the total dose), but is approved for use with any jet nebulizer.[7] This can result in an inhaled mass ranging from 3% to 18% depending on the system used (Figure 13.2).

The frequency of aerosol administration influences the choice of nebulizer characteristics such as portability and speed of administration. For daily and twice daily administration (when treatments are taken at the beginning and/or end of the day) it may be reasonably convenient to have the aerosol device reside at home. More frequent (i.e. 3–4 times daily or as and when required) administration necessitates greater portability for the aerosol device. Lack of portability and long administration times are major impediments to adherence with prescribed therapy.

Patient characteristics

The patient's diagnosis and condition will dictate both the drug and the specific devices which will best meet their individual needs. Lung deposition will vary between individuals due in part to airway caliber.[8]

265

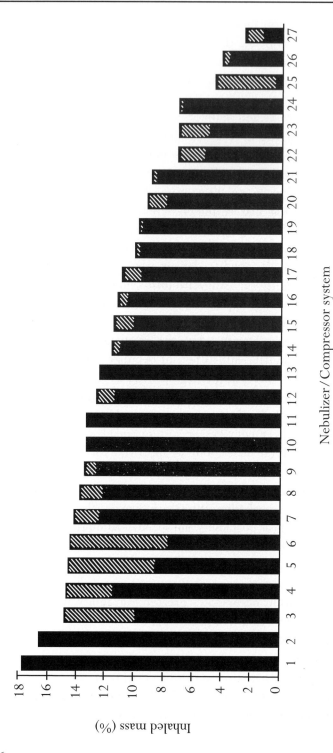

Figure 13.2 *Inhaled mass as a percentage of the nebulizer charge versus nebulizer/compressor system. The black bars represent output over the first 5 min and the shaded bars represent additional output to dryness. The nebulizer charge consists of 1.0 mg of budesonide in 2.0 ml solution. (From Smaldone GC et al. J Aerosol Med 1998; **11**:113–25.[7])*

Disease

The condition of the airways affects how much and where aerosol will deposit in the lungs. Smokers, asthmatics and patients with obstructive lung disease tend to have higher pulmonary aerosol deposition for some aerosols than normal subjects (Figure 13.3).[9] The more obstructed a patient's airway, the more hyperinflated the lungs, elevating residual volume and functional residual capacity. However, distribution patterns in the lungs are less homogeneous in patients with obstructive disease than in normal subjects. While overall efficiency of aerosol delivery may be higher with obstructive lung disease, there is a greater challenge to get the aerosol beyond the obstructed airways to the desired site of action. In such cases, aerosol characteristics such as particle size can play an important role, with smaller particles having a better chance of accessing obstructed airways.

Severity of disease will influence deposition.[10] The more affected the airways and the breathing pattern are by a disease, the greater the impact on deposition of the drug. Owing to the increased obstruction of the airway the breathing pattern is also changed. Patients with severe lung disease may have increased deposition in the central and upper airways associated with increased breathing frequency. Secretions in the airways contribute to further obstruction of the airway and increased turbulent inspiratory flow. A large amount of inspired aerosol is deposited on the secretions within the airways. During severe exacerbations with dyspnea, a mouthpiece may be uncomfortable and difficult for the patient, so that face masks might be preferred.[11]

Dosing requirements are disease dependent. The label dose of a bronchodilator via a pressurized MDI or DPI may be sufficient for mild and moderate asthmatics to receive sufficient therapeutic benefit. However, during severe exacerbation, it is not uncommon for patients to require up to 20-fold more drug before the desired bronchodilator effect is achieved.[12] While pressurized MDI and valved holding chambers have been shown to be effective in the treatment of severe asthma in the emergency department setting, it has been estimated that less than 5% of emergency departments in the USA utilize this pressurized MDI strategy, preferring to administer high doses with solutions using intermittent or continuous nebulizers. While clinical evidence suggests that there is no difference between pressurized MDI with valved holding chambers and nebulizers in treatment of severe asthma (Figure 13.4),[13] factors such as provider time, cost for materials, ease of administration and patient comfort should, and often do, guide device selection.

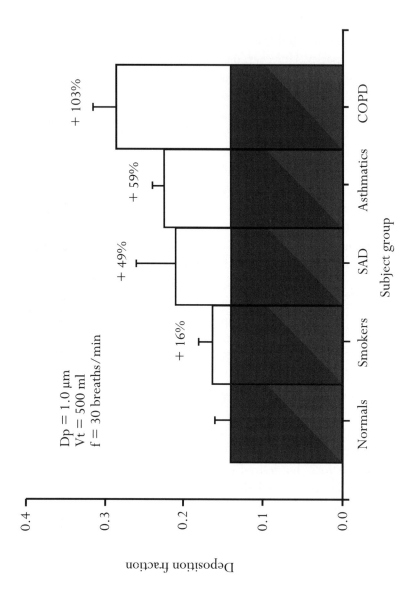

Figure 13.3 *Total lung deposition of a fine aerosol in healthy adults and subjects with obstructive airway disease. The numbers shown over the bars indicate percent increase above normal values. SAD, smoker with symptoms of small airway disease; COPD, patients with chronic obstructive pulmonary disease; Dp, particle diameter; Vt, tidal volume; f, respiratory rate. (From Kim CS. Respir Care 2000; 45:695–711[9] with permission from Daedalus Enterprises.)*

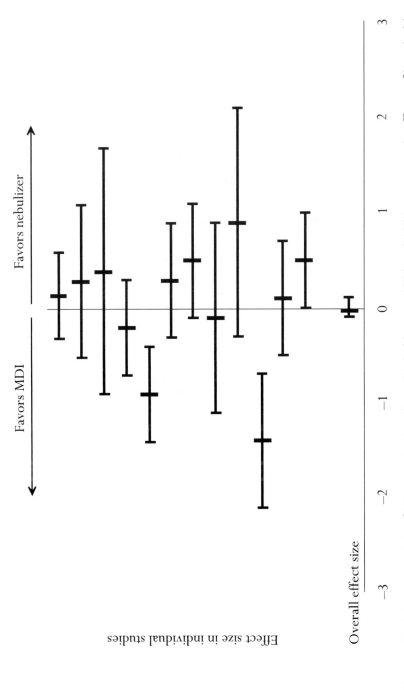

Figure 13.4 *A meta-analysis of 12 randomized studies published between 1978 and 1993 comparing the efficacy of bronchodilators administered with nebulizers or metered dose inhalers (MDI) in a total of 507 patients with acute airflow obstruction due to asthma or chronic obstructive pulmonary disease. (From Turner MO et al. Arch Intern Med 1997; **157**: 1736–44.[13])*

Mobility
The mobility of the patient should be mirrored by the portability of the nebulizer. Heavy compressor nebulizer systems may be fine for patients who are confined to bed or home, while patients who are more mobile, may benefit from systems that are lighter, more compact and hand or battery operated.

Age
Children differ from adults in more than just size (Figure 13.5).[14] The relative proportions of the airway, the anatomy and structure of the lung and upper airway, as well as lung function change during childhood and affect the deposition and response to inhaled therapy in children.[15] There are areas of uncertainty such as the effect of different inhalation patterns on the deposition of nebulized drugs for infants, children and adults (Figure 13.6).[16] Nebulizers have been considered to be the aerosol delivery system of choice for the very young and the very old. On the surface, continuous nebulization requires less active involvement and breath coordination than pressurized MDIs or DPIs for the patient to breathe the aerosol, but the nebulizer requires considerably more preparation, cleaning and maintenance.

Valved holding chambers have emerged as an important accessory device option for administration of aerosol via pressurized MDI to infants and small children as well as the elderly. In the emergency department both pressurized MDIs with valve holding chambers and nebulizers provide comparably efficacy.[12] Leversha and colleagues found that use of pressurized MDI with a spacer was as effective in the emergency treatment of children with moderate to severe asthma as the nebulizer for clinical score, respiratory rate and oxygen saturation but produced a greater reduction in wheezing ($p = 0.03$), while the nebulizer was associated with greater increase in heart rate (11.0/min vs 0.17/min for spacer, $p < 0.01$) and required admission. The mean cost of each emergency department presentation was NZ$825 for the pressurized MDI spacer group and NZ$1282 for the nebulizer group ($p = 0.03$); 86% of children and 85% of parents preferred the spacer.[17]

DPIs currently have severe limitations in children under the age of 6 years due to their size-related inability to reliably generate sufficient inspiratory flow of ≥ 60 l/min required to release the drug from the device. Fok and coworkers reported that both the pressurized MDI with a non-valved aerochamber and an ultrasonic nebulizer with a small medication cup were both more efficient than jet nebulizers in preterm infants.[18]

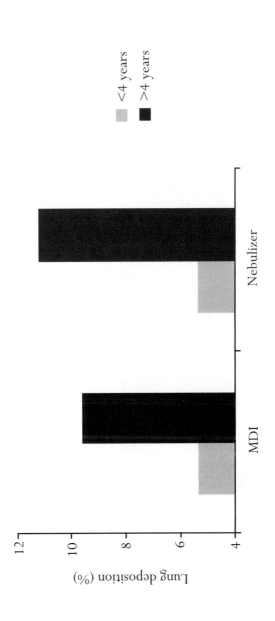

Figure 13.5 *Age-dependency of lung deposition of nebulized or metered dose inhaler (MDI)-administered radiolabeled albuterol in children.[14] (From Roche N, Huchon GJ, J of Aerosol Med 2000, 13(4): 393–404.)*

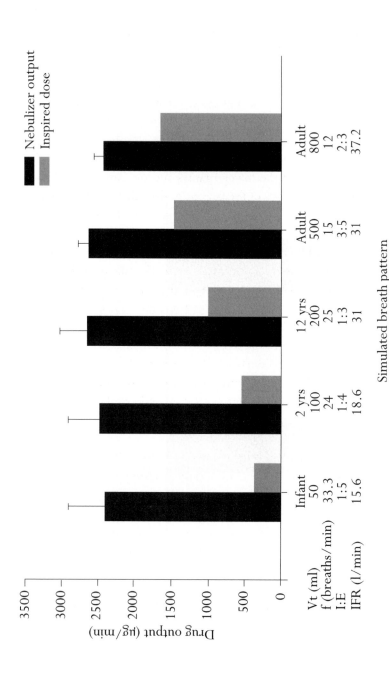

Figure 13.6 *In vitro measurement of the dose of cromolyn sodium available with the Pari LC Star (Pari, Monterrey, CA, USA) nebulizer, for infant, child and adult breathing patterns. The amount of drug delivered to a filter per minute of nebulization time increases with tidal volume and inspiratory flow rate, approaching the per minute output of the nebulizer when driven continuously, but only for the adult breathing pattern. Vt, tidal volume; f, breathing frequency; I:E, inspiratory:expiratory ratio; IFR, inspiratory flow rate. (From Dolovich MB. Respir Care 2002; 47:1290–301[16] with permission from Daedalus Enterprises.)*

Nebulizers are generally prescribed for those not tolerating spacer devices. More recent designs, such as the open vent nebulizer systems deliver the drug more rapidly to adults. The breath-enhanced open vent systems have the advantage of delivering significantly more drug to older patients. These systems rely on the relatively large tidal volumes of older patients. As a result of their smaller tidal volumes, young children are unlikely to benefit as greatly from these devices. The open vent system may result in some young children receiving less drug than from a conventional nebulizer.[19]

Extremes in age are associated with problems in using a mouthpiece for aerosol administration. In theory a mouthpiece is preferable to a face mask when drug delivery is aimed at the lower airways and the patient is able to use it in a sealed fashion.[11] The age of the patient or disabilities can influence whether a mouthpiece or face mask is used. Masks are actually the device of choice in treatment of infants (who are obligate nose breathers) and small children who can not reliably use a mouthpiece. It is interesting to note that patients of any age with moderate to severe exacerbation of asthma or COPD tend preferentially to breathe through their mouth as a natural mechanism to reduce work of breathing. In such patients use of an aerosol mask has similar efficacy as the mouthpiece (Figure 13.7).[20] To be effective, masks should be properly fitted to the face. Poorly fitting masks, as much as 1–2 cm off the face, greatly reduce aerosol inhaled by the patient.[22] Similarly, the practice of 'blow-by' administration of aerosols to infants by pointing the aerosol stream toward the face is remarkably inefficient.[23]

Skills

Can the patient (or care provider) reliably operate and maintain the device? No aerosol device is foolproof. Proper use of even the simplest device must be learned, and it is amazing how many patients have difficulty performing what appears to be the simplest of techniques.[24] Most patients learn best with demonstration and return demonstration. It is important that the patient has the opportunity to be instructed in use and maintenance of the device and the opportunity to perform the manuevers before a trained observer. Only through this observation of the successful return demonstration can the clinician be sure that the patient has the coordination and physical ability to operate the device successfully.

Cognition

Does the patient understand how and when to take their medication? Do they consistently use the device as directed? These are difficult questions for

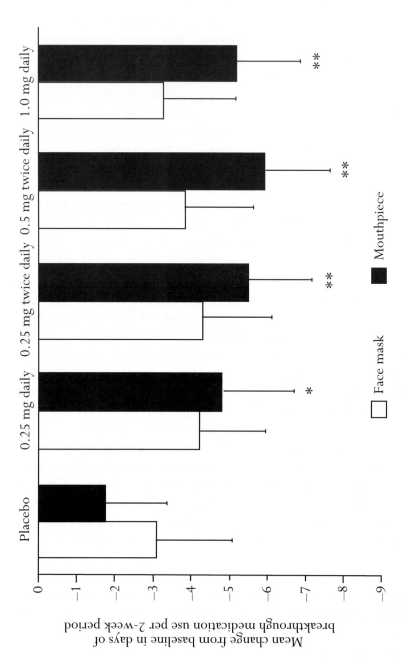

Figure 13.7 *Adjusted mean changes from baseline in days per 2-week interval of breakthrough medication use.* $*p = 0.0008$ *for budesonide at 0.25 mg daily versus placebo;* $**p < 0.001$ *for budesonide at 0.25 mg twice daily, 0.5 mg twice daily and 1.0 mg daily versus placebo. Face mask and mouthpiece were similar at each dose. (From Mellon M et al. Am J Respir Crit Care Med 2000;* **162:**593–8.[21])

many patients and clinicians to answer. The most effective way to assure what the patient knows, is to have the patient demonstrate their technique. It is recommended to repeat this. In addition, questions such as 'What is your biggest problem with your aerosol device?' may help identify issues that affect compliance. Identifying what the patient likes and dislikes about their aerosol device is vital to device selection.

Motivation

Will the patient tolerate the inconvenience of the device to benefit from the medication? This is a common problem with all medication forms, as many patients, even physicians[4] fail to complete their full course of oral antibiotics once the severity of symptoms has subsided. The vast majority of patients who require aerosol therapy have chronic long-term needs for the therapy. The less convenient the device, the more frequent the dosing, the more complicated and longer the time for administration, the less likely that the patient will consistently adhere to their prescribed therapy over time.

A major problem exists with long-term use of anti-inflammatory drugs in asthmatics. The longer the patient takes the drug, the less the perceived need for the expense and inconvenience of regular dosing. Clinicians need to reinforce the benefits and causal relationship of adherence to therapy and of avoiding exacerbation. In addition, the device and dosage forms chosen should have minimal costs for the patient and the number of treatments per day, and require the least time for administration with the least amount of cleaning and maintenance. Another major concern with the use of inhalers is psychological dependence and over-reliance. This is seen frequently in patients with COPD. Interventions such as pulmonary rehabilitation should be attempted before nebulizer treatment is prescribed.[25] Nebulizers for home use must be accompanied by clear guidelines, both written and verbal, as to their use and when to seek medical help.

Payor

The economics of health care have to be considered in device and drug selection. If medications and devices are not affordable to the patient, they simply will not be used as prescribed. Payor reimbursement procedures and policies directly impact the choice of devices available for use by many patients. In some countries, such as the USA, up to 30% of the population does not have health insurance. All too often the working poor have to directly pay for their visits to the doctor and medications, and often must balance the ongoing cost of therapy with other competing priorities such as food and shelter. It is not uncommon for the patient who has to choose between medication and food for the family to cut corners, and only use the least expensive of the prescribed drugs, e.g. albuterol/salbutamol versus budesonide, sacrificing the use of the more beneficial therapeutic agent.

For patients who do have health insurance, whether through private or government programs, coverage varies by specific payor. For example, historically the USA Medicare coverage for senior citizens would not pay for inhaled medications administered through pressurized MDI or DPI, but would pay for nebulizer solutions. Consequently, the payor has inadvertently driven many senior citizens to use of nebulizers for inhaled medications.

A reimbursement cap, or maximum payment, for nebulizers has created a financial incentive for home medical equipment companies to supply the cheapest device that qualifies for the reimbursement cap. Higher quality, more expensive nebulizer compressor systems may erode the profits for the equipment provider. In response to the Montreal Accord, banning the use of chlorofluorocarbons by the year 2000, some government funded healthcare systems will only approve use of DPIs for its citizens, eliminating the drug/device options available only in pressurized MDIs.

Choice of home nebulizer device may reduce healthcare costs
Home nebulizer use has been associated with reduced hospital admissions and inpatient days for some.[26] Hospital inpatient units and emergency departments which have the ability to dispense a home nebulizer, have an additional therapeutic option available for selected patients who may benefit from it. Home nebulizers are a cost effective means of providing home nebulized albuterol for selected outpatients. Medical insurance companies should fully support (i.e. pay for) home nebulizers for patients who have been assessed by a respiratory specialist according to agreed protocols because for these patients it is cost effective. If there is any concern about the reliability of the patient to follow-up with their primary care physician, the latter should be contacted to discuss the feasibility of discharging the patient with a home nebulizer.[27]

Nebulizer use by inner-city children with asthma is higher than anticipated but is not associated with reduced asthma morbidity. This group of high-risk children were undertreated with inhaled corticosteroids for long-term control of asthma despite reports of adequate monitoring by a primary care physician.[28]

Providers

Successful device selection begins and ends with the prescribing clinician as well as the resources brought into play to support the patient. Rational device selection requires a fairly extensive knowledge of the device options and their relative merits. Unfortunately, aerosol therapy is not a major component of the physician or nursing core curriculum. In a recent informal review of 40 general textbooks used for training medical students, only two contained a detailed list of steps to use a simple pressurized MDI.

There are several reasons why most clinicians have been ambivalent towards the characteristics of nebulizer systems. For the past several decades, with many of the available medications, the relative efficiency of the available systems seems to not really matter. When dose does not matter, any device may be technically adequate. The most common respiratory drugs, i.e. bronchodilators with low toxicity profiles such as albuterol/salbutamol and ipratropium, require only minute amounts deposited in the lungs to produce a substantial clinical response in the majority of patients and have a broad range of dose tolerance for most patients.

Simply put, if providers do not possess the knowledge, they can not apply it to their practice, or teach it to their patients. This results in a situation in which most clinicians are more proficient with those inhalers that have been in the market for the longest time, and less familiar with the most recently introduced devices. Lack of familiarity regarding device options leads to poor selection and inability to educate the patient properly in the use of the prescribed device. We suggest that aerosol device selection should be a formal part of medical and nursing training. Even pharmacists, assumed to be responsible for first-line patient education in the use of the nebulizers and inhalers, have minimal training in aerosol devices, and seldom actively provide demonstration of proper technique to new patients.[29]

Knowing how to use the device is important, but of little value unless adequate time is allocated to teach the patient. Time should be allocated to provide proper education, and allow for a demonstration with return demonstration at both initial and follow-up clinic visits. This time allocations should be insisted upon by clinicians, required by regulators and reimbursed by payors.

In Italy, a large survey of 1257 respondents reported that 40% of patients over 60 years of age use nebulizer at least once a day, 60% received no information on correct usage of their nebulizer and 75% received no information from healthcare workers on the nebulizer. Patients who received information on the use and maintenance of their nebulizer from care givers more commonly attended to proper treatment and maintenance practices ($p<0.01$).[30,31]

A periodical check-up of user-related aspects and technical quality of jet nebulizers is necessary. Struycken et al reported that the suppliers of home nebulizers often did not provide clear instructions on user-related aspects and technical maintenance of the jet nebulizer resulting in use of damaged and poorly functioning, contaminated jet nebulizers. The operating pressure of compressor and nebulizer was below the requirements in more than 50% of the jet nebulizers, resulting in particle sizes >5 μm.[32]

Cleaning is key to nebulizer performance. Standaert and co-workers reported that when properly maintained, there was no trend of deterioration of performance with repeated use of disposable nebulizers. However, unwashed units containing tobramycin started to fail by 40 runs.[33]

Device providers have largely differentiated devices by cost, providing the least expensive system that is capable of meeting the perceived need for the patient. Nebulizer services need to be properly organized and staffed to assure that patients receive thorough instructions, and can demonstrate their ability to administer the prescribed therapy and maintain the equipment.

Device performance

Nebulizer selection criteria

A variety of device characteristics should be considered (Table 13.2). Nebulizers vary in terms of particle size and mass output. It is not clear how these differences impact clinical response, especially with bronchodilators, where label doses are of an order of magnitude greater with nebulizers than

Table 13.2 Characteristics of nebulizers for upper airway, bronchial or deep lung disease according to particle size.

MMAD	Upper airway disease*	Bronchial disease	Deep lung disease
>10	Yes	No	No
10–7	Yes	No	No
6–4	++	Yes	No
3–2	No	Yes	++
1	No	++	Yes

MMAD, mass median aerodynamic diameter; *except for sinusitis; Yes, adequate; ++, acceptable; No, non-acceptable. (From Dautzenberg B et al. *Eur Respir Rev* 2000; **10**:545–8[11] with permission from European Respiratory Society Journals Limited.)

with pressurized MDIs or DPIs. Although the dose of a drug inhaled by a patient from a device may vary by up to 400%, such information is not usually available to the prescribing doctor.[34]

The three main factors that determine where in the respiratory tract a nebulized drug droplet will deposit are: droplet size, breathing pattern and the age or condition of the lung. Amongst these, the easiest to control is the size of the droplets.[25] The majority of particles emitted from a nebulizer should be in the respirable range. Particle size is commonly determined by use of either impactors or laser diffraction technology. Particles considered to be in the respirable range can be dependent on the measurement technique used. Respirable range, measured with an Anderson Mark II Cascade Impactor (Graseby Anderson, New Smyrna, GA, USA) measuring at 28.3 l/min, has been described as 1–5 μm MMAD (mass median aerodynamic diameter). The MMAD of the aerosol determined with the drug is an important criterion for the choice of nebulizer. A classification based on particle size and disease is shown in Table 13.2 and Figure 13.8.

Emitted dose is the volume or mass of drug that leaves the mouthpiece of the nebulizer as an aerosol. The difference between the drug placed in the nebulizer and the emitted dose is the residual or dead volume. The residual volume or mass of drug remaining in the nebulizer after nebulization is complete varies with type and model of nebulizer (range 0.1–2.0 ml). The fine particle fraction is the proportion of emitted aerosol particles that are in the respirable range. The larger the fine particle fraction, the greater the chance that aerosol will deposit in the lungs.

Inhaled mass is the amount of aerosol that is inhaled by a patient. Respirable mass is the portion of inhaled mass that actually deposits in the lung. Respirable mass can be demonstrated in vivo with scintigraphy and calculated in vitro by multiplying inhaled mass by the fine particle fraction.

Matching a drug to the appropriate nebulizer is becoming increasingly important. Drugs such as TOBI and Pulmozyme (Genentech, South San Francisco, CA, USA) were approved for use with specific nebulizers, while Pulmocort has a label allowing use with a broad range of jet nebulizers. Ultrasonic nebulizers have been identified as inefficinet nebulizers for delivery of suspensions, generate enough heat to be of concern with antibiotics and proteins, and have residual volumes similar to those of jet nebulizers (up to 1.5 ml). Newer technology, such as the electronic micropump (Aerogen, Mountain View, CA, USA) efficiently nebulizes a full range of solutions and suspensions, generating no noise or heat, with residual volumes as low as 100 μl.

Particle size (µm)	Regional deposition	Efficacy	Safety
>6	Mouth/oesophageal region	No clinical effect	Absorption from GI tract if swallowed
2–6	Upper/central airways	Clinical effect	Subsequent absorption from lung
<2	Peripheral airways/alveoli	Low local clinical effect	High systemic absorption

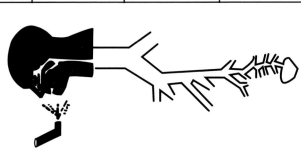

Figure 13.8 *Regional deposition of inhaled particles of different sizes and their pharmacodynamic effects. (Modified from Pritchard JN. J Aerosol Med 2001; 14(Suppl 1):S19–S26.)*

Portability

For the vast majority of patients requiring aerosol therapy outside of the acute care setting who are mobile and active, it is important that their aerosol devices are portable. The more convenient the device is to transport, the more likely that the device will be there when the patient needs it. While most nebulizers claim to be portable, the degree of portability depends on weight, size and power source. Although the majority of nebulizers require standard AC power, a growing number of nebulizers can operate off 12 volt DC power (e.g. automobile power outlets) and alkaline or rechargeable batteries. While batteries add convenience, they also can add expense to operation, and it is important to consider nebulization time with batteries. A set of batteries should provide at least 1 week of nebulizer treatments.

Noise associated with nebulizer therapy can be disruptive in home and school environments, drawing attention to the fact that the nebulizer is in use, and disrupting other activities in the vicinity such as conversations and entertainment. A loud compressor results in regular nebulizer treatment taking place in an area away from the rest of the family or other group activities for prolonged periods each day, and can negatively impact prescribed use of the device.

Finally, cost is a major factor in device selection. Reimbursement rates are often limited to the cost for standard compressor nebulizers. Unfortunately, many of the preferred attributes that make devices more accessible for patient use and integration are only available at a premium, and may require additional out of pocket expense for the patient. In summary, a device that efficiently delivers a high respirable dose of medication is a foundation upon which a variety of attributes can improve the patient/device interface, and better integrate use of that device into the patient's daily life.

Device options

Device selection should be based upon the ability of the device to reliably administer consistent respirable doses under the range of environmental conditions in which the patient will use it.[36,37] Drugs such as albuterol and abuterol, which are available as solution for nebulizer, pressurized MDI or DPI are the exception, with many formulations developed initially for use with only one type of device. Figure 13.1 compares deposition patterns with standard doses of albuterol from DPI, MDI (with and without holding chamber) and nebulizer. It is important to realize that albuterol doses range from 200 μg to 2.5 mg between devices, so that 10% lung deposition with each device can result in delivery of 20–250 μg of drug. Both pressurized MDI and DPI results in large oropharyngeal deposition. Use of valved holding chambers with the pressurized MDI serves to reduce oropharyngeal deposition, and reduce the negative impact of poor hand–breath co-ordination.[38] Currently, more formulations are available for the pressurized MDI than other aerosol delivery devices.[4]

The cheapest and most common handheld inhaler device is the pressurized MDI. Simple as the pressurized MDI seems, this device is often used incorrectly by patients[2,24,39] and many physicians, nurses, respiratory physiotherapists and pharmacists have been shown to be unable to demonstrate its proper use.[40,41] The pressurized MDI's clinical efficacy is technique dependent, and proper use requires education, the ability to follow instructions and coordinate breathing with the actuation of the device.[40] Nebulizers are very versatile and can deliver a variety of drugs. They also have the advantage of requiring minimal coordination of inhalation or effort.[42] Possible benefits may include changes such as the humidification action of the nebulized aerosol, improved mucociliary clearance and changes in small airway caliber that are not always detectable using simple spirometric techniques.[43]

Each aerosol device has different operational parameters and instructions. DPIs require rapid high inspiratory flows, while pressurized MDIs provide better pulmonary deposition with slow deep inspiration. While pulmonary deposition ranges from 6% to 27% with pressurized MDIs and DPIs, pharyngeal deposition can be greater than 85%. Patient confusion between devices reduces available dose to the lung by as much as 70%.[4,44,45]

The patient's ability to perform maintenance and clean devices is a key factor for optimal device performance and minimal risk of infection or insufficient medication delivery. Pressurized MDI and DPI have not been associated with significant risk of bacterial contamination between treatments. While manufacturers may recommend periodic cleaning/washing of the actuator, no reports exist of the risk of infection from use of pressurized MDIs and DPIs. In contrast, nebulizers have long been associated with bacterial contamination, in part due to the relatively large residual volume of medication that remains in the nebulizer reservoir at the end of and between treatments. The residual medication and humidity that remains in typical nebulizers between treatments provides an excellent environment for bacterial growth. While there is a possibility of contamination by airborne pathogens[46] the most common source of contamination is oropharyngeal bacteria.[32,47]

Rosenfeld et al cultured *Staphylococcus aureus* from 55% and *Pseudomonas aeruginosa* from 35% of returned nebulizers.[48] Concordance between nebulizer and sputum cultures was poor. Consequently, nebulizers that can be easily disassembled, washed and completely air dried between treatments minimize risk of bacterial proliferation. To minimize bacterial growth in nebulizers that can not be easily disassembled, rinse with sterile water and run with dry gas until completely dry. Unfortunately, this can require an addition 10–30 min to achieve. The Centers for Disease Control recommends that between uses by the same patient nebulizers be rinsed with sterile water, air dried or washed, and sterilized or disposed of between uses by different patients.[49]

The AARC (American Association of Respiratory Care) Aerosol Consensus Statement recommends that device features and limitations guide device selection, with the caveat that we should always select the most cost effective device that will meet the needs of the individual patient. For many patients, with proper training and adequate competence, the selection of pressurized MDI (often with valved holding chamber) or DPI is appropriate.

Misconceptions regarding the efficiency of nebulizers

Many patients and indeed some healthcare professionals have the view that nebulizers are more efficient than other forms of inhalers. In fact, pressurized MDIs with valve holding chamber and DPIs have similar or greater efficiency compared with standard nebulizers.[25,51–58] Nebulizers are no more effective than other delivery systems, provided a similar dose is given by each method, and proper administration technique is used (Figure 13.9).

In clinical practice we too often reinforce beliefs that nebulizer treatment is the superior delivery system and frequently replace 'ineffective inhalers' with the nebulizer. This approach teaches patients that when they get into trouble with their breathing they cannot rely on their 'inhaler' and makes them feel they need to be treated with the best medication to make them feel better.[4,58] The use of handheld inhalers, such as pressurized MDI with valve holding chamber, in the emergency department, or hospital wards, whenever possible may help reduce this problem and alter patients' expectations regarding nebulizer therapy.

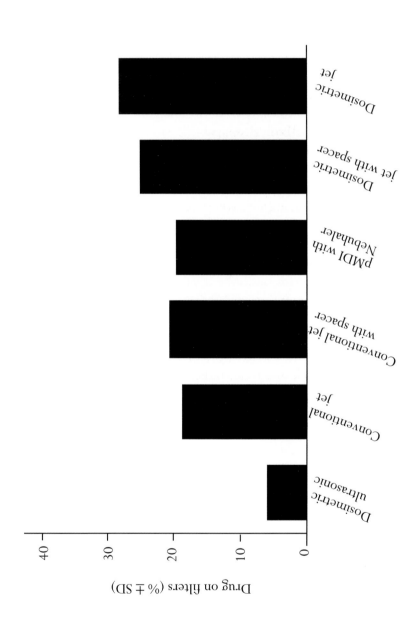

Figure 13.9 *Budesonide output of a range of nebulizers. pMDI, pressurized metered dose inhaler; SD, standard deviation. (From Smaltdone GC. J Aerosol Med 1998; 11:113–25.[7])*

The provision of home nebulizers for patients with COPD is increasing in the United Kingdom (UK).[59] It is not uncommon for patients to purchase their own compressor and nebulizer without the appropriate medical advice. This causes several problems. First, instruction and education may not have been given regarding this form of treatment. Second, patients may develop an overreliance on the nebulizer and delay seeking potentially important medical assessment and treatment. Third, patients will also be responsible for servicing arrangements, which can be costly.

Indications for nebulizer therapy

Nebulizer therapy is usually given for the following reasons:

- Drugs are not available in any other form (e.g. mucolytics such as recombinant human deoxyribonuclease (rhDNase) or antibiotics).[25,50,60]
- High-dose medication is needed, e.g. beta-agonists,[1,25,50] antibiotics and mucoactive agents.
- Patient is too sick to cooperate with other devices, e.g. during a severe asthma attack.[25,50,61]
- Target treatment where it is needed.[25,50]
- Patients are unable to use other devices, e.g. handheld inhalers.[25]
- Practical convenience or economics.[25,61] In busy emergency departments or wards it may be more convenient to apply a nebulizer mask to a patient and come back in 10 min rather than to instruct and watch a patient use an inhaler for up to 24 puffs per hour.[55]
- Where drug delivery to the alveoli is needed.[61]
- Reimbursement bias for nebulizer medication versus MDI or DPI.

Nebulizers may be classified as jet, ultrasonic and vibrating mesh based on how they produce aerosol.

Type of nebulizer

Jet nebulizers

Three types of jet nebulizer are currently available: constant output nebulizers, breath-enhanced nebulizers and dosimetric or breath actuated nebulizers.

Constant flow nebulizers are generally the least expensive and most commonly used jet nebulizers. They generate aerosol constantly, so that aerosol is available to the patient during the inhalation phase of the breathing cycle, but wasted to atmosphere through the remainder of the respiratory cycle.

Subsequently, up to 60–70% of the drug generated as aerosol is wasted.[62] These nebulizers retain 1–2 ml of medication as residual in the device, so that less than 50% of the drug is available as aerosol. Breath-enhanced or vented nebulizers produce more aerosol during the inhalation phase, resulting in less waste to atmosphere, making them marginally more efficient with adult breathing patterns,[3,63] but potentially less efficient with pediatric breathing patterns.[15] Breath actuated nebulizers, generating aerosol only during inspiration, eliminate some of the waste associated with continuous nebulization. These devices are limited by the flow limitations required to actuate which may be a limitation with children, and the inefficiency of residual drug remaining in the nebulizer at the end of nebulization.

Disposable or durable jet nebulizers are available, impacting the frequency for recommended replacement. Disposable units may be replaced on a weekly basis, while the more durable device may be recommended for quarterly replacement. The literature does not support clear criteria for nebulizer replacement. It is clear that frequency of cleaning impacts consistency of operation, and number of treatments for which nebulizers remain within their aerosol generation specifications.

Driving gas: The pressure of compressed gas driving the jet nubulizer will influence the delivery of drug to the lung.[64] The shape and size of the baffles and flow rate of gas have important roles to play in determining the particle size, with higher flow rates producing smaller particles[15] (Figure 13.10). The type of driving gas can also influence lung deposition. For example Heliox (He:O_2) has the theoretical advantage of causing less turbulence and therefore increasing drug delivery[66,67] and humidified air will cause less evaporation of the solution than dry piped oxygen.[64] Whether oxygen or air is used will depend on the clinical situation rather than drug delivery issues. If oxygen is to be used it should be prescribed.

Marked variability exists in the flow rates among different commercially available compressors used for home nebulization of inhaled pulmonary medications. Different nebulizer/compressor combinations have markedly different performance characteristics which could result in different efficacy and safety profiles of the medications being administered via these devices. We recommend that this type of information be used as a starting point for selecting different nebulizer/compressor combinations.[68]

The performance of a nebulizer is affected by the compressor or gas flow used to aerosolize the solution. Low flow compressors generate larger particle size, high flow compressors produce smaller aerosols, high

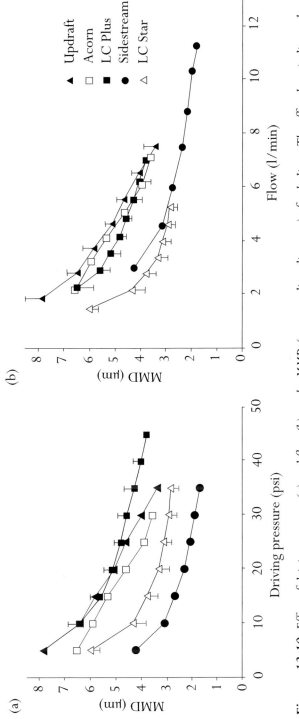

Figure 13.10 *Effect of driving pressure (a) and flow (b) on the MMD (mean median diameter) of nebulizer. The effort bars indicate the standard deviation; n = 6–11 samples per model. PSI, pounds per square inch. (Adapted from Standaert TA et al. J Aerosol Med 2001; 14:31–42.[65])*

rates of delivery and variable effects on the residual or dead volume (see Figure 13.10).[69-71] Several investigators have shown that the gas flow or compressor significantly affects nebulizer performance.[45,72] The output and droplet size are directly related to flow of gas through jet nebulizers.[73]

Manufacturers of aerosolized medications approved by the Food and Drug Administration (USA), specify the nebulizer(s) and compressor to be used with their product, in an attempt to achieve efficacy comparable to that obtained in the clinical trials. The need to limit the compressor to that used in the trials has not been investigated in detail. However, for any specific compressor–nebulizer combination there is a unique flow and pressure, and the nebulizer generates a given MMD. Standaert et al suggest an in vitro technique to determine the equivalency of different compressors such that a chosen nebulizer's performance is not significantly altered.[65]

Once approved for clinical use, switching to a different nebulizer system requires extensive testing. If a new system delivers 100% more drug as respirable dose, it is tempting to consider that only as much as 50% drug need be used to achieve comparable results, with substantially reduced treatment times. However, it is reasonable to caution that changes in respirable mass may not correlate with changes in serum levels, pulmonary microbiology or pulmonary function.[74]

Ultrasonic nebulizers

Ultrasonic nebulizers generate an aerosol by means of a rapidly vibrating piezoelectric crystal. The heat of the crystal can denature some medications (particularly proteins), and the crystal can develop coating or cracking that can be difficult to detect and undermines reliable performance.[73] In those units producing small particles, delivery of suspensions can be problematic, with the aerosol particle being smaller than the particles in suspension, resulting in inefficient nebulization (Figure 13.11). Currently available small volume ultrasonic nebulizers have residual medication volumes of up to 1.2 ml remaining in the reservoir after nebulization is complete. Ultrasonic nebulization is less effective and efficient at bronchodilator delivery than other devices.[76] However, some ultrasonic nebulizers have been shown to be more efficient than jet nebulizers when three medications, tobramycin, colistin and amiloride, were nebulized with volumes ranging from 1.5 ml to 13 ml. The variation of concentration due to nebulization was independent of the type of apparatus.[77] In contrast, Le Brun and colleagues compared the performance of 14 jet and ultrasonic nebulizers nebulizing a 10% tobramycin solution. The output rate ranged from 0.06 ml/min to

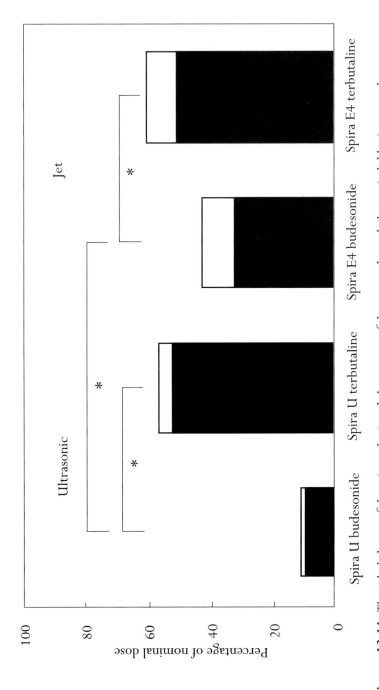

Figure 13.11 *The inhaled mass of drug (open bar) and the amount of drug wasted to exhalation (solid bar) expressed as percentage of total dose for each nebulizer and drug. *p <0.001. (Adapted from Nikander K et al. J Aerosol Med 1999; 12:47–53.[75]) Spira U is an ultrasonic nebulizer, Spira E4 is a jet nebulizer (Respiratory Care Center, Hameenlinna, Finland).*

0.50 ml/min emitting tobramycin at a rate of 1.2–39.5 mg/min. Only three of the jet nebulizers nebulized 300–600 mg of 10% tobramycin within 20–30 min.[78]

Newer vibrating mesh and electronic micropump technology has been introduced in recent years, which uses a piezo element, at lower frequencies than the ultrasonic nebulizers, to vibrate an aperture plate or mesh to create an electronic pumping action in which particle size is dictated by the diameter of the aperture. These nebulizers produce consistent particle sizes with a relatively high output (0.2–0.5 ml/min) and low residual volumes of <0.2 ml. Unlike the ultrasonic nebulizers, the vibrating mesh nebulizers do not heat or denature medications, and can efficiently nebulize suspensions.[79] These nebulizers are silent and portable, but are more expensive than standard compressor nebulizer systems.

Choosing an effective nebulizer

Effective nebulizer therapy requires a device that repeatedly and quickly delivers sufficient drug to the site of action, with minimal wastage, at a low cost.[52] The current system of nebulized drug delivery is largely uncontrolled; drug solutions and suspensions are delivered using a great range of nebulizer systems and driving gases, often depending on the vagaries of local availability and pricing, mixing different drug formulations with different nebulizer systems, many of which have not been adequately evaluated, either in vitro or in vivo.[25]

The ideal nebulizer system
In practice it is difficult to choose 'the ideal nebulizer system'. Many of us have received limited training, if any, regarding this form of treatment. We generally learn as we go along. There is also a bewildering range of inadequate or misleading information, making it difficult to make an informed choice. When choosing a nebulizer it would be useful to consider the points in Box 13.2 and Table 13.3

Device conforms to international standards
Use of a consistent analytic method to characterize device performance, which conforms to international standards allows comparison of devices. Medical devices for single patient use in Europe should be manufactured by a CE marked manufacturer (European Standard). European manufacturers are now required to test each of their nebulizer systems with a reference solution according to the European Standard EN 13544–1. Standard information

290

Box 13.2 Factors to consider when selecting a nebulizer.

Clinical benefit

Ease of use

   assembly, cleaning, portability

   face mask versus mouthpiece

Rate of drug delivery

   treatment time

   frequency of treatments

Cost and convenience

   cost of competing nebulizers

   use with all drugs

   replacement parts, accessories

Dose delivered

   dose dependency on inspiratory flow rate

   breathing pattern required for optimal dosing

   breath actuated, synchronization with actuation

Aerosol characteristics

   mass median aerodynamic diameter

   fine particle fraction

   fine particle mass

Upper and lower respiratory tract deposition

   efficiency versus other aerosol systems

   adverse effects

(Modified from Dolovich M. *Respir Care* 2002; **47**:1290–301[16] with permission from Daedalus Enterprises.)

should be supplied with every nebulizer. Methods used for this standard are designed to reflect clinical conditions as closely as possible so meaningful comparisons can be made between different nebulizer systems. There are some important limitations in interpreting test data supplied by manufacturers complying with the European Standard.[25] First, the data relate to drug solutions that have properties similar to saline. Test data cannot readily be extended to suspensions (e.g. budesonide) or to solutions that have a significantly greater viscosity than saline (e.g. some antibiotics). It is advisable to ask suppliers for additional information on the specific drug solutions and suspensions that are to be used by a particular patient, and alternative breathing patterns.[25] Second, the rates and amounts of aerosol delivery have been obtained using a simulated adult healthy breathing pattern and these cannot be readily transferred to pediatric patients or to adults with lung disease.[25]

For bronchodilator drugs it is recommended that a system with a good CEN performance (output and droplet size) should be chosen. This would require

Table 13.3 Criteria for an ideal nebulizer.

Criteria	Common	Preferred
Particle size	<9 μm	<5 μm
Fine particle fraction	≤0.50	>0.70
Output rate	≤0.15 ml/min	≥0.3 ml/min
Residual (wasted) drug volume	0.8–2.0 ml	≤0.2 ml
Respirable dose (% of dose)	4–12%	10–35%
Concentration of medication	Increases during treatment	No change
Temperature	Decreases (jet) or increases (USN)	No change
Delivery of suspensions	Decreased efficiency	Efficient delivery
Orientation for operation	Vertical	Any
Reservoir	Open to patient airway	Separated from airway
Sound levels	High: >50 db	Low: <35 db
Power options	Limited to AC	Battery, manual or AC
Portability	>5 pounds	≤0.5 pound
Size	>200 in³	<20 in³
Cost	$100–500	≤$150
Treatment time (3 ml)	7–20 min	≤6 min
Ease of cleaning	Hard to dry between treatments	Easy to dry between treatments
Dosing	Single dose	Multiple doses
Dose indicator	No indicator	Doses remaining
Reservoir/mouthpiece	Open	Valved
End of dose	Sputtering	End of dose indicator
Exhaled aerosol	Open to atmosphere	Filtered

USN, ultrasonic nebulizer; db, decibels; AC, alternating current; DC, direct current.

lower doses of medication, or shorter treatment times, that may be more convenient for patients and also yield savings in overall treatment costs.[25]

Drugs
Drugs approved for nebulization by national regulatory authorities differ from country to country. In some countries, a number of drugs approved by

292

other routes of administration such as intravenously are used 'off label' for nebulization (e.g. certain antibiotics).

It is common practice for prescribers to specify the amount of drug to be placed in the nebulizer (i.e. albuterol 2.5 mg) rather than to prescribe a dose delivered to the lung (e.g. 250 μg target dose). Rarely do prescriptions specify the nebulizer system (so delivered dose could range from 100 μg to 1000 μg). The choice of drug should alert the user to choose an appropriate nebulizer not only for particle size and efficiency, but for the need for a filter system to reduce second hand aerosol (i.e. antibiotics and gene therapy). Some drugs are not suitable for use in ultrasonic nebulizers (e.g. drug suspensions such as steroids and proteins).

Location or site of nebulization

Nebulization may be required in the home, community, clinic or hospital setting. Some compressors are more portable than others so the weight and size should be considered. Battery operated nebulizers are also available for travel, and should be able to provide at least 1 week of nebulization on a fresh set of readily available standard disposable batteries, or with a fully charged rechargeable system.

In the hospital or clinic with piped compressed gas systems, nebulizers should be chosen that produce optimal particle size with the pressure used in those systems (up to 55 psi (pounds/square inch)). The same nebulizer would typically produce a larger particle when driven by a compressor producing less pressure (10–15 psi). In the hospital, large volume jet nebulizers may be employed for long-term continuous administration of aerosol, typically bronchodilators, in the emergency or critical care departments. These devices are designed for use with the high pressure piped gas systems, and are not suitable to be driven by the typical home compressor system. Oxygen should only be used to drive a jet nebulizer when specifically prescribed.

In clinic, hospital and home, time to administer a dose to non-intubated patients is important (Figure 13.12). The shorter the treatment time, the less patient and provider time required. For intubated patients receiving mechanical ventilation, time of administration is less critical than the particle size and impact of nebulizer on ventilator operation. Nebulizers that produce smaller particle sizes deliver a greater proportion of emitted aerosol to the patient. Additional gas flow into the ventilator circuit from the nebulizer tends to increase delivered volumes and inspiratory pressures, which should be adjusted during administration. Nebulizers that do not require additional flow are preferable for aerosol delivery during mechanical

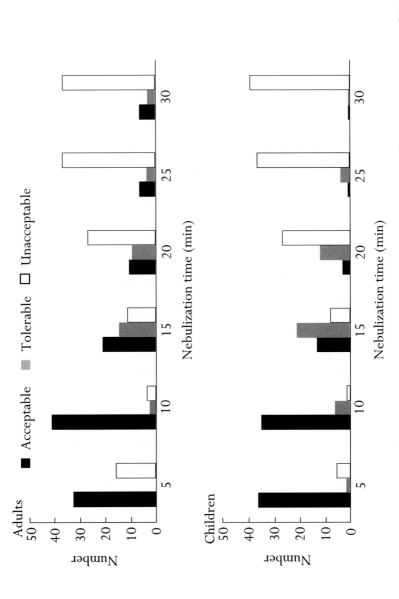

Figure 13.12 *Patient acceptability of different durations of nebulizer treatment. Most patients preferred a treatment time of 10 min or less. (From Kendrick AH et al. Thorax 1997; 52(Suppl 2):S92–S101[80] with permission from the BMJ Publishing Group.)*

ventilation, especially with neonates. For clinic or hospital use, nebulizers should be disposable or sterilized between patients.

Another key issue, especially in the hospital treatment of infants, is the sound level generated by the nebulizer. Jet nebulizers used in the nursery have been shown to generate greater than 85 db (decibel) often into an enclosed hood system. This noise level has been associated with long-term hearing loss. It is recommended that systems with less than 60 db be utilized in that setting.

Long- or short-term use
Disposable or durable equipment is available. For short-term use, such as a limited series of treatments in the clinic or emergency department, disposable equipment may be more suitable. Durable equipment may be more cost effective for long-term use. However, even durable nebulizer chambers require periodic replacement in the home setting.

Duration of nebulization
Clear information should be given regarding how long each treatment with a specific medication should take. Commonly this is about 6–20 min, which is usually acceptable to most patients.

Cost of device
Sadly, economic constraints often guide the choice of equipment used. The best device is a cost effective one with characteristics that are acceptable to the patient's need.

Policy guidelines
Within nebulizer therapy certain parameters can be standardized (see Table 13.2). These could be used to form a standard operating policy for each nebulizer system in used.

Nebulizer service

If nebulizer therapy is provided to a patient, a nebulizer service should be available. Nebulizer services throughout the world serve different populations and vary considerably in their organization.[64] In the UK, it is the responsibility of the National Health Service (NHS) to provide and maintain nebulizer equipment if the prescribing physician decides that it is a necessary part of NHS treatment.[81]

In practice, standards, experience and engagement vary considerably from one unit to another. It is therefore important that there are guidelines in place to satisfy local needs but also lead to a standardized, effective and efficient service, which encompasses within it internationally recognised standards.[82]

Providing a nebulizer service

The service is best organized and administered centrally by a designated consultant or group of consultants.[51,64] A named and appropriately trained individual, such as a respiratory nurse specialist, physiotherapist, physiological measurement technician, respiratory therapist or medical scientist could supervise the day to day management of the service. Clerical support may be beneficial.[51]

Components of a nebulizer service

The components of nebulizer services may vary but are likely to include the following.

Patient assessment and trials of nebulized therapy: The need for this form of treatment varies depending on the purpose of the treatment and, as such, assessment criteria will vary. Good instructions from the prescribing doctor or good communication between the doctor and the nebulizer service are required. The important considerations include the age of the patient, the respiratory condition and the purpose of the treatment. Adult patients with cystic fibrosis may have a trial of nebulized antibiotics. Spirometry will usually be recorded pre- and posttreatment (to detect any bronchoconstriction) before nebulized therapy will be prescribed. In comparison, a patient with COPD would have a trial of therapy over a longer period of time and the results may be compared with alternative treatment, i.e. bronchodilators via a spacer device. Improvements in quality of life may also be considered.

Registration: All patients prescribed nebulizer therapy should be registered. This includes patient details, prescribing physician data, current prescription and may also include a consent form if the equipment is on loan to the patient. This allows for follow-up and servicing of equipment.

Provision of nebulizer system: Whole nebulizer systems, where the driving source and the nebulizer are delivered in one piece from the same manufacturer are preferable, since the aerosol quality and drug output can then be guaranteed by the manufacturer. The choice of nebulizer, i.e. ultrasound or jet nebulizer, and its capacity depends on the drug being prescribed, the respiratory condition and individual circumstances. If jet nebulizers are used, the driving source can either be a compressor or compressed gas in a cylinder. If compressed gas is used the flow/pressure regulator needs to be checked at regular intervals. The method of supplying refilled cylinders needs to be established and financed.

Compressors should be certified by a recognized testing authority to conform to European standards. Light, quiet, reliable and robust equipment that is easy to maintain is preferable.[51] Current guidelines suggest a maximum duration of nebulization of 10 min for patient convenience.[51] If using disposable or durable devices, the nebulizer unit should be matched with a compressor that will deliver an adequate output in an acceptable period of time with a suitable particle size distribution to provide adequate deposition to give a therapeutic response.[79] Durable nebulizers may be more cost effective for domiciliary use. When drugs such as antibiotics are nebulized, a filter system should be used to reduce the risk of side effects.

Other equipment: The nebulizer service, the manufacturers or the department at which the prescribing doctor works (if required) can provide syringes, sharps container and sundries, e.g. needles. The patient also needs to be aware of how to dispose of the equipment safely.

Exchange and servicing system: Usually there should be a recall system for servicing.

Out of hours back-up service: An alternative device can be given for emergency use, e.g. a metered dose inhaler and a large volume spacer. Or additional equipment should be available at specified sites, e.g. accident and emergency departments or a designated ward or primary care center.

Patient education and support: This should include a practical demonstration and return demonstration with verbal and written instructions which include:

- Why nebulized therapy is required.
- What medication is to be used including the dose and frequency of the treatment and what strategy if more medications or airway clearance is prescribed.

- How much medication to use in the nebulizer, whether to dilute and with what (and how to mix drugs if required).
- The expected side effects of the drug treatment.
- How to take the nebulizer apart and put it together.
- How to connect the equipment.
- Training regarding the proper inhalation technique to optimize the effect of the treatment and to avoid side effects, e.g. from hyperventilation.
- How long nebulization will take, i.e. a maximum of 10 min in most cases.[51]
- Written instructions for patients regarding the use, cleaning and maintenance.
- How to identify malfunctions.
- Contact telephone numbers for queries or emergency replacement.
- Clear management plans about any additional measures that may be needed and when to seek medical advice.[83]

After equipment is issued, patients should be reviewed after 3 months and thereafter regularly, at least annually.[51] By whom the patient is reviewed is likely to vary depending on local policy. Patients should be asked to bring their equipment for checking when attending for follow-up.

Audit
Nebulizer therapy and the quality of local care should be audited.[84] Basic requirements are given in Box 13.3.

Box 13.3 Basic requirements of nebulizer therapy.

Written protocols are established and updated

Patients are registered and monitored through a nebulizer service

Arrangements are made to reduce nebulizer prescription outside the agreed local protocol
  (especially by non-specialist prescribers)

Patients are given verbal and written instructions regarding nebulizer use and care

Servicing arrangements are completed yearly or as per manufacturer recommendations

Side effects monitored

Arrangements are in place for sundries and equipment to be replaced

Patient satisfaction and outcomes are audited

Views of primary care teams and other healthcare personnel are monitored

---

Conclusion

Nebulizer therapy is useful in the delivery of inhaled medication to children and adults. Although nebulizer therapy is commonly used there remain many variations in practice. Where nebulizers are used, careful attention should be paid to optimizing delivery by selecting an appropriate nebulizer and correct use of equipment. Developing local nebulizer services following European standards should help eliminate current bad practice and improve the efficiency of nebulizer use. Audits may be performed to ensure these standards are maintained.

References

1. Nikander, K. Some technical, physicochemical and physiological aspects of nebulization of drugs. *Eur Respir Rev* 1997; **7**:168–72.
2. Brocklebank D, Ram F, Wright J et al. Comparison of the effectiveness of inhaler devices in asthma and chronic obstructive airways disease: a systematic review of the literature. *Health Technol Assess* 2001; **5**:1–149.
3. Pederson S. Inhalers and nebulizers: which to choose and why. *Respir Med* 1996; **90**:69–70.
4. Lewis RM, Fink JB. Promoting adherence to inhaled therapy: building partnerships through patient education. *Respir Care Clin North Am* 2001; **7**:277–301.
5. Finley WH, Stapleton KW, Zuberbuhler P. Variations in predicted regional lung deposition of salbutamol sulphate between 19 nebulizer types. *J Aerosol Med* 1998; **11**:65–80.
6. Fink JB. Metered-dose inhalers, dry powder inhalers, and transitions. *Respir Care* 2000; **45**:623–35.
7. Smaldone GC, Crux-rivera M, Nikander K. In vitro determination of inhaled mass and particle distribution for budesonide nebulizing suspension. *J Aerosol Med* 1998; **11**:113–25.
8. Lipworth BJ, Clark DJ. Effects of airway calibre on lung delivery of nebulised salbutamol. *Thorax* 1997; **52**:1036–9.
9. Kim CS. Methods of calculating lung delivery and deposition of aerosol particles. *Resp Care* 2000; **45**:697–711.
10. Saari SM, Vidgren MT, Koskinen MO et al. Regional lung deposition and clearance of 99mTc-labeled beclomethasone-DLPC liposomes in mild and severe asthma. *Chest* 1998; **113**:1573–9.
11. Dautzenberg B, Nikander K. Choice of a device for each disease and medicine. *Eur Respir Rev* 2000; **10**:545–8.
12. Fink J, Dhand R. Bronchodilator resuscitation in the emergency department, Part 1: device selection. *Respir Care* 1999; **44**:1353–74.

13. Turner MO, Patel A, Ginsburg S, Fitzgeral JM. Bronchodilator delivery in acute airway flow obstruction. A meta-analysis. *Arch Intern Med* 1997; **157**:1736–44.

14. Wildhaber JH, Dore ND, Wilson JM, Devadason SG, Le Sonef PN. Inhalation therapy in asthma: nebulizer or pressurized metered-dose inhaler with holding chamber. In vivo comparison of lung deposition in children. *J Pediatr* 1999; **135**:28–33.

15. Barry PW, O'Callaghan C. Drug output from nebulizers is dependent on the method of measurement. *Eur Respir J* 1998; **12**:463–6.

16. Dolovich MB. Assessing nebulizer performance. *Respir Care* 2002; **47**:1290–301.

17. Leversha AM, Campanella SG, Aickin RP, Asher MI. Costs and effectiveness of spacer versus nebulizer in young children with moderate and severe acute asthma. *J Pediatr* 2000; **136**:497–502.

18. Fok TF, Lam K, Ng PC et al. Delivery of salbutamol to nonventilated preterm infants by metered-dose inhaler, jet nebulizer, and ultrasonic nebulizer. *Eur Respir J* 1998; **12**:159–64.

19. O'Callaghan C. Delivery systems: the science. *Pediatr Pulmonol Suppl* 1997; **15**:51–4.

20. Lowenthal D, Kattan M. Facemasks versus mouthpieces for aerosol treatment of asthmatic children. *Pediatric Pulmonol* 1992; **14**:192–6.

21. Mellon M, Leflein J, Walton-Brown K et al. Comparable efficacy of administration with face mask or mouthpiece of nebulized budosenide inhalation suspension for infants and young children with persistent asthma. *Am J Respir Crit Care Med* 2000; **162**:593–8.

22. Amirav I, Newhouse MT. Aerosol therapy with valved holding chambers in young children: importance of the face mask seal. *Pediatrics* 2001; **108**:389–94.

23. Everard ML, Clark AR, Milner AD. Drug delivery from jet nebulizers. *Arch Dis Child* 1992; **67**:586–91.

24. Crompton GK. Problems patients have using pressurized aerosol inhalers. *Eur J Respir Dis* 1982; **119**(Suppl):S101–S104.

25. Boe J, Dennis J, O'Driscoll BR et al. European Respiratory Society guidelines on the use of nebulizers. *Eur Respir J* 2001; **18**:228–42.

26. Ryan CA, Willan AR, Wherrett BA. Home nebulizers in childhood asthma. Parental perceptions and practices. *Clin Pediatr (Phila)* 1988; **27**:420–4.

27. Yamamoto LG, Okamura D, Nagamine J et al. Dispensing home nebulizers for acute wheezing from the hospital is cost-effective. *Am J Emerg Med* 2000; **18**:164–7.

28. Butz AM, Eggleston P, Huss K, Kolodner K, Rand C. Nebulizer use in inner-city children with asthma: morbidity, medication use, and asthma management practices. *Arch Pediatr Adolesc Med* 2000; **154**:984–90.

29. Mickle TR, Self TH, Farr GE et al. Evaluation of pharmacists' practice in patient education when dispensing a metered-dose inhaler *DICP* 1990; **24**:927–30.

30. Melani AS, Sestini P, Aiolfi S et al. Associazione Italiana Pneumologi Ospedalieri (AIPO) Educational Group. GENebu Project: home nebulizer use and maintenance in Italy. *Eur Respir J* 2001; **18**:758–63.

31. Murphy D, Holgate ST. The use and misuse of domiciliary nebulizer therapy on the Isle of Wight. *Respir Med* 1989; **83**:349–52.

32. Struycken VH, Tiddens HA, van den Broek ET et al. [Problems in the use, cleaning and maintenance of nebulization equipment in the home situation] *Ned Tijdschr Geneeskd* 1996; **140**:654–8.

33. Standaert TA, Morlin GL, Williams-Warren J et al. Effects of repetitive use and cleaning techniques of disposable jet nebulizers on aerosol generation. *Chest* 1998; **114**:577–86.

34. O'Callaghan C. Delivery systems: the science. *Pediatr Pulmonol Suppl* 1997; **15**:51–4.

35. Pritchard JN. The influence of lung deposition on clinical response. *J Aerosol Med* 2001; 14(Suppl 1):S19–26.

36. Fink JB. Aerosol device selection: evidence to practice. *Respir Care* 2000; **45**:874–85.

37. Dolovich MA, MacIntyre N, Anderson P et al. Consensus statement: aerosols and delivery devices. *Respir Care* 2000; **45**:589–96.

38. Wilkes W, Fink J, Dhand R. Selecting an accessory device with a metered-dose inhaler: variable influence of accessory devices on fine particle dose, throat deposition, and drug delivery with asynchronous actuation from a metered-dose inhaler. *J Aerosol Med* 2001; **14**:351–60.

39. Goodman DE, Isreal E, Rosenberg M et al. The influence of age, diagnosis and gender on proper use of metered-dose inhalers. *Am J Respir Crit Care Med* 1994; **150**:1256–61.

40. Fink J. Flawed paradigms drive aerosol device selection. *Chest* 1997; **112**:447–9.

41. Guidry GG, Brown WD, Stogner SW et al. Incorrect use of metered dose inhalers by medical personnel. *Chest* 1992; **101**:31–3.

42. Knoch M, Sommer E. Jet nebulizer design and function. *Eur Respir Rev* 2000; **10**:183–6.

43. Hosker HSR, Teale C, Greenstone, Meurs MF. Assessment and provision of home nebulizers for chronic obstructive pulmonary disease (COPD) in the Yorkshire region of the UK. *Respir Med* 1995; **89**:47–52.

44. Mathys H, Kohler D. Pulmonary deposition of aerosols by different mechanical devices. *Respiration* 1985; **48**:269–76.

45. Smith EC, Denyer J, Kendrick AH. Comparison of 23 nebulizer compressor combinations for domiciliary use. *Eur Respir J* 1995; **8**:1214–21.

46. Kelsen SG, McGuckin M, Kelsen DP, Cherniack NS. Airborne contamination of fine-particle nebulizers. *JAMA* 1977; **237**:2311–14.

47. Popa V, Mays CG, Munkres B. Domiciliary metaproterenol nebulization: a bacteriologic survey. *J Allergy Clin Immunol* 1988; **82**:231–6.

48. Rosenfeld M, Emerson J, Astley S et al. Home nebulizer use among patients with cystic fibrosis. *J Pediatr* 1998; **132**:125–31.

49. Department of Health and Human Services, Centers for Disease Control and Prevention: Guidelines for prevention of nosocomial pneumonia. Part 1. Issues on prevention of nosocomial pneumonia. Part 2. Recommendations for prevention of nosocomial pneumonia: Notice of comment period. *Am J Infect Control* 1994; **2**:247–92.

50. AARC (American Association of Respiratory Care) clinical practice guideline. Selection of an aerosal delivery device for neonatal and pediatric patients. *Respir Care* 1995; **40**:1325–35.

51. British Thoracic Society. Current best practice for nebulizer treatment. *Thorax* 1997; 52(Suppl 2):S1–S106.

52. O'Callaghan C, Barry PW. The science of nebulized drug delivery *Thorax* 1997; 52(Suppl 2):531–44.

53. Wildhaber JH, Dore ND, Wilson JM et al. Inhalation therapy in asthma: nebulizer or pressurized metered-dose inhaler with holding chamber? In vivo comparison of lung deposition in children. *J Pediatr* 1999; **135**:28–33.

54. Schuh S, Johnson DW, Stephens D et al. Comparison of albuterol delivered by a metered dose inhaler with spacer versus a nebulizer in children with mild acute asthma. *J Pediatr* 1999; **135**:22–7.

55. Evitt MA, Gambrioli EF, Fink JB. Comparative trial of continuous nebulization versus metered-dose inhaler in the treatment of acute bronchospasm. *Ann Emerg Med* 1995; **26**:273–7.

56. Idris AH, McDermott MF, Raucci JC et al. Emergency department treatment of severe asthma: metered-dose inhaler plus holding chamber is equivalent in effectiveness to nebulizer. *Chest* 1993; **103**:665–72.

57. Dewar AL, Stewart A, Cogswell JJ, Connett GJ. A randomised controlled trial to assess the relative benefits of large volume spacers and nebulisers to treat acute asthma in hospital. *Arch Dis Child* 1999; **80**:421–3.

58. Levy M, Hilton S. *Asthma in Practice*. London: Royal College of General Practitioners, 1993.

59. O'Driscoll R. Home nebulized therapy – is it effective? *Respir Med* 1991; **85**:1–3.

60. Dodd ME, Hanley SP, Johnson SC, Webb AK. District nebuliser compressor service: reliability and costs. *Thorax* 1995; **50**:82–4.

61. Muers M. Overview of nebuliser treatment. *Thorax* 1997; **52**(Suppl 2):S25–S30.

62. Dennis JH, Hendrick DJ. Design characteristics for drug nebulisers. *J Med Eng Technol* 1993; **16**:63–8.

63. Wilson AM, Nikander K, Brown PH. Drug device matching. *Eur Respir Rev* 2000; **10**:558–66.

64. Wison RSE, Muers MF. Running a domiciliary nebuliser service. *Thorax* 1997; **52**(Suppl 2):S104–S106.

65. Standaert TA, Bohn SE, Aitken ML, Ramsey B. The equivalence of compressor pressure-flow relationships with respect to jet nebulizer aerosolization characteristics. *J Aerosol Med* 2001; **14**:31–42.

66. Hess DR, Acosta FL, Ritz RH et al. The effect of heliox on nebulizer function using a beta-agonist bronchodilator. *Chest* 1999; **115**:184–9.

67. Goode ML, Fink JB, Dhand R, Tobin MJ. Improvement in aerosol delivery with helium-oxygen mixtures during mechanical ventilation. *Am J Respir Crit Care Med* 2001; **163**:109–14.

68. Reisner C, Katial RK, Bartelson BB et al. Characterization of aerosol output from various nebulizer/compressor combinations. *Ann Allergy Asthma Immunol* 2001; **86**:566–74.

69. Ramsey BW, Pepe MS, Quan JM et al. Intermittent administration of inhaled tobramycin in patients with cystic fibrosis. *N Engl J Med* 1999; **7**:23–30.

70. Coates AL, MacNeish CF, Meisner D et al. The choice of jet nebulizer, nebulizing flow and the addition of albuterol affects the output of tobramycin aerosols. *Chest* 1997; **111**:1206–12.

71. Phipps PR, Gonda I. Droplets produced by medical nebulizer, Some factors affecting their size and solute concentration. *Chest* 1990; **97**:1327–32.

72. Weber A, Morlin G, Cohen M et al. Effect of nebulizer type and antibiotic concentration on device performance. *Pediatr Pulmonol* 1997; **23**:249–60.

73. Newman SP, Pellow PG, Clarke SW. In vitro comparison of DeVilbiss jet and ultrasonic nebulizers. *Chest* 1987; **92**:991–4.

74. Standaert TA, Vandevanter D, Ransey BW. The choice of compressor effects the aerosol parameters and the delivery of tobramycin from a single model nebulizer. *J Aerosol Med* 2000; **13**:147–53.

75. Nikander K, Turpeinen M, Wollmer P. The conventional ultrasonic nebulizer proved inefficient in nebulizing a solution. *J Aerosol Med* 1999; **12**:47–53.

76. Nakanishi AN, Lamb BM, Foster CF, Rubin BK. Ultrasonic nebulization of albuterol is no more effective than jet nebulization for the treatment of acute asthma in children. *Chest* 1997; **111**:1505–8.

77. Faurisson F, Dessanges JF, Grimfeld A et al. [Comparative study of the performance and ergonomics of nebulizers in cystic fibrosis] *Rev Mal Respir* 1996; **13**:155–62.

78. Le Brun PP, de Boer AH, Gjaltema D et al. Inhalation of tobramycin in cystic fibrosis. Part 1: the choice of a nebulizer. *Int J Pharm* 1999; **189**:205–14.

79. Dhand R. Vibrating mesh technology. *Respir Care* 2002; **47**:1406–16.

80. Kendrick AH, Smith EC, Wilson RSE. Selecting and using nebulizer equipment. *Thorax* 1997; **52**(Suppl 2):S92–S101.

81. Department of Health. Safety of electrical, medical and laboratory equipment. Safety Action Bulletin 1991; 784' SAB [91], 57.

82. NHS Management Executive. Provision of NHS Equipment. EL(92) 20, 1992.

83. Gregson RK, Warner JO, Radford M. Assessment of the continued supervision and asthma management knowledge of patients possessing home nebulisers. *Respir Med* 1995; **89**:487–93.

84. Milroy R, Caldwell N, McCabe J, Banham SW, Moran F. An audit of nebulisation techniques in a major teaching hospital: scope for improvement. *Thorax* 1990; **45**:817–18.

14. EDUCATION AND STAFF TRAINING

Karen Heslop and Louise Lannefors

Introduction

Inhalation therapy is developing rapidly and many improvements in nebulizer technology have been made. However, the success of nebulizer treatment is dependent on the operator.[1] Unfortunately, there is increasing evidence that the understanding of the use of nebulizer treatment among healthcare professionals who operate such equipment is poor.[2–13] This may lead to inappropriate and suboptimal use. Most clinicians have received limited training or guidance regarding the use of handheld inhalers and nebulizer therapy. The standard of training regarding nebulizer treatment remains variable. Training is often provided for nurses, physiotherapists, respiratory function technicians, pharmacists and clinical scientists. Despite this, there is often a lack of knowledge regarding many areas of nebulized treatment (Box 14.1).

Many professionals do not update themselves in advances of inhalation treatment even if it is commonly used in their clinical area. As a result examples of bad practice are common (Box 14.2).

Box 14.1 Areas of nebulizer treatment where knowledge is often lacking.

Why nebulizer systems are to be used

How efficient nebulizer systems are

Type of nebulizer system needed

How to store and mix the drugs

Fill volume required

Whether disposable or durable nebulizers should be used

Driving gas required

Flow rate or driving pressure needed

Whether a mouthpiece or face mask is best

Correct inhalation technique including breathing pattern and position of patient

Timing of nebulizer therapy including when the drug should be given and how long the treatment should take

How equipment should be cleaned

Box 14.2 Examples of bad practice in nebulizer therapy.

Inappropriate assessment and prescribing of a nebulizer system without assessing the patient's ability to use a handheld inhaler

Unsupervised use of nebulizer systems (often self-purchased without appropriate medical assessment or advice)

Incorrect use of the equipment such as inadequate fill volume, drug mixture or flow rates

Unsuitable nebulization time, i.e. too long. Patients have been known to tolerate nebulization times of more than 30 min. This is unacceptably long

Infrequent or inappropriate provision, service and maintenance of equipment such as compressors

Use of nebulizer therapy for conditions where this form of treatment is not indicated, e.g. heart failure or lung fibrosis

Use of nebulizers for hypoxic patients who would be better treated by oxygen therapy

Prescribing nebulizer therapy without appropriate education, support and follow-up

Use of nebulizers to justify claims for disability or welfare benefits (common in the United Kingdom)

Training

Education of those involved in prescribing, supplying and supervising nebulizer treatment is essential.[1] This should include the hospital and community setting. A named healthcare professional should have the responsibility of organizing a training program at local level and implementing appropriate guidelines. This individual should have the required knowledge and expertise to undertake this role. Topics which could be included in the training program are discussed below.

Indications for nebulizer therapy

These are listed in Box 14.3. There is a clear need to educate staff and patients regarding the indications for nebulized treatment. Patients and indeed healthcare professionals hold the view that nebulizer systems are more efficient than other forms of inhaled therapy despite the fact that there is a wealth of evidence supporting the view that this is not the case.[2,13,16–21] Nebulizers are no more effective providing the same dose is given in another device such as a metered dose inhaler or dry powder.

Devices

Staff should understand the basic principles of common devices used and how to use them correctly. They should be able to choose a suitable device

---

Box 14.3 Indications for nebulizer therapy.

Drugs are not available in any other form, e.g. recombinant human deoxyribonuclease (rhDNase)[2,13,14]

Patient is too sick to cooperate with other devices, e.g. during a severe asthma attack[2,13,14]

Target treatment where it is needed[2,13]

High doses of medication are needed, e.g. beta-agonists and other methods of administration would be inconvenient[2,13,15]

Patient is unable to use other devices, e.g. handheld inhalers[2]

Practical convenience.[2,14] In busy emergency departments or wards it may be more convenient to apply a nebulizer mask to a patient and come back in 10 min rather than watch a patient use an inhaler. Practical convenience is a poor indication for nebulizer treatment. If the patient is unfamiliar to the staff or very sick, it may be far better to stay with the patient during treatment

Where drug delivery to the alveoli is needed[14]

---

for the patient's needs and abilities. It is useful to be aware of the advantages and disadvantages of each device.

Technical details

This should include the aim of nebulization and technical terms used such as particle size, fill volume, residual volume and driving source, e.g. oxygen, air or compressor and flow rate. Healthcare professionals using nebulizer systems should be able to differentiate between the types of systems available and understand the principles of use, the variation in output between the different nebulizers and the pattern of respiratory tract deposition. Staff should know the characteristics of a good nebulizer system, maintenance and servicing requirements.[13]

Pharmacology

Staff should understand which drugs are available in the common types of inhalers. They should have a sound knowledge base regarding the nebulizer drugs available, their mode of action and dosage, aerosol deposition in the airways and side effects. Knowledge of storage requirements is also needed (e.g. drugs stored in the refrigerator could take longer to nebulize compared to drugs at room temperature). Certain drugs can be mixed together, others cannot. A good understanding of the timing of treatment is important, e.g. giving a bronchodilator before physiotherapy followed by an inhaled antibiotic after physiotherapy.

Patient factors

The patient's breathing pattern and position may have a profound effect on the amount of drug delivered to the lungs. Normal relaxed breathing during inhalation of a good quality aerosol in fully developed and well-functioning lungs gives therapeutic pulmonary deposition with most drugs and a deposition pattern that is satisfactory. However, the more affected the airways and the breathing pattern are by a disease, the more this influences lung deposition. On the wards, patients are often seen slumped in their beds during nebulizer therapy and are generally given limited advice, if any, on their position or breathing pattern.[22]

Cleaning

All personnel using nebulizer equipment need education on microbial risks, effects of malfunction of equipment and proper cleaning, disinfection and maintenance. There is very little literature available regarding the cleaning of equipment and practice may vary between individual clinical areas and amongst staff in one area. Regular education and practical instructions in proper handling of the whole procedure should help patients and staff understand this form of treatment.[17] Staff hygiene remains important, along with choosing nebulizer systems that are washable and can be disinfected. There are several clinical concerns regarding the cleaning of nebulizers. First, problems of bacterial contamination could arise if the nebulizer is not cleaned correctly (or indeed at all) after each treatment.[23] Equipment can either be sterilized according to the manufacturers recommendations or single-use equipment can be used. Single-use or single patient nebulizers should not be re-used for different patients.

Patient assessment and education

A good knowledge of how patients should be assessed for inhalation treatment is important and various guidelines are available to practitioners. It is recommended that an appropriately trained specialist such as a chest physician, pediatrician, respiratory nurse specialist, pulmonary function technician or physiotherapist should assess whether nebulizer treatment is indicated using a standard protocol.[24]

Conclusion

Although nebulizer treatment is widely used in clinical practice there remain many variations in practice. Many clinicians have had limited training and guidance regarding their use. There is a great need to improve technical standards and clinical practice regarding inhalation therapy. It is especially important to target healthcare professionals such as doctors, nurses, physiotherapists, pharmacists, pulmonary function technicians and paramedics who may be involved in administration of nebulized treatment. Clinicians need to acquire the necessary knowledge to make decisions about which nebulizer system is the most appropriate for their clinical area and what problems could be expected to occur. Developing local nebulizer services following European or International Standards may help eliminate current bad practice and improve the efficiency of nebulizer use.

References

1. Smith EC, Kendrick AH, Brewin A. Staff education. *Thorax* 1997; **52**:(Suppl 2):S102–S103.
2. British Thoracic Society. Current best practice for nebuliser treatment. *Thorax* 1997; **52** (Suppl 2):S1–S24.
3. Lane, DJ. Chronic persistent asthma: nebulisers and therapy additional to inhaled B-agonists and steroids. *Respir Med* 1991; **85**:359–63.
4. Laroche CM, Harries AVK, Newton RCF, Britton MG. Domicillary nebulisers in asthma: district survey. *BMJ* 1985; **290**:1611–13.
5. Milroy R, Caldwell N, McCabe J, Banham SW, Moran F. An audit of nebulisation techniques in a major teaching hospital: scope for improvement. *Thorax* 1990; **45**:817–18.
6. Childs HJ, Dezateux CA. A national survey of nebuliser use. *Arch Dis Child* 1991; **66**:1351–3.
7. Mansfield K. Evaluating a nebuliser service to improve patient care. *Nurs Times* 1996; **92**:27–9.
8. Critchley D, Roulsten J. Nurses' knowledge of nebulised therapy. *Nurs Standard* 1993; **8**:37–9.
9. Godden DJ, Robertson A, Currie N et al. Domiciliary nebuliser therapy – a valuable option in chronic asthma and chronic obstructive pulmonary disease? *Scottish Med J* 1998; **43**:48–51.
10. Caldwell NA, Milroy R, McCabe J, Banham SW, Moran F. An audit of nebulisation techniques in a major teaching hospital: scope for improvement. *Pharmaceut J* 1991; **247**:706–8.

11. Gregson RK, Warner JO, Radford M. Assessment of the continued supervision and asthma management knowledge of patients possessing home nebulizers. *Respir Med* 1995; **89**:487–93.

12. Heslop K, Harkawat R. Nebulizer therapy from a practical perspective. *Eur Respir Rev* 2000; **10**:213–15.

13. Boe J, Dennis J, O'Driscoll BR et al. European Respiratory Society guidelines on the use of nebulizers. *Eur Respir J* 2001; **18**:228–42.

14. Muers M. Overview of nebuliser treatment. *Thorax* 1997; **52**(Suppl 2):S25–S30.

15. Nikander K. Some technical, physicochemical and physiological aspects of nebulization of drugs. *Eur Respir Rev* 1997; **7**:168–72.

16. Wildhaber JH, Dore ND, Wilson JM et al. Inhalation therapy in asthma: nebulizer or pressurized metered-dose inhaler with holding chamber? In vivo comparison of lung deposition in children. *J Pediatr* 1999; **135**:28–33.

17. Schuh S, Johnson DW, Stephens D et al. Comparison of albuterol delivered by a metered dose inhaler with spacer versus a nebulizer in children with mild acute asthma. *J Pediatr* 1999; **135**:22–7.

18. O'Callaghan C, Barry PW. The science of nebulized drug delivery. *Thorax* 1997; **52**(Suppl 2):S31–44.

19. Levitt MA, Gambrioli EF, Fink JB. Comparative trial of continuous nebulization versus metered-dose inhaler in the treatment of acute bronchospasm. *Ann Emerg Med* 1995; **26**:273–7.

20. Idris AH, McDermott MF, Raucci JC et al. Emergency department treatment of severe asthma: metered-dose inhaler plus holding chamber is equivalent in effectiveness to nebulizer. *Chest* 1993; **103**:665–72.

21. Dewar AL, Stewart A, Cogswell JJ, Connett GJ. A randomised controlled trial to assess the relative benefits of large volume spacers and nebulisers to treat acute asthma in hospital. *Arch Dis Child* 1999; **80**:421–3.

22. Lannefors L. Specific problems relating to restricted airways and patient adherence. *Eur Respir Rev* 2000; **10**:216–19.

23. Barnes KL, Rollo C, Holgate ST et al. Bacterial contamination of home nebulizers. *BMJ* 1987; **295**:812.

24. Heslop K, Lannefors L, Dautzenberg B. Local nebulizer services. *Eur Respir Rev* 2000; **10**:549–51.

15. SUMMARY AND GUIDELINES FOR USE

Jacob Boe, John H Dennis and Ronan O'Driscoll

It is hoped by the authors that every reader of this book will have found information within the book that will help them to provide safer and more effective treatment for their patients. The success of the book will rest on achieving this goal. The reader should have a sound grasp of the principles of nebulizer use and an understanding of how to apply these principles to the treatment of individual patients.

After having read this handbook, the reader will realize that nebulizer treatment is very different from other inhaled treatments. In the case of metered dose inhalers (MDI) and dry powder inhalers (DPI), the product is sold as a drug–device combination and the operating characteristics of the systems are standardized. In the case of nebulized treatments, the inhalation device (nebulizer), the power source, accessories and drugs are all sold separately and the healthcare provider must decide which combination to use and how to use it. Depending on the drug, device, disease and patient characteristics, drug delivery to the patient's lungs can vary by a factor of 10 or more. Some nebulized treatments are not even licensed for use by the inhaled route but have been shown to be beneficial in clinical trials. We hope that this book contains the answers to readers' questions about how to select and use appropriate nebulizer equipment and how to care for it and that the reader will find shelf space in their clinic, laboratory or office so that the book can be referred to again and again as more questions arise. It is not proposed that this book will answer every possible question about nebulizer use but the reader should find within the book the principles underlying most aspects of nebulizer therapy.

What was not covered and why

This book is designed for use by busy healthcare professionals so it was essential to keep it focused on common and basic issues. The research scientist may find that particular research issues are not covered in depth but the basic principles have been covered and the researcher will find guidance toward a solution for his or her problem.

The book has not given a list of all available nebulizer equipment or a price list. This is because there is a large number of manufacturers indeed and many products are marketed in only a few countries or at different prices in different countries. Furthermore, the price and product characteristics are likely to be out of date within a few months of publication of the book. However, the reader can use the principles described in this book to decide which type of product will meet the needs of each individual patient. It is hoped that other countries will follow the European model of describing the product characteristics in a standardized format. This will allow the reader to select the best device(s) for each patient.

The book has not given didactic advice about how to run a local nebulizer service or how to clean and service nebulizers. The requirements of readers and patients will vary widely depending on which country and healthcare system are involved. It is hoped that this book will allow the reader to develop best practice locally and to enhance the local service further in the future as confidence and experience grows and as new nebulizer equipment becomes available.

Advantages of nebulizer therapy: why use a nebulizer?

There are many situations where a handheld device is much more convenient and efficient for a patient to use that a nebulizer. Most patients with asthma and chronic obstructive pulmonary disease can take all of their inhaled therapy using MDI or DPI devices which are smaller, lighter, quicker and cheaper to use than a nebulizer. However, there are some situations where a patient needs high-dose inhaled therapy which may best be given by a nebulizer and there are other situations, e.g. inhaled antibiotic therapy, where the drug cannot be given in any other way. Some of the advantages of nebulizer therapy are listed in Box 15.1.

Problems with nebulizers

Nebulizers have certain disadvantages compared with MDI and DPI devices in situations where the inhaled medication is available in each type of device.

Box 15.1 Advantages of nebulizer therapy.

High doses can be delivered

Independent of patient's inhalation technique or activation of device

Ease of administration to babies, elderly patients, confused patients or in emergency situations

Inhaled therapy can be driven by oxygen in medical emergencies

Can administer drugs such as antibiotics or DNase which are not available in MDIs or DPIs

Box 15.2 Disadvantages of nebulizer therapy.

Cost to patient or health service

Time taken to administer treatment

Noise

Pollution of air by drug residues

Complexity of treatment/equipment

Need for cleaning, maintenance and servicing of equipment

Misconceptions by patients and healthcare workers

Abuse (e.g. use of nebulizers to obtain or justify social welfare payments)

Difficulty replicating the exact nebulizer system used in successful clinical trials

The smaller devices are far more convenient for everyday use by those patients who need standard doses of bronchodilator drugs (and much cheaper too). Existing nebulizers have a number of additional disadvantages as shown in Box 15.2.

The future

The reader will, by now, be familiar with the sometimes subtle advantages and disadvantages of each treatment modality and more confident in choosing the best treatment for their patient. However, will this situation change in future? The answer is that change is certain and some of it is almost upon us (see Chapter 3). There will be incremental improvements to existing nebulizer systems and a host of novel systems will appear over the next 10 years or so. Some of these devices will be as small and light as a MDI or DPI and some of the distinctions between the systems are already being blurred (e.g. the Respimat system is effectively a handheld miniaturized multidose nebulizer).

However, the reader can apply the principles of this book to any new nebulizer equipment which they might need to use. The differences between the new and the old devices should be clear and the reader will be in a position to decide whether the advantages of the new system are applicable to and whether any higher cost is offset by benefits to the patient.

INDEX

Note: page numbers in bold refer to illustrations, boxes and tables